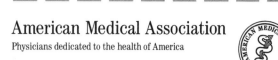

American Medical Association

Physicians dedicated to the health of America

# The Physician as Learner

## Linking Research to Practice

Edited by

*David A. Davis, MD*

*Robert D. Fox, EdD*

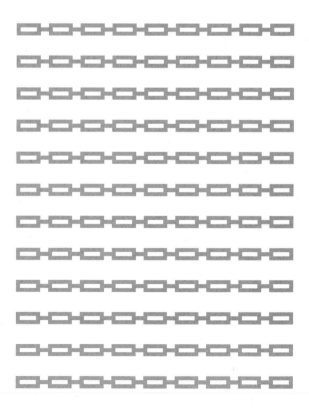

*This book is dedicated to*

- *Our wives, M. D. and K. C.*

- *Colleagues and thought leaders in physician life-long learning*

  *and*

- *A role model and father, D. O.*

# The Physician as Learner: Linking Research to Practice

*Supervising Editor*:    Dennis K. Wentz, MD
*Managing Editor*:    Ashish Bajaj
*Assistant Editor*:    Dan Reyes
*Graphics*:    Karen Costie
*Proofreading*:    Constance Manno
*Desktop Publishing*:    Dan Reyes

This work was supported in part by a grant from the Upjohn Company.

**Library of Congress, Cataloging in Publication Data.**

The Physician as Learner:  Linking Research to Practice,
edited by David Davis and Robert Fox
  Includes bibliographies and index.
  ISBN 0-899-70-627-4
  Library of Congress 94-072102

EA36: 94-313: 1.5M: 7/94

# Foreword

In this time of change in health care and medicine in the United States of America, all aspects of medicine are undergoing analysis. The forces driving reform— including access, cost, and quality—are joining the genetics revolution to profoundly challenge current medical education thoughts. It is clear to even the most casual observer that a new paradigm for education is required to accommodate these developments. Focusing on undergraduate medical education (UGME) alone, or even in conjunction with graduate medical education (GME), will not suffice in the future.

It is time for the medical community to adopt the *continuum of medical education* covering medical school, residency training, and continued learning throughout a physician's life. It is no longer necessary or defensible to think that all basic science information can or should be taught in medical schools, or that residency training provides all the skills required to function throughout 40 to 50 years of "practice." Educators must begin to plan educational experiences so that the content is spread across a physician's lifetime.

It must be recognized that all physicians learn in different ways at different times. It is also clear that the behavior of lifelong learning must be calculated into a physician's behavior early in his or her training, and it must be continually reinforced.

It is equally clear that, while we know some about adult learning, much research must be done to expand our competency in this area. This volume contains superb updates on the status of continuing medical education (CME) research. While this field is in its infancy, it offers exciting opportunities for study as we enter the "Golden Age of CME."

*M. Roy Schwarz, MD*
*Senior Vice President,*
*Medical Education and Science*
*American Medical Association*

# CONTENTS

Preface

# From Banff
# to
# Beaver Creek:

## Consensus
## building in CME

*David Davis*
*Robert Fox*

# From Banff to Beaver Creek:
## Consensus building in CME

**First**, this is a book *about* the science of physician learning. It has, at its core, an emphasis on the third and, arguably, most complex phase of medical education—the phase which occurs after the completion of formal training, and which takes place in the context of the practicing physician.

While a concentrated study of this construct goes by a number of names, the phrase, continuing medical education, or CME, is by far the most commonly used. However, in order to acknowledge its linkages to practice, and because of the perception that "CME" consists primarily of didactic activities or programs unrelated to clinical settings or outcomes, other phrases describing the activity have drawn support—medical practice education, dissemination strategies, and physician enhancement are only random samples. To date, none has replaced the common usage of the acronym "CME."

Whatever the field is called, it is the domain in which reside serious questions related to three, until the last decade, relatively discrete fields: the personal development, competence, and satisfaction of physicians as learners; the assessment of physician competence and performance and of health care outcomes; and optimal CME delivery methods or systems. Each of these areas is explored as separate sections in this book, with increasing focus on relational and mutually interactive issues, and the development of a "topography" of research in physician learning as the text progresses.

We believe that this book is also about an intellectual and virtual journey—from Banff, Canada, to Beaver Creek, Colorado (the sites of two extensive conferences on the research in and delivery of CME). This journey has permitted an exploration of the terrain of physician learning and change, and its close relationship to practice and health care outcomes, based on the best research evidence available to those who took this "journey."

Lastly, this book is about imbedding the best available evidence about physician learning and change into a new "discipline" or practice of CME, and into the practices of physicians. This movement, incorporating evidence about outcomes, cost-effectiveness, and efficacy of interventions, has just as much a place in the world of the CME provider as it does in the world of the clinician. However, while the text uses the literature and evidence related to CME and physician learning extensively, it is not intended to be a comprehensive document of all research relevant to this emerging discipline. Rather, we see its role as providing thoughtful, literature-driven essays in a variety of relevant topics. Its liberal use of postsection annotations is, however, an attempt to provide further references in this field, and to delineate the body of knowledge which drives it.

**Second**, based on our experience in CME, this is a book written *for* an important audience, whose representatives increasingly form significant agents in the development of new health care delivery systems. These agents include:

1) *Those in the medical and other health care professions, either as individual practitioners, or as members of more global, comprehensive organizations with responsibility for assuring, maintaining, or enhancing professional competence. These organizations include professional specialty societies, licensing bodies, and credentialing agencies.*

2) *Those "partners" in the ongoing education of physicians with significant interest in the outcomes of physician learning, competence, and performance, namely, those individuals and organizations in the fields of quality assurance, utilization review, competency assessment, in the burgeoning field of health services research, and increasingly, governments.*

3) *Educators and students of adult education, including: educational psychologists, those interested in continuing professional education, and educators across the continuum of medical education, undergraduate, (post) graduate, and continuing medical education.*

4) *Lastly, the most usual recipients of this information, those interested in the production and delivery of CME programs and activities. Increasingly, this includes individuals, often in clinical settings, interested in developing and testing new practice-based interventions designed to increase physician knowledge and skills, to change their clinical performance, and, thereby, alter patient outcomes.*

We note that members of this "audience" have traditionally seen their role as discrete and relatively nonoverlapping. In this sense, they are not unlike the members of audiences of traditional CME events—noninteractive, passive recipients of information.

It is the major thesis of this book that, to effect change in the delivery, outcome, and evaluation of appropriate physician learning systems, major efforts in intersectoral collaboration and research between these fields or disciplines must occur. Thus, while the book may appear to perpetuate, by its sections, some of the discreteness of the fields of inquiry represented by these sources, section bridges and introductory or concluding chapters attempt to develop common themes, recommendations, and perspectives. We hope these themes will provide a substrate, both theoretical and practical, on which research directions and firm practices in optimal physician learning may be forged.

**Third**, this is a book derived *from* the literature of CME and those related fields explored above.

That literature is varied, complex, and difficult to access. The variety of fields from which it originates speaks to the need for a collaborative, systematic approach to the themes and directions of this book. Those originating fields include the biomedical literature, educational or social psychology, adult or continuing professional education, and other areas including health services, dissemination, and adoption of innovation research. Each of these fields possesses a significant focus on the alteration of physician learning or behaviors by persuasive and educational means, asks different sets of questions, and gives different kinds of answers to the complex issue of physician learning and behavior change. Moreover, each field has its own unique nomenclature, paradigms, and constructs on which to base theory and practice.

Struck by the wide and diverse nature of literature in this area, and interested in capturing, categorizing, and analyzing it, a group of researchers at McMaster University, Hamilton, Canada, developed an annotated bibliography in CME in the early 1980s, now existing as the more useful, computer-stored database, the Research and Development Resource Base in CME. The database, funded by the American and Canadian Medical Associations, the Alliance for CME, the Society of Medical College Directors of CME, and corporate sponsors indicated elsewhere, has formed the substrate on which most of the references and literature driving each of the chapters in this book has been established. At the time of the writing of this book, more than 4000 references supplied the database of articles used to build the themes, policies, and recommendations of this book.

**Fourth**, this is a book *by* colleagues in CME, and in some of the parallel fields referred to in the preceding paragraphs, derived from a process of meeting, collaborating, and synthesizing ideas and knowledge in CME. While the names and biographical sketches of the conference participants are captured elsewhere, a characterization of their common purposes and the process of writing this book requires a description of a "journey."

## Foundations in CME Research: The Banff Conference

The first mention of a need for a conference to discover more about the future of CME came at a Research in CME meeting (now called RICME), in the mid 1980s. It was hoped that such a conference would give participants an extended period of time in which to consider issues and questions in CME. Following a period of planning, a week-long meeting of 20 participants was held in Banff, Canada, in July 1989.

The flow of the meeting, the exchange of ideas, and the meeting's outcomes were the responsibility not of the planners, but of the Banff conference participants themselves—they shaped the content and format of the meeting. It was an exercise in group process, the products of which were believed to have the potential for changing the provision, delivery, research, and development of the growing and evolving field of CME. The Banff conference employed nominal group process extensively, recognizing that institution-specific concerns tend to fall to the bottom of any list of priorities established by this process, and interdisciplinary and interinstitutional issues tend to rise to the top. This is a technique which values the opinion of the group more than the opinion of the individual. In addition to its advantages for planning, it also provided opportunities for building working teams by creating a sense of equality and common purpose.

The summary statement produced by the Banff conference proves a useful starting point for this text.

> *To be effective, Continuing Medical Education, the third, and arguably the most important phase of medical education, can no longer be seen solely as a unidirectional educational delivery system. It must be aware of, and responsive to, the needs of the practitioner/learner, derived both from understanding of the principles of adult education, and from educational and cognitive psychology; must understand, work with, and even begin to direct the realities of practice and health care delivery, including patient forces, practice environment, exigencies; and continue to develop the delivery systems of continuing education in order that they be practice-based, appropriate, effective, and integrate with the practice and professional life of the physician. In order to accomplish this goal, it may be that a new phase is required in order to describe the vacuum which CME researchers and providers may fill—that between areas of the learner, practice environment, and educational delivery systems. This common domain may be called "medical practice education," or the discipline of CME, but it is the expanding and intersectoral nature of the purview of continuing education which is most important to grasp.[1]*

## From Banff to Beaver Creek: Articulating the Questions

To describe the "journey" that led from the Banff to the Beaver Creek conferences requires an exploration of the opportunities and challenges the group faced following Banff. First, it was apparent that knowledge and information sources about CME, both from the group and beyond it, were within grasp, derived in large part from the Research and Development Resource Base in CME. Second, there was the opportunity of moving participants' institutions, associations, and immediate colleagues to a position of fuller understanding of the full ramifications of CME/ medical practice education. Third, there was the opportunity to define, articulate, and nurture the development of a "discipline" of CME in research, presentations, writing, and practice. Fourth, there was the opportunity to move systems relating to the maintenance of competence, health care providers, government or private insuring agencies, licensing bodies and others, and the diverse world of medical education. Fifth, the period between Banff and Beaver Creek provided the opportunity to work in a more concentrated, focused, and collegial manner on larger research and developmental questions relative to CME.

We believe that the Beaver Creek conference was a milestone in that movement—the product of reflection on, and work in, seizing the opportunities explored above, assisted by the American and Canadian medical associations. Here, the agendaless, nominal group style of Banff gave way to a more directed, literature-driven attempt to answer questions in the realm of the discipline of CME or medical practice education. These questions were:

*1) About Physician Learning:*

- *What are the factors that motivate physicians to self-directed learning?*

- *What are the characteristics of self-directed learning?*

- *How do physicians adopt innovations?*

- *What are the effects of age or stage of development on physician learning?*

- *How do physicians learn from clinical encounters?*

*2) About the Assessment of Physicians:*

- *How effective are chart audits in performance assessment?*

- *How effective are standardized patients and structured clinical examinations in competency assessment?*

- *How may incompetency be identified?*

*3) About the Provision of CME:*

- *How do CME providers differ?*

- *How effective are formal CME activities?*

- *What are the factors influencing physician motivation to participate in CME activities?*

- *What is the nature of individualized CME?*

- *How does the practice environment affect learning?*

While at the conference, working groups explored the parameters of the questions, reviewed and synopsized the literature at hand, discussed the questions using the resources of group members, and presented their findings to the full group at concluding sessions. These reports then became working documents which formed the basis for the chapters contained in this book—refined and reworked, and added to by new literature sources, with the themes and topics collapsed where necessary. The results of this work are captured in this text and outlined below.

# The Record of Beaver Creek: Incorporating Evidence About Physician Learning into CME and Health Care Practice

In the introduction, Dennis Wentz and Alexandra Harrison provide a North American perspective of the practice, professional, and political environment in which CME exists. Robert Fox, David Davis, and Dennis Wentz establish the beginning framework of research in the discipline of physician learning, "The Case for Research on Continuing Medical Education."

The first section focuses on the physician as learner. Karen Mann and Judith Ribble, and Penny Jennett and colleagues discuss the nature of, and drive to take part in, self-directed learning. Jocelyn Lockyer provides the perspective of the adoption of innovation, while Nancy Bennett contributes a review of age and stage of developmental issues and their role in physician learning. A concluding chapter by Robert Fox and Jennifer Craig outlines other research directions and models in physician learning.

The second section is a bridge, tying issues relative to the learner to those of the CME delivery "system." It elaborates the notion of assessing the gap between what physicians know and what they do—in CME jargon this is called "needs assessment." Terrill Mast and David Davis provide the reader with an overview of competence, and outline two sorts of measures—tests of competency delivered in the test environment and measures of performance assessed in the practice site. As an example of the former, Murray Kopelow describes the use of standardized patients in competency assessment; while Van Harrison and Jocelyn Lockyer discuss the role of chart review in performance-based assessments.

The third section is devoted to issues relevant to the provision of CME interventions, programs, and strategies. This section begins with an exploration by John Premi of individualized CME, linking the learner and assessment issue to the delivery of CME. Motivational factors relative to participation in CME programs are outlined in a chapter by Donald Moore, et al. The effectiveness of the formal short course and other interventions falling under the rubric of CME are explored by David Davis, Elizabeth Lindsay, and Paul Mazmanian. A concluding chapter on the enterprise of CME, and the size, scope, and future of the industry-like provision of CME in North America is provided by Paul Mazmanian and Willard Duff.

Finally, we conclude with a section leading to the development of a "science" of physician learning, physician performance change, improved health care outcomes, and CME. That science derives from an integrated construct of these fields, has implications for the organization and delivery of CME, and, moreover, becomes a significant impelling factor driving further research into this complex, iterative and compelling field.

## Reference

1.  Proceedings of the Banff Conference, Banff, Canada. *Exploring new frontiers in CME.* McMaster University Pub: Hamilton, Canada; 1989.

# Acknowledgments

## Authors

**David A. Davis, MD** Currently, Associate Dean, Continuing Education, University of Toronto. He participated for many years in the development of continuing education at McMaster University, Hamilton, Ontario. His research interests include effective continuing medical education interventions, problem-based learning, and competency assessment. He is a primary care physician with special interest in HIV and AIDS.

**Robert D. Fox, EdD** Director, Research Center for Continuing Professional and Higher Education and Professor, Adult Education and Higher Education and Family Medicine, University of Oklahoma, Norman. He has served as a consultant and principal investigator or co-principal investigator on projects sponsored by the Royal College of Physicians and Surgeons of Canada, the American Medical Association, the American Institute of Architects, the Bureau of Health Professions of the Department of Health and Human Services in Washington, DC, and the American College of Veterinary Pathology, among others. His research has focused on how and why physicians learn and change clinical practices.

**Nancy L. Bennett, PhD** Director of Educational Development and Evaluation, Department of Continuing Medical Education and Lecturer in Medical Education, Harvard Medical School, Cambridge, Massachusetts. Her interests include defining stages of the professional development of physicians, and understanding how they go about learning.

**Jennifer L. Craig, RN, PhD** Honorary Associate Professor, University of British Columbia, Vancouver, she has worked in undergraduate and continuing medical education for 12 years. She is also the Regional Director for the TIPS program which offers workshops on effective teaching techniques in Canada and the Commonwealth. Her main professional interest is to help health professionals learn how to teach.

**Willard M. Duff, PhD** Dr Duff died on June 17, 1994. Formerly, he was the Associate Dean of CME, Medical College of Wisconsin, Milwaukee. He also served for many years as a member of the Accreditation Review Committee of the ACCME and as an accreditation and research consultant to the ACCME.

**Kathleen Egan, PhD** Currently, Senior Associate for Research & Development, American College of Physicians, Philadelphia, Pennsylvania. At the time of the conference, she was with the Office of CME, University of Pennsylvania School of Medicine. Her research interests are self-directed learning, the relationship between continuing education and practice change, and issues associated with recertification and retraining.

**Alexandra Harrison**  Currently doing doctoral studies at the University of Calgary in the Department of Community Health Sciences in the Faculty of Medicine and the Management of Organizations and Human Resources in the Faculty of Management. She was Director of Educational Services, Canadian Medical Association, Ottawa, Ontario at the time of the conference. Her present research interests include health system organization, management, and evaluation.

**R. Van Harrison, PhD**  Director, Office of Continuing Medical Education and Assistant Professor, Department of Postgraduate Medicine, University of Michigan Medical School, Ann Arbor. His training as a social psychologist emphasized individual behavior in organizational settings. For several years, his primary research interests have been the evaluation and improvement of physician performance and the operation of medical school CME units.

**Penny Jennett, PhD**  Associate Professor, Director, Office of Medical Education and Chair, Medical Education Research Group, University of Calgary. She spent many years studying how physicians and future physicians practice and learn. Some of her research interests include curriculum design and evaluation, learning and teaching methods, lifelong learning, and self-directed learning.

**Martyn O. Hotvedt, PhD**  Independent Consultant and current President, Alliance for Continuing Medical Education. He spent a number of years as Director, Center for Research and Education with the Health Corporation of America. His main research interest is in individualized learning.

**Deborah L. Jones, PhD**  She has been active in CME since 1981. Her most recent appointment was Director, Office of CME, Jefferson Medical College, Philadelphia, Pennsylvania. Her writing and research interests include student-centered and problem-based learning, gender issues in medical education, and medical humanities.

**Alan B. Knox, EdD**  Professor, Adult Education, University of Wisconsin, Madison. His research interests include lifelong self directed education, assessing the impact of continuing education, influences on continuing education participation, and strengthening adult and continuing education.

**Murray Kopelow, MD**  Associate Dean for Continuing Medical Education, Faculty of Medicine, University of Manitoba, Winnipeg. He is particularly active in the development of programs directed at the assessment of professional competence. He has worked for several years developing standardized patient examinations as evaluation tools within medical schools and national credentialing organizations, both in Canada and the United States.

**Robert E. Kristofco, MSW**  Executive Director for Health Affairs, Continuing Education, University of Alabama, Birmingham. His interests and experience in CME focus on strategic planning, needs assessment, expanding delivery systems for lifelong learning, and the role of CME in health system reform.

**Elizabeth A. Lindsay, PhD**  Associate Professor, Department of Epidemiology and Community Medicine and Co-Director, The Community Health Research Unit, University of Ottawa.  Her CME research interests have grown out of the study of individual and community change and have focused on the development and evaluation of programs designed to alter clinical health promotion practices.

**Jocelyn Lockyer, MHA**  Director, Continuing Medical Education and Adjunct Associate Professor, University of Calgary.  She has been involved in the development of CME at the University of Calgary for many years.  She also contributes many hours to the Alliance for CME, the SMCDCME, and the Standing Committee for CME of Canada.  Her research and development interests lie in the adoption of innovation, needs assessment, and outcome measurement.

**Karen V. Mann, PhD**  Assistant Director for Research, Division of Continuing Medical Education, and Associate Dean for Undergraduate Medical Education, Dalhousie University, Halifax, Nova Scotia.  She has a background in nursing, health education, and patient education.  Her research interests include the effectiveness of different educational approaches to changing physician behavior, particularly in the area of preventive activities in their practice, and the application of recent educational techniques and adult learning principles to continuing professional education, and to medical education right across the continuum.

**Terrill A. Mast, PhD**  Assistant Dean for Continuing Medical Education, Professor, Department of Medical Education, and head of the international relations program, Southern Illinois University School of Medicine, Springfield, Illinois.  He was also the founding editor and is still editor of *Teaching and Learning in Medicine; An International Journal.*

**Paul E. Mazmanian, PhD**  Assistant Dean of Medical Education and Professor, Preventive Medicine and Community Health, School of Medicine, Virginia Commonwealth University, Richmond.  Involved in planning and evaluating projects throughout the continuum of medical education, his current research interests include technologies for change in teaching, learning, health care, and health policy.

**Donald E. Moore, Jr, MD**  Currently, Director, Health Education Services, Saint Thomas Hospital, Nashville, Tennessee, he has devoted a considerable amount of his professional career to examining, writing, speaking about, and doing needs assessment.  Recently, he has devoted an increasing amount of time on applying Continuous Quality Improvement to the health care setting.

His research interests also include physician participation in CME and the impact of CME on health care outcomes.

**John Premi, MD**  Director, Practice-Based Small Group Learning Program, Director of Research and Development in CME, Professor Emeritus in the Department of Family Medicine, McMaster University, Hamilton, Ontario. His CME interests are in the development and evaluation of learner-centered CME models.

**Judith G. Ribble, PhD**  Director of CME, GeoMedica Networks, New York, New York. GeoMedica is the successor to Lifetime Medical Television, which produced CME programming on the Lifetime Channel from 1983 to 1993. Her research interests include distance learning in medical settings with an emphasis on multimedia technology.

**Dennis K. Wentz, MD**  Director, Division of Continuing Medical Education, American Medical Association, Chicago, Illinois. He also chairs the Task Force on CME Provider/Industry Collaboration and has spent many years working with the ACCME and the SMCDCME. His areas of interest are developing rational long-term funding for CME and CME research, feedback to physicians of clinical outcomes linked to recognition of the role of self-directed learning in physician's lives, establishing CME as an important academic discipline, and the creation of a National Institute for Continuing Physician Education.

# Other Contributors and Conference Participants

**Bart W. Galle, Jr, PhD** Director of CME, University of Minnesota, Minneapolis.

**Michael I. Gannon**  Associate Director, Division of CME, American Medical Association, Chicago, Illinois.

**Martin P. Kantrowitz, MD**  Director, Office of CME, University of New Mexico, Albuquerque.

**George D. Lundberg, MD**  Editor in Chief, *Journal of the American Medical Association*, Chicago, Illinois.

**Phil R. Manning, MD**  Professor of Medicine, Paul Ingalls Hoagland Professor of Continuing Medical Education, Associate Vice President of Health Affairs, Associate Dean for Postgraduate Affairs, University of Southern California School of Medicine, Los Angeles.

**John Parboosingh, MB, FRCSC**  Currently, Professor, Medical Education, University of Ottawa, Ontario.  At the time of the conference, he was Assistant Dean, CME, University of Calgary.

**Sharifah H. Shahabudin, MD**  Professor and Head, Department of Medical Education, University Kebangsaan Malaysia, Kuala Lumpur, Malaysia.

**Henry B. Slotnick, PhD**  Director, Medical Education & Research Services, University of North Dakota School of Medicine, Grand Forks.

**Kenneth S. Warren, MD**  Currently, Chief Executive Officer, Comprehensive Medical Systems, Inc., New York, New York.  At the time of the conference, he was Director for Science, Maxwell Communications Corporation.

## Staff

The editors would especially like to thank the following people for their help with the Consensus Conference and this book:

**Barbara J. Fletcher**, a long-time member of the AMA's Chicago staff, died unexpectedly in February 1993.  She was very active in planning and coordinating the conference.

**Marlene Rogers**, secretary to David A. Davis, MD, spent countless hours working with the chapter authors, the editors and the publishers to make this book a reality.

## Organizations

The **American Medical Association** and the **Canadian Medical Association** wish to acknowledge **Marion Merrell Dow** and the **Upjohn Company** for their educational grants in support of the conference at Beaver Creek. The editors and the staff at the AMA's Division of CME would like to thank the **Upjohn Company** for a special educational grant which assisted in the publication of this book.

Introduction

# Forces for Change in the CME Environment

*Dennis Wentz*
*Alexandra Harrison*

# Forces for Change in the CME Environment

The field of CME has become a significant subject for investigation over the last decade. CME studies have expanded dramatically as a result of a need to know why and how physicians learn, and how formal and informal education contribute to the medical practice of competent clinicians. As the knowledge base encompassing CME has grown larger and more varied, there is also a need to coalesce new knowledge, to develop useful research models for CME providers, and to set priorities for future investigation.

In light of this expanding knowledge base, a mechanism for integrating diverse research and experiential findings and for projecting directions for the future seemed essential. Thus, the American Medical Association (AMA) and the Canadian Medical Association (CMA) hosted a 3-day invitational workshop in Beaver Creek, Colorado, from July 27-31, 1991, the Consensus Building Workshop in CME. We believe it provided the mechanism for, and was a pivotal event in, the emergence of CME as a full-fledged discipline of study.

## The Environment for Continuing Medical Educators

While multiple and complex pressures and challenges for the field of CME have existed for decades, a host of new forces have developed within the past 20 years. Some of these are shown in the accompanying diagram (see Figure), developed by Michael Gannon of the AMA. It graphically illustrates the interdependence of these forces by the use of three concentric, semipermeable circles, operating with constant flux between them. Represented are forces within CME, forces driving the CME system (the players on the CME scene), and forces outside of CME.

## Forces Driving CME

The innermost circle illustrates the forces driving the discipline of CME in the early 1990s. A decade ago, leaders in the field of CME identified the need for CME to become a discipline, and suggested that the proper study of the discipline is medical practice, from a physician's individual practice to the aggregate system of health care. Published CME literature now demonstrates that CME activities can affect an individual physician's practice and, in turn, change the delivery of health care as a whole. Other researchers have identified factors that motivate physician learners and have proposed ways to better design effective CME. Faculty used in CME, often drawn from academic medical centers or large tertiary teaching hospitals, have been asked to reexamine not only how they teach practicing physicians, but whether they have any conflicts of interest. Another force stems from their "parent"

# Forces outside CME
(External Environment)

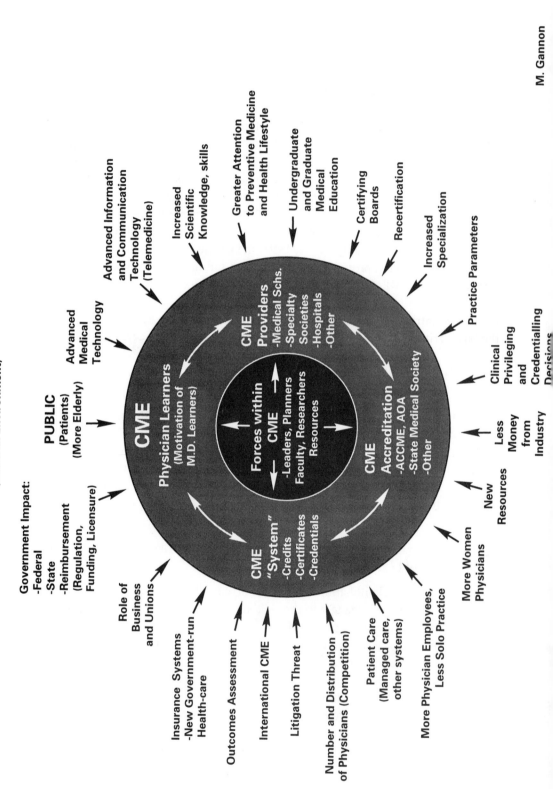

M. Gannon

academic institutions, who are examining potential conflicts of commitment which keep faculty from carrying out other duties owed the institution. Pervading all of these factors is the lack of a dependable financial base for CME, including the limited resources available to continue pilot projects or fund new research.

## The Players on the CME Scene

The middle circle represents the interactions defining the current practice of CME. At the top of the circle are physician learners whose preferred learning styles change constantly, depending on their clinical needs, past learning experiences, and a host of other variables. In the United States, over half of the practicing physicians are age 44 or younger and, with every passing year, physicians newly in practice represent individuals with different learning preferences from previous practitioners. Virtually all new physicians are comfortable with computer technology and have experienced the advantages of video and other information delivery techniques.

There are approximately 2500 CME providers in the United States, an enormous number compared to the 126 medical schools accredited in the United States and the 16 CME-accredited schools in Canada. The accreditation of CME varies between the two countries. In the United States, CME providers are accredited if they fulfill the basic criteria of national accrediting bodies, such as the Accreditation Council for Continuing Medical Education (ACCME). Since this is not restricted to organizations and institutions whose primary mission is education, a host of CME providers exist, ranging from medical schools, to major specialty societies, to small subspecialty-oriented groups, to hospitals of all sizes, as well as voluntary health agencies. In addition, a number of pharmaceutical and medical device manufacturers have become accredited providers of CME, as well as entities organized on a for-profit basis.

In Canada, the only accredited providers are the schools of medicine. The Committee on Accreditation of Canadian Medical Schools accredits undergraduate and CME programs, while residency training programs are accredited by the Royal College of Physicians and Surgeons of Canada or the College of Family Physicians of Canada. In the United States, accreditation is specific for CME, is voluntary, and is directed at institutions and organizations, not specific, individual CME activities. It functions largely under the ACCME. The ACCME accredits about 517 "national" sponsors of CME. The Committee for Review of Recognition of the ACCME provides recognition of (and thus accrediting authority for) the state medical societies, which in turn accredit the approximately 1912 largely local providers of CME. Accreditation for osteopathic physicians is provided under the auspices of the American Osteopathic Association (AOA) which accredits individual programs under a system of recognized CME providers. Still another system operates through the American Academy of Family Physicians (AAFP), which reviews and accredits individual programs felt to be especially appropriate for family physicians.

Accreditation permits the awarding of CME credits, which, in turn, are used to provide certificates and awards and to assist in credentialing. The oldest system in the United States was developed by the AAFP in 1947, when it described a system of "prescribed" and "elective" credit. In 1968, the AMA announced its Physician's Recognition Award, by which was established a series of credit categories. Currently, these are AMA PRA category 1 and category 2. Another system of credit has evolved through the AOA also labeled categories 1 and 2. Finally, some individual state licensing boards have provided differing individual definitions of CME, often also designated category 1. The area of credit remains confused, at least in the United States, and the AMA is currently beginning a national effort to unify CME credit systems.

The outer circle represents forces for change outside CME in the external environment. Again, the circle is semipermeable, with flux in all directions. The world of CME will be greatly affected by the changing environment of health care for both Americans and Canadians. To be fully prepared to function in an increasingly complex environment, those interested in CME and physician learning must understand the major systems in both countries. The common denominator in both remains the financial one, related to the overall costs of health care and the source of the funding.

# Changes in the North American Health Care Environment

The probability is high that major changes in the system of health care in the United States are forthcoming. However, as of the date of publication of this book, no one knows that exact nature of the changes. Perhaps even more than in Canada the overriding concern in the United States is the dramatically escalating cost of medical and health care in the face of a declining economy and an increasing federal debt. In 1992 the United States spent more than $839 billion on health care, according to federal estimates, and this is expected to escalate to $1 trillion by 1995. As a result, more than 60 health reform bills are currently under consideration by the US Congress.

The election of President Bill Clinton, together with major changes in Congress, virtually guarantee that health systems reform will receive priority attention in 1994. A special White House Task Force on Health Systems Reform, headed by Hillary Rodham Clinton, crafted a plan for reform that was presented to the nation in September 1993. The plan calls for a major restructuring of the current system and has attracted some support but also fostered strong opposition from certain players, especially the insurance industry. Congressional committees were beginning hearings on the plan, together with the other bills in the legislative hopper, in March 1994, with the hope of reaching agreement and a compromise bill by the time of the 1994 fall elections.

# Health Care Issues to be Addressed

One of the huge issues facing American society is the provision of a basic level of health care to everyone. While estimates vary, and exact data are difficult to come by, in 1993 at least 34 000 000 people were not covered by health insurance of any kind—government-provided, employer-purchased, or privately purchased coverage. Many have stressed that a careful distinction needs to be made between "access" to health care and the actual presence or absence of health insurance, since most American physicians and hospitals have a solid tradition of providing needed care first, then assigning the charges. As a result, costs are often shifted to those insured patients and providers who can pay.

Another problem in the American system is medical liability costs. Liability claims rose from three claims per 100 physicians in 1981 to 10 per 100 in 1985. Almost 78% of obstetricians and gynecologists have been sued at least once, the number of career suits per ob/gyn physician averaging three. In 1989, total professional liability costs related to physician services alone were $20.7 billion, or 17.6% of total US health expenditures. Of this $20.7 billion, reliable data suggests that $15.1 billion was not related to patient needs, but to defensive medical practices. Liability premiums alone cost $5.6 billion in 1989.

Still another challenge to North American health care is the cost of administering a complicated and often uncoordinated system, which has been reported to represent more than 20% of all US health care expenditures. These figures are in dispute and, since the system is so fragmented, the exact percentage may never be known. The Clinton plan calls for an immediate simplification of the system with estimated major cost savings.

Another important change of significance to CME is the number, age, and distribution of physicians. The number of female physicians in the United States has grown at four times the rate of male physicians over the past 8 years; it is projected that within 10 years more than 50% of practicing physicians will be female. In addition, studies of medical school graduates suggest that physicians are less apt to be in solo practice and more willing to work in groups, or to be employed by managed care systems. Group practices have increased by 54% from 1980 to 1988 (from 10 762 to 16 579), and the number of individual physicians in solo practice has declined dramatically. Both countries are also experiencing a generation change. In the United States, for example, half of the 615 000 licensed physicians in 1992 were 44 years of age or younger.

The allocation of resources is changing. Medical care spending in the United States is highly concentrated among small portions of the population. For example, 10% of the population accounts for more than 75% of medical expenditures, in both the under and over-65 age groups. In fact, 25% of the population accounts for 90% of health expenditures, suggesting to some that the US health care dollar is being spent on illness treatment. Medical statistics from the government reveal that, while Medicare beneficiaries comprise only 12% of the population, they account for 36%

of total personal health care spending. Fully half of total Medicare payments go to 4% of Medicare enrollees. While hospital services account for 40% of the national health care expenditures, only 11.5% of the population is hospitalized each year. Spending on physician services accounts for about 19% of national health expenditures. Although percentages may vary in the Canadian system, the issues of resource allocation are the same.

Many have raised the issue of advances in medical technology as a basic cost issue. However, recent studies at the AMA Center for Health Policy Research have demonstrated that it is not a basic force behind increasing volume or intensity. Using Medicare cost data, new technology procedures for Medical beneficiaries accounted for 25% of all new physician services between 1986 and 1989. Other research shows that the use of technology has not been concentrated on the terminally ill or "high-cost" patients in general. Thus, rising medical costs cannot be blamed fully on advancing medical technology. Nevertheless, society is beginning to ask key questions about new technology. "Who should use it"; "When should it be used"; "Is it effective?" CME providers are increasingly drawn into this debate, which has also focused on appropriate clinical credentialling and privileging.

The population of North America is aging dramatically; health care spending increases significantly with age. Per capita costs for individuals 65 years and older are three times the US national average, while for those under 65 years of age they are 72% of the average. The "old-old" are also increasing, and the per capita spending on individuals 85 and over is 7.5 times the national average.

## Medical Practice and Physician Issues

Finally, there are a wide variety of other factors influencing the practice of medicine. They include recertification in all specialities, tensions between specialities, subspecialization versus training in primary care in graduate medical education and in practice, the development of practice parameters (or practice guidelines), and increased demand for measurement of patient care outcomes and individual "physician profiling." Organizations such as hospitals, ambulatory surgical centers, systems of managed care or "managed competition," and others are responsible for credentialing physicians and have heightened their review of basic credentials and granting of specific clinical privileges. Other key impactors on physicians, and subsequently on the meaning and outcomes of their learning, are licensing bodies, professional associations, and peer review organizations, among others.

There are a number of factors that are applying pressure to cause a shift in physician behavior from autonomy to accountability. Not only are physicians expected to "do the thing right," economic pressures are demanding that they "do the right thing." Health care facilities are becoming increasingly sophisticated in monitoring the performance of individuals or groups of physicians to determine appropriate resource utilization, manage risk, and assure quality. Many hope that these systems will allow physicians to be aware of actual outcomes of patient care. Several

Canadian provinces have legislation that allows the medical licensing authorities to randomly review physicians' offices and charts. Problems identified by the medical licensing authorities can be dealt with in a number of ways, most severe of which is withdrawal of the physician's license. In the United States, peer review organizations (PROs) under Medicare have been key players in physician review. Under health system reform, the PROs may be phased out and replaced by regional entities focusing on educational issues.

The public, in both the United States and Canada, still rates physicians highly relative to ethical and professional standards. Part of this trust is the expectation that physicians will maintain their professional competence. The College of Family Physicians of Canada requires 50 hours of CME per year to maintain certification. The American Board of Family Practice has required periodic recertification since its beginning in 1969; 50 hours of CME per year are required, in addition to successful completion of an examination and review of a sample of office records. Twenty-one of the 24 boards of the American Board of Medical Specialities have endorsed recertification; most of these require evidence of CME as well. The Royal College of Physicians and Surgeons of Canada, which accredits educational programs in 52 specialities as well as certifying graduates of these programs, has introduced a Maintenance of Competence Program (MOCOMP). This is at the pilot stage at present, but it is likely that in the near future all specialists will need to document and report their CME activities in Canada.

These factors contribute to a milieu which demands more than physician attendance at CME activities; a new standard of actual change in performance may be expected. Such environmental changes will lead to increased pressure on physicians to maintain and demonstrate their professional competence and to CME providers and professionals to assist in this process.

# Impact of Health System Reform on CME

Continuing medical education is one of the areas thus far omitted from the US debate on health systems reform. The ability of the system to provide the best possible quality of care for patients would seem to be dependent on competent, well-informed physicians and other health professionals, as well as educated patients. Many would argue that a societal goal should be the best-educated patients and physicians possible.

Many issues arise for the discipline of CME as a result of health systems reform. Dependent on the nature of the changes ahead, some of these issues are:

- the creation of individual physician profiling, with CME linked to practice needs,

- drastic changes in the methods and format of CME, eg, refocusing CME to individual practice settings, using interactive telecommunications and information technology,

- restructuring of the CME accreditation process,

- development of a variety of suggested curricula for physicians in the practice years, to assist them in more rational planning and for purposes of self-assessment,

- the retraining of physician-specialists into physicians providing primary care services,

- a need for CME to focus on the learning needs of increased numbers of primary care providers,

- education to assist physicians in coping with managed care and other new health delivery systems,

- education to assist physicians in understanding and using practice parameters/guidelines,

- development of information systems to provide ongoing feedback to doctors about patient outcomes and other patient care issues,

- education to teach physicians new skills for teamwork and relationships in teams, with the expectation that a new system may use multiple levels of health care professionals working as a team,

- education of physicians to be more effective "teachers" of patients, on "wellness" strategies focusing on public health and prevention of disease, and to provide culturally sensitive care,

- a CME enterprise responsive to unprecedented diversity of physicians, other health care professionals, and patients, and

- a CME enterprise capable of dealing with a changing interface between graduate medical education and education during the practice years.

This total agenda would suggest that the development of more rational, planned financing systems for CME are needed. This is especially timely as industry funding, once a very important source for CME, is withdrawn due to changes in the business plans of both the pharmaceutical and the medical device industries.

## The Role of the AMA and the CMA in Changing the Shape and Impact of CME

The activities of the CMA serve its mission: "to provide leadership for physicians and to promote the highest standards of health and health care for Canadians." Further, the mission statement of the CMA Council of Medical Education is to "provide leadership at the interface between practicing physicians and the academic medical community to facilitate high standards of education for physicians and service for patients, throughout the lifelong continuum of medical learning." Roles to accomplish this mission statement include:  "a catalyst for establishing and maintaining high standards of medical training and practice, consensus builder, and honest broker."

Similarly, the CME mission statement of the AMA articulates the overall goal of the AMA:  to "promote the art and science of medicine and the betterment of the public health to the benefit of all people."  The AMA carries out the educational parts of this mission through its Council on Medical Education and the Council's CME Advisory Committee (CMEAC).  Upon recommendation of CMEAC and the Council, the AMA has committed itself to two CME roles: (1) continued leadership in the field of CME; and (2) the development of individual learning activities that enhance and expand the knowledge and skills of physicians, in concert with the medical specialty, state and territorial medical societies, and other physician organizations dedicated to improved CME.  Because it is the national association that includes almost all of the major groups and interests of organized medicine in its constituency, the AMA is in a unique position with regard to CME in the United States.  For many years, the AMA has encouraged voluntary participation of physicians in CME, in part through its AMA Physician's Recognition Award, the AMA PRA.  Celebrating its 25th anniversary in 1993, the AMA PRA has been awarded to over 600 000 physicians.

In 1990, the AMA's Council on Ethical and Judicial Affairs (CEJA) issued an important Ethical Opinion on "Gifts to Physicians from Industry" which profoundly affected many providers of CME, as well as physician participants.  The concern of the profession about various abuses in CME led the AMA to further issue two specific guidelines for physicians regarding their participation in CME.  The first, developed through the Council on Medical Education, was entitled "Physician Commitment to Life-long Learning," followed by a CEJA "Ethical Opinion on Continuing Medical Education," which addresses the ethical responsibilities of physicians as attendees, faculty, and as sponsors of CME.

In 1994, the AMA announced the formation of a new foundation, the Institute for Continuing Physician Education, to explore many of the major issues facing the field of CME, to foster collaborative problem-solving and research, and to perhaps forge the basis of a proud new discipline.

Thus, the cosponsorship of the consensus building conference by the CMA and the AMA is a concrete example of the commitment of both associations to serve these stated roles.

# The Development of Consensus in CME

The purpose of the conference was to advance understanding and research activities in the discipline of CME and to build a consensus on three important areas of research and scholarly activities in the field.

Agreement about the areas of emphasis of the conference was achieved as a result of a 1989 invitational meeting of leaders in CME research convened at Banff, Canada, subsequently known as the Banff Conference. The convening of the Beaver Creek conference 2 years later represented an evolution of ideas in CME research and channeling of forces set in motion in 1989.

The Beaver Creek workshop was by invitation only. A core group of key individuals from across Canada and the United States were identified from their previous scholarly activities in CME. The invited individuals were associated with schools of medicine, hospitals, medical association, or medical journals; some had been present at the 1989 Banff Conference. In addition, nominees were sought from societies and organizations with a major commitment to advancing the discipline of CME. Invitations were mailed to 60 individuals; about half accepted and participated in the workshop. Participants paid their own travel expenses, and the AMA and the CMA provided the meeting arrangements.

## Objectives of the Conference Participants in the Workshop:

- Review and summarize significant literature related to major questions in the study of CME and related areas.

- Develop a synopsis for major questions related to CME.

- Refine a nomenclature related to CME to foster greater consensus and communication for practitioners and scholars concerned with CME.

## About the Workshop

In advance of the workshop, working groups were identified to address questions in physician learning, competency assurance, and the delivery of CME. Participants were sent material collated from the Research and Development Resource Base in CME related to their questions.

This database (and this book) make available for the first time many ideas and publications about CME that can best be characterized as "fugitive." They have been lost to the mainstream of CME researchers and often appear in indexes not commonly used by biomedical researchers. Participants reviewed the material related to their assigned questions in preparation for the discussions relating to the questions, and were formed into several working groups. These groups were composed of between four and six people, at least one of whom had special expertise or experience related to the question addressed by that group. Each group was assigned a leader and nominated a recorder.

The consensus building conference was thus targeted at those with research experience, those with publications, and those with demonstrated knowledge and scholarly activities in the field. As such, the Beaver Creek workshop was the first major effort to coalesce opinions of known experts about the significant literature in CME, physician learning, and its place in North American health care delivery.

## About this Book

The new concepts and linkages that developed as a result of the discussion and reflection at the consensus building conference provided stimulation and new insights for participants. Participants indicated the importance of capturing these discussions for those who were not able to be present at the workshop. Subsequently, the group leaders agreed to work with representatives of their group to expand and synthesize the information that had been developed during the workshop into a book. It is our hope that the publication of this book will permit other scholars, planners, and policy makers to identify new directions in the provision of CME and to target other areas for further research.

Chapter 1

# The Case
# for
# Research
# on
# Continuing
# Medical
# Education

*Robert Fox*
*David Davis*
*Dennis Wentz*

# The Case for Research on Continuing Medical Education

Frustrations abound when simple questions are applied to complex processes. CME is such a process. It involves physicians, practice environments, learning resources, and interventions designed to improve the ability of physicians to provide better medical care to patients. Many have viewed the process of learning and its relationship to changes in clinical practices as a simple and direct causal relationship without paying attention to the many ways that CME may be viewed. The simple view of CME is as a seminar or out-of-town conference, full of lectures, perhaps using the occasional workshop, stimulation, or case study, but always dominated by the teaching of medical school faculty or other experts. From this perspective, physicians who participate absorb the new knowledge and skills that these CME programs promote, return to their practices, and immediately change their procedures, thoughts, and decisions accordingly. In this definition of CME physicians are rational; experts know better; practice settings are malleable; education is organized, purposeful, and meaningful; and practices are easily changed.

Traditionally, this narrow view has confined CME to a static system built of faculty-controlled objectives, didactic teaching, and "did you like the coffee?" evaluations. This view does not reflect the state of knowledge as to the nature of learning in practicing physicians. It does relate often to the inadequate efforts of CME providers who may lack the commitment or capability to help physicians learn and change. However, this view of CME, with all of its shortcomings, has organized the thoughts and actions of program planners as well as CME researchers until the 1980s.

Research based on simple but inadequate assumptions about the relationship between historical CME programs and change in medical practices should have found it easy to document that, after participating in a CME program, medical practices change and patients improve. However, this set of assumptions has led to a long history of foiled attempts to successfully answer the question, "Does CME make a difference in medical practices and patient care?"

Our purpose is not to question all the attempts to solve this problem, but to examine the basic assumptions underlying the simple view of CME. If questions are poorly formed, answers will be hard to identify. If questions are based on false assumptions, the answers usually will be inconsistent and misleading. Better questions formulated from more thoughtful explanations and based on an ample body of literature are necessary if research is to capture the role of CME and continuing learning as they relate to changes in medical practices.

The case in support of the value of CME should be built on what is known about how physicians change and learn and the role of CME in the practice of medicine. CME must not be seen as medical science. It is not a prescription written by educators to counteract some disease plaguing physician performance and patient outcomes. Physicians' performances may be inadequate, but disease models do not form an appropriate analogy. Moreover, the basic science underlying the understanding of health and illness is older, more robust, and more definitive than the body of theory related to understanding physicians' knowledge, competence, performance, and the processes that underlie these critical determinants of clinical outcome. Just as prescriptions are written from a body of knowledge of medical science, CME should be based on research and theory from the behavioral and social sciences and studies of the learning and performance of professionals.

Unfortunately, many of the attempts to document the effectiveness of CME have not considered that CME should be rooted in its own basic science—the knowledge of how and why physicians change their performance. In fact, many studies have failed to consider that the way the CME intervention is formulated and administered can vary dramatically—from well founded and consistent with what is known about education and learning to whimsical and spontaneous. Effective CME is based on sophisticated understandings of physicians' needs and motives, clinical problems, the context of care, theories and principles of human behavior, learning, education, and theories of planned change. It is not based on qualified and entertaining speakers.

In the last 10 years, the knowledge base of CME has expanded rapidly. Students of the process of CME have begun to understand the characteristics of learning and the qualities of education that foster learning. Two kinds of information have begun to emerge from these studies, each developed from unique intellectual traditions. First, there have been studies that seek to illuminate, by rigorous qualitative methods, the natural process by which change and learning occur in medical practices. The second set of studies has used equally rigorous quantitative methods to document the effects of high-quality CME on medical performance. Each of these approaches has contributed uniquely to explanations of the ways that education and learning in practice affect physicians' performance.

## Studies of Change and Learning in Physicians

Over the last 5 years, debates over the effects of CME on knowledge, competence, and performance have stimulated a new line of investigation that draws from methods of anthropology, sociology, and biology. Although controlled studies of the effects of new drugs or new procedures are most common to contemporary methods of investigation in clinical medicine and the basic sciences, these methods depend on theories that were originally generated from careful observations, classifications, and associations among categories. For example, Darwin's efforts to generate a theory of natural selection can be viewed as a process involving description, classification, association, and interpretation of similarities and differences observed in specimens he collected. Most would be reluctant to criticize the methods Darwin used to collect and classify his specimens now, but many criticize these same qualitative approaches to understanding human behavior. Yet, without this kind of description and analysis, new theories cannot be developed for testing by more controlled studies.

Theory-building studies are essential ways to organize research around hypotheses that warrant investigation because they have been carefully constructed from systematic observation and analysis. Without underlying theory, hypotheses are no more than ill-informed guesses.

In 1984 the Society of Medical College Directors of Continuing Medical Education and a number of organizations and agencies recognized the need for systematic analysis of the process of change and learning in medical practice.[1] Data on 775 cases of change were collected in interviews with 340 physicians in proximity to 26 medical centers in the United States and Canada. The study used extensively trained interviewers and focused interviews to collect and analyze data on the reasons physicians changed their practices and the means by which they learned in order to make these changes. The assumptions that guided this study were that change in practices are common and readily observable, and that many of the changes made in clinical practices require that the physician learn new information and develop new skills. Careful questioning of a random sample of physicians would provide insights and explanations relating the process of change to the ways and means physicians learn new knowledge and skills. This data could then be organized and classified into a theory that would lead to hypotheses for future experimental and correlational studies.

In this sense, the "change study" met its objectives. It demonstrated that physicians engage regularly in systematic processes to change their practices. The causes of changes were classified and labeled according to the force for change experienced and described by these physicians. Some forces were personal (such as curiosity) or a desire for a sense of well-being. Some were social, such as regulations and relationships with peers. By far, most changes in clinical practices were driven by the desire to be more competent in the delivery of health care to patients.

Once a force for change initiated the process of change, physicians described how they developed a mental image of the outcome of changing. When this image of the outcome was clear, the process of change tended to be shorter and more efficient. When the image was unclear, change took longer and followed a more erratic course. A physician's image of the outcome of changing practices predicted how directly and efficiently learning and changing occurred.

After the outcome of changing was imagined, physicians described an internal process of self-assessment of the abilities they needed to make the change. They described examining and comparing how capable they were of performing the new or different practice in light of what they imagined was required to perform success-fully. For some who sought a level of excellence, their estimates of what was required in terms of knowledge and skills were quite high. For others who sought to be competent but not necessarily expert, estimates of desired knowledge and skill were not so high. Comparisons of their current knowledge and skills with the knowledge and skills necessary to make the change predicted whether or not they would learn, and the way they would learn in order to make the change. When the discrepancy between what was known and what was required was large, efforts to learn were more common than when the gap was small.

Thus, learning varied according to the force for, and the image of, the change and the knowledge and skill necessary to make it. When the force for change was the desire to be more competent, learning was more likely to be directed toward solving clinical problems and to depend on direct experiences.

## Figure 1.1

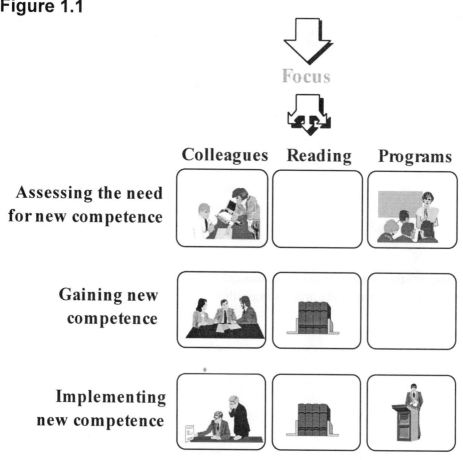

In follow-up studies,[2-4] it was discovered that, when physicians learned as part of changing practices, they usually used three different kinds of learning resources in tandem. This triangulation of information usually included CME programs as one of the three sources of information. Although CME programs seldom caused a change, or represented the only resource used to learn in order to make the change, they were an important part of learning associated with making changes in practice. They played a role in preparing to change, making the change, and integrating the change into ongoing procedures for care of patients. The figure depicts this self-directed curriculum for change. Although the figure shows CME in specific places, this is only an illustration. CME programs could play a part in each or all of the three stages of the learning associated with making a change in practice.

Formal CME also served as a trigger, releasing the energy to make changes in practices. Sometimes, it served as a means for self-assessment, enabling better decisions about the kind of formal and informal learning that was necessary to make a change. In some cases, it helped physicians develop a clearer image of the kinds of changes that were necessary.

These initial and follow-up studies of change and learning in the lives of physicians confirmed that change was a ubiquitous feature of clinical practice, and that the most prevalent means of making a change was to engage in systematic learning. Although a substantial portion of this learning was from informal means, CME programs and activities were common tools used in the overall self-directed curriculum for change.

# The Specific Effects of CME in Producing Change

A second means by which the effect of CME may be assessed is the quantitative or controlled trial study, a more common and familiar research design in the biomedical world. Such studies form a significant part of the Research and Development Resource Base in CME documented in the preface and elsewhere.[5,6] A complete review of the hundreds of reports of CME interventions (eg, courses, programs, activities, or other methods) in this database would be impossible. Instead, an overview of a subset of these articles may illuminate the features of successful behavior-modifying educational activities.

Selected for discussion, and illustrative of well-crafted CME or physician-change interventions, is a relatively recent "convenience sample" of randomized trials found in the Research and Development Resource Base. These 50 studies have, as their dependent variables, changes in physician performance and/or health care outcomes. While they are explored more fully in chapter 12 and elsewhere,[7] a review provides an example of this type of research and argues for further exploration of the components of successful CME interventions. Strategies used by the authors of this trial represent a wide-ranging use of methods to change physicians' behavior and included: didactic, traditional methods (such as lectures or courses) and other practice-linked methods such as academic detailing, reminders, and feedback based on audit, materials and methods, chart review, and clinical opinion leaders. Of the 50 studies, 43 examined physician behavior and 18 examined health care outcomes (11 studies assessed both measures). Of the first group, the majority showed changes in at least one major measure in such clinically diverse areas as counseling patients, health promotion, preventative medicine, resource utilization, and the general management of medical conditions. Of the latter 18 studies eight demonstrated improvements in at least one major outcome measure of health care.

An extraction and review of those factors that appeared to be responsible for the degree to which were achieved outcomes illuminate some of the characteristics of effective CME, at least in the studies and populations selected for analysis. They provide models for those committed to changing physician performance or health care outcomes.

First, the frequency, intensity, and timing of interventions appears to be critical to changing physician behavior. Second, interventions based on reminders or feedback (and thus intimately linked to practice needs) are more successful in changing performance than those that are more remote from the learner's needs. Third, changes in physician performance appear to vary with the degree to which the physician learner is committed to, and capable of, making the change. For example, Palmer et al[8] indicated that physicians commit to change when they perceived a relatively straightforward process without the need to alter non-physician-dependent variables. Fourth, in studies that showed no changes following CME interventions, note may be made of the "ceiling effect"—the assumed degree to which physicians volunteering to take part in CME or quality-of-care studies may already be operating at higher or optimal levels of performance. Finally, if a change in health care outcomes is a desirable objective of CME, the results of these studies may appear, at first glance, disappointing. This disappointment may be tempered somewhat by the considerable gap between physician performance and patient outcomes as influenced by such factors as patient compliance and by treatment ineffectiveness. Furthermore, reasons for physician attendance at formal CME events may not be tied directly to learning and changing in some cases. Such participation may reflect a desire to socialize with others of like interest, or to fulfill a desire for professional development.

These studies, and other reviews of the efficacy of CME (from that of Bertram and Brooks-Bertram[9] in 1977 to Beaudry[10] in 1990), provide a window on the relationship between individual CME activities and physician or patient outcomes. Their conclusions are relatively consistent—well-designed CME interventions, when consideration is given to environmental (practice site) and internal (physician as learner) variables, can effect changes in physician performance. The questions of what constitutes CME, which variables affect which physician outcomes, and what factors affect the translation of physician performance into patient outcomes, are eloquent representatives of the imperative of research into CME and its place in health care.

## Implications for the Life-long Development of Physicians

Although CME is a vital part of the process by which physicians build and refine their practices, new information suggests that learning and education for practicing physicians is more complicated and important than has been assumed in the past. Medical practices must change constantly as patients, conditions of practice, and requirements of clinical care change. For the present (and even more so for the future), physicians must have the skills and resources to manage the process of change. CME is an important tool in the workshop of change. Other forms of learning are also necessary, as physicians construct and reconstruct their practices to respond to the needs of individual patients and societal demands in health care.

As with any tool, CME can be well constructed, efficient, and effective, or it can be poorly constructed, inefficient, and ill suited to the task. Knowledge of the ways it may be used, and the principles of design and construction are necessary precursors to developing CME that meets needs. When the principles of education are applied systematically in the design and construction of CME, the tool for change works. When they are ignored, CME is less likely to be effective and efficient. Even when CME is well made, it is only one of many resources for change. Nevertheless, without good CME, learning and changing is difficult and less likely to be successful.

Clinical performance is a complex outcome of change and learning. Good clinical performance is also the keystone to optimal medical care. Little is known about the means that may be used to construct good clinical performance. Continuing improvement of CME depends on continuing growth in understanding of the predictors of physicians' performance of their role as health care providers. It also depends on more understanding of the processes physicians use to alter their practices. Understanding the predictors of performance, and the processes by which performance changes, will enable CME to be more useful in the continuous growth and development of clinicians.

In the future, undergraduate and graduate medical education must join CME in recognizing that learning and change are necessary ingredients in effective medical practice over the life span of physicians. Education at all levels must consider that it is the performance of the medical role that is the purpose of medical education, and that performance changes routinely. Performance in the clinical setting should be returned to the center of attention. Information, knowledge, and skill must be organized around performance requirements rather than around taxonomies, hypotheses, and models of research. This is not to say that the basic science is unimportant. It is vital and necessary, but it is not sufficient. It is the raw material of clinical decisions, but it is not adequate for making decisions, or reasoning through the complexities of modern practices.

From its position in the continuum of the medical career, CME has begun to explore predictors of practice performance and change in practice performance through learning. It should be connected to others across the wide range of learning and changing that shapes medical performance.

In the early part of the 20th century, Flexner[11] studied and reported on the status of medicine and the role of medical education. He called for the integration of science into the process of medical education. This changed medicine and medical education in a way that would contribute to the eventual successes over most of the infectious diseases that dominated the turn of the century. Flexner saw that, by systematic study, a focus on science could benefit medical education and health care.

In an era of increasing rates of change in clinical problems, scientific information, and social conditions, it is time for another review of the state of medicine and the role of medical education from admission to retirement. What better object for such a study than performance and change in performance. Perhaps it is time for undergraduate and graduate medical education to join CME in focusing on the behavior of physicians as the organizing principle of medical learning. Perhaps it is time for another landmark study, this one devoted to building education on the factors and processes that enable effective medical performance and foster the skills to change when and where it is appropriate and necessary to quality health care. Perhaps this text, its ensuing chapters, and annotated bibliographies, will facilitate this process.

### References

1.  Fox RD, Mazmanian PE, Putnam RW, eds. *Change and Learning in the Lives of Physicians.* New York, NY: Praeger Publishing; 1989.

2.  Putnam RW. A further analysis of the change data in prescribing practices. Presented at the Fourth Research in CME Conference; April 4, 1990; San Antonio, Tex.

3.  Blanchard D, Fox RD. A profile of nonurban physicians from the study of changing and learning in the lives of physicians. *J Cont Ed Health Prof.* 1990;10:329-338.

4.  Crandall SJS. The role of continuing medical education in changing and learning. *J Cont Ed Health Prof.* 1990;10:339-348.

5.  *The Impact of CME: An Annotated Bibliography of Continuing Medical Education.* Hamilton, Ontario, Canada: McMaster University; 1984.

6.  Haynes RB, Davis DA, McKibbon A. A critical appraisal of the efficacy of continuing medical education. *JAMA.* 1984;251:61-64.

7.  Davis DA, Thomson MA, Oxman AD, Haynes RB. Evidence for the effectiveness of CME: a review of 50 randomized controlled trials. *JAMA.* 1992;268:1111-1117.

8.  Palmer RH, Louis TA, Hsu EN, Peterson HF, Rothrock JK. A randomized controlled trial of quality assurance in 16 ambulatory care practices. *Med Care.* 1985;23:751-770.

9.  Bertram DA, Brooks-Bertram PA. The evaluation of continuing medical education: a literature review. *Health Ed Monog.* 1977;5:330-362.

10. Beaudry JS. The effectiveness of continuing medical education: a quantitative synthesis. *J Cont Ed Health Prof.* 1990;10:285-307.

11. Flexner A. *Medical Education in the United States and Canada: A Report to the Carnegie Foundation for the Advancement of Teaching: Bulletin No. 4.* Boston, Mass: Updyke; 1910.

# Section I

# The
# Physician
# as
# Learner

"If physicians are to change, their education will have to encourage reflection, personal development, and the growth of self-knowledge. Medical scientists sometimes make reference to 'the frontiers of knowledge.' I think they have in mind a frontier that is 'out there.' The newest and most challenging frontier may be within us."

McWhinney, ER.
Through Clinical Method to a More Humane Medicine.
In: *The Task of Medicine-Dialogue at Wickenberg*.
Menlo Park, Calif:
JH Kaiser Found Pub;
1988.

# Introduction to Section I

This first section reflects a restructuring of thought about CME.

In the early 1980s, CME was seen by practitioners and scholars as a disorganized array of individual educational efforts offered as remedies for the problems that plagued practitioners. The principal problem, they felt, was simply remaining current. Offerings of medical schools and hospitals focused on the principle that knowledge was changing rapidly. Educational programs that resembled the basic fare of undergraduate education (eg, lectures, printed material, and occasional discussion periods) were the treatment for laggards who had not kept up-to-date or for competent practitioners who needed to add new facts and concepts to their fund of knowledge. The underlying beliefs that guided this pattern of CME were:

- *Physicians were rational; with the acquisition of new or updated knowledge, their practices would also change.*

- *If physicians did not change, it was because CME programs were poorly done.*

- *The goal of research in CME was to attempt to identify CME programs that changed behavior and hold these up as models for other CME efforts.*

This set of beliefs formed the intellectual underpinnings of a plethora of studies directed at demonstrating effectiveness in CME programs. If they were successful, we felt that CME "worked." These assumptions led to an ever-expanding interest in instructional design and evaluation methodology. Rather than expanding the knowledge base, however, this movement narrowed attention to investigations and debates centered on the proper way to state objectives, the benefit of slides or presentation skills, and the proper format for maximum effect on knowledge and skill. CME grew ever smaller as a concept as attempts to show its direct effects on competency grew more numerous.

A sample of the literature of that era was this study, conceived by the late Jack Sibley[1] and his colleagues in the late 1970s.

> *Volunteer family physicians in Ontario were randomly allocated to one of two groups—a control, receiving no intervention, and an experimental group that received printed educational packages, or a variety of family practice topics. The physicians chose the majority of the topics. Hours were spent on selecting the format and presentation, and, of course, the content of the packages. Following the sequential mailing of the material over several weeks, chart audits by carefully trained nurse record abstractors were performed on the charts of patients in both groups. There was no difference between them—at least none that reached statistical significance [with the exception of one difference which we'll discuss in the*

*introduction to section II]. The authors concluded [something like] 'CME doesn't work,' 'work' in this case, meaning changing physician performance.*

It is not difficult to imagine the impact of this study on the CME community. It provoked a response, characterized by Goldfinger[2] as the "case for contamination," which elaborated the concept that physician learning took place by a variety of routes (formal CME being only one of them). It also provoked a considerable response in the editors. One of us (D. D.) became more interested in designing effective CME interventions and trials. The other (R. F.) viewed learning as the result of the interplay of a variety of forces and resources. The Change Study[3] (explored in greater detail in this section) is the product of that thinking.

And so providers, scholars, and researchers in CME have begun to change their point of view from a tight focus on education to a broader and more inclusive focus on learning and the learner. This transition is reflected in this section. Each of the authors contributes to this larger view of the physician as learner by describing a variety of theoretical models of the process of learning. Each of them provides evidence to support the assertion that education is a contribution to the more global phenomenon of learning in practice.

An imaginary but not atypical scenario might help us focus on the applications of this theoretical base:

*Ten years ago, Blumenthal-Nipon, Inc. developed panoxyldimethyliodorone, proven by epidemiologically sound studies to be the most effective agent in the prevention of ventricular tachycardia, a potentially lethal cardiac arrhythmia. Five years ago, Blumenthal-Nipon, Inc. licensed a North American firm, J. S. MacLean Pharmaceuticals, to distribute the product. While worldwide sales of the drug have been impressive, North American sales have been sluggish. A recent marketing report shows these findings:*

- Some physicians prescribed the drug within the first year after its release; others prescribed it over the last 4 years.
- Two distinguishing characteristics of the physicians not prescribing the drug appear to be that they are either solo practitioners or physicians over 60 years of age.
- Some "communities" (eg, groups of physicians in hospitals) have high prescribing rates; the prescribing rates of other physicians are quite low. High-prescribing communities appear to be marked by one or more of the following: physicians interested in their own learning, one or several highly respected clinicians who used the drug early on, a large proportion of well-educated patients (especially those who have health backgrounds), and an active sales force.

Many of the issues that are raised in this scenario are explored in this section. The first chapter in this section (chapter 2 by Jocelyn Lockyer) describes theory and research related to the natural process of diffusion of innovations in medicine from its research base to clinical practice. Ensuing chapters reflect a growing interest in the power that physicians hold over their own learning. Chapter 3, by Penny Jennett and her colleagues, outlines the characteristics of self-directed learning. Karen Mann and Judith Ribble contribute understanding about motivating factors in self-learning in chapter 4. The concluding chapters describe emerging ideas and theories about the effects of maturation across the span of life and career (by Nancy Bennett), and the complexities of learning from the practical, everyday experiences embedded in the practice of medicine (by Robert Fox and Jennifer Craig).

Each of these contributions predicts a future full of complexities for investigators and providers of CME. Each describes for us the foundations for a new CME, and adjunct to patient care, designed to fit smoothly and evenly into the practice of medicine, rather than occupying a place on the periphery. It is an expanding universe rather than a collapsing one. It provides lots of challenges for the next generation of investigators. These challenges lie within the assumptions of a new era in CME research that operates under new assumptions:

- *Although physicians are rational, they are also subject to forces from within themselves, their colleagues, and the environment of health care; these factors play a role in learning and changing medical practices.*
- *Although there is a set of design principles or curricula at work, it is in the hands of learners and not teachers.*
- *Learning is a natural and continuous process that must be facilitated rather than directed by CME providers.*
- *Research should be organized around the formal explanations and predictions contained in scientific theories related to physicians as learners.*

These assumptions represent new perspectives reflected in this section.

### References

1. Sibley JC, Sackett DL, Neufeld VR, et al. A randomized controlled trial of continuing medical education. *N Engl J Med.* 1982;306:511-515.

2. Goldfinger SE. Continuing medical education: the case for contamination. *N Engl J Med.* 1982;306:540.

3. Fox RD, Mazmanian PE, Putnam RW, eds. *Changing and Learning in the Lives of Physicians*. New York, NY: Praeger Publishers; 1989.

**Chapter 2**

# The
# Adoption
# of
# Innovation

*Jocelyn Lockyer*
*Paul Mazmanian*
*Donald Moore*
*Alexandra Harrison*
*Alan Knox*

# The Adoption of Innovation

The study of physician adoption of innovation has fascinated researchers for at least four decades, beginning with the first study of drug adoption in the midwestern United States.[1]

> *A better understanding of the dynamics of how physicians adopt new drugs, begin using different investigational protocols, and train for new surgical procedures should make it possible to design CME interventions in such a way that variation in medical and surgical management is reduced, and health care, based on the best evidence available, is realized.*

The purpose of this chapter is to describe models for adoption of innovation within medicine; examine, describe, and critique the research that has been conducted in this area; and suggest a number of practical implications for CME providers. Rogers' definition of innovation, namely that it is "an idea, practice or object that is perceived as new by an individual or other unit of adoption,"[2] will be used throughout this chapter. Thus, innovation applies equally to newly released pharmaceutical compounds as well as to the acceptance and use of laparoscopic surgical techniques. It also encompasses an evolving reconceptualization of a disease. Asthma, for example, is now recognized by contemporary clinicians as a continuum and not simply a problem of problem intermittent bronchial constriction.

## Theoretical Models of Change

Most studies examining physician change have built on the concepts developed by theorists Rogers[2] and Geertsma et al[3] who suggest that change is a multistage process. Rogers'[2] synthesis of adoption in all fields, including medicine, outlined a five-stage process. In the first two phases, the individual learns about innovation and is then persuaded to think about it. In the third phase, a decision to try the change is made. Following implementation, the individual confirms that the change was the appropriate one and continues to use it or discontinues using it.[2] Geertsma et al[3] identified a similar five-stage process including priming, focusing on the innovation, rationalizing the innovation, using the innovation, and, finally, evaluating it.

A number of factors govern the process. According to Rogers,[2] these include considering the relative advantage of the innovation over other practices, the compatibility of the innovation with contemporary practices, the complexity of the innovation, the ability of the individual to try out the innovation prior to full adoption, and the opportunity to observe others using it. Generally, an innovation that is fairly simple, similar to current practices, able to be incorporated into practice with little or no cost, and visible, will be adopted more quickly than an obscure innovation that requires an intensive period of training and extensive resources to initiate.

Both Rogers[2] and Geertsma et al[3] have based their theories on autonomous individuals who possess the ability to initiate change within their own environment. That model of physician adoption is helpful for changes in which the physician is not dependent on organizational resources to facilitate change. Generally, adoption of a new drug, simple surgical techniques, and the requisitioning of a new lab test fit this model of individual diffusion of innovation.

However, when the changes physicians wish to effect are made within the context of a hospital, university, or large group-practice environment, it is helpful to complement individual change models with others relevant to organizational change. Reflecting the reality of complex environmental changes, Fennell and Warnecke[4] have criticized classic innovation diffusion theories which characterize the innovative physician as a lone scientist or solo practitioner, as being inadequate for understanding innovation in the modern medical setting. Organizational models, by contrast, underscore the importance of understanding the environment,[5] particularly the social culture of an organization. Similarly, Nowlen's theory of professionals' performance, namely that their performance is a function of both the individual and the group in which they work,[6] identified and analyzed those variables that most affect individual and group performance: life skills, environmental and cultural influences, and personal dimensions. These variables, when creatively orchestrated, can enhance both individual and collective performance.

Fennell and Warnecke[4] examined seven regional networks designed to promote state-of-the-art treatment for head and neck cancer and which displayed wide variation in adoption profiles. Each network in this study had evolved very different strategies for patient management, depending on its culture and organization. Innovations such as those involving laparoscopic surgical techniques, the purchase of new expensive technologies, and the creation of new service units (in which many people are involved in the decision to proceed) all require an understanding of organizational dynamics.

## A Review of the Literature

Adoption of innovation has been studied in virtually every discipline of medicine. Researchers have done extensive analyses of the acceptance of new drugs,[1,7] innovative protocols for preventive medicine,[8,9] new surgical procedures,[10,11] and computer information systems.[12,13] A variety of research tools has been used to assess adoption—network analysis,[12,13] mail surveys,[14,15] interviews,[16,18] data from third-party paying agencies,[19,20] and chart reviews.[21,22]

A number of patterns emerge in these investigations. Most studies suggest that multiple pieces of information from different sources are required before physicians will make a change in their clinical practices.[7,17,23] For simple changes, fewer sources of information are required and the adoption process is generally faster.[17,18] Major changes that require learning a highly complex procedure require a longer period of time and employ more sources of information.[17,18] Thus, it is not surprising that acceptance of new pharmaceutical products requires less adoption time than does the acquisition of skills for new surgical procedures.[17]

While the literature is not conclusive, it does suggest that some sources of information appear earlier in the adoption process than others. Manning and Denson[7,23] identified medical journals as the first source of information. Another study found that such journals, along with CME courses and communication with colleagues, were most often initial sources of information.[17] The conclusion of the adoption process is dependent on collegial communication, particularly among specialists who represent local professional opinion.[1,3,24,25]

There is some evidence to suggest that physicians encounter innovations first in the literature since this learning resource is easily available and accessible to physicians.[26] However, difficulties with the literature (including inadequate indexing and retrieval systems) and the inability to quickly synthesize articles or studies[26,27] rule out its use in the final stages of adoption when a physician needs to clarify and confirm that innovation is appropriate.[26]

Changes are, however, made constantly. Small, fairly simple innovations make few demands on the physician. Frequently, the physician simply accepts the change without a major conscious effort. On the other hand, when the change is a significant departure from traditional practice, Fox et al[18] found that a number of conditions must be met in order for change to occur. First, the physician has to make a personal commitment to the change. Further, a conceptual base is necessary, as is time to deliberate over the change and its implications for both physician and patient. As might be expected, this requires a lengthy process with multiple experiences of learning and reinforcement.[18] When one looks at the adoption of new consensus statements and guidelines among large numbers of physicians, greater compliance is further associated with high levels of agreement within a specialty group.[28] Further, the addition of incentives or the removal of disincentives may be needed to effect rapid change in actual practice.[29] Greer[24] discusses the intrinsic difficulty in knowledge emanating from external sources to affect local medical behavior; physicians must feel that an innovation is valid, and relevant to and attainable within their local communities.[24]

Despite the influence of these external forces, physicians do not adopt innovations at the same rate. Rogers[2] envisions adopters along a continuum from "early adopters" to "laggards." Early work identified early adopters as those physicians having the most extensive personal and professional ties.[1] The physicians to whom others refer or ask advice, or who serve on major committees, tend to be early adopters independent of background and practice characteristics.[12] Recent work suggests that early adoption of complicated products will be more likely if the physician has had previous experience with a therapeutic agent (possibly through a referral to a consultant). This is particularly the case if the physician perceives difficulties with the product's administration and side effects.[30]

Several studies have drawn associations between early adoption and physician characteristics. These include age of less than 50 years, board certification, association with a group practice, involvement with teaching programs, publication in the medical literature, holding an academic appointment, and managing busy practices.[14,25,31,32] Conversely, older age, solo practice, and lack of board certification have been associated with adoption of fewer new procedures.[14,31] Researchers who have examined adoption within the context of large organizations have also noted that the clinical setting (particularly larger size and teaching hospital status) facilitates earlier adoption.[33]

The latest direction for adoption studies involves examination of high volume or very expensive procedures to discern patterns of adoption. These studies, which have encompassed cesarean section, carotid endarterectomy, and endoscopy, show that overuse of one technique in an area does not predict overuse of other modalities in the same area.[10,11,20,34] While utilization rates for specific diagnostic and treatment procedures and alternative treatments for the same condition vary, the differences cannot be explained by the actions of a small number of physicians, differences in case mix, or inappropriate use.[10,20] Some researchers have suggested that variation in approach may be due to lack of agreement about optimal treatment between local and national authorities.[24,28,34]

A number of studies have been conducted with the purpose of accelerating adoption of an innovation.[21,35] Others have studied "natural adoption."[14,18] While there does not seem to be one method of dissemination that works in all circumstances, it is clear that dissemination and adoption require validation by trusted experts.[24,29,35]

Research into techniques for promoting better prescribing of drugs has demonstrated that effective dissemination strategies included engaging the physician in two-way communication and targeting programs to specific physicians who are known or suspected to be at high risk for inappropriate practices.[36,37] Well-designed graphic aids for face-to-face encounters were found to be helpful, provided they contained clinically relevant and understandable recommendations for positive alternative actions by physicians.[8] Some repetition and reinforcement over time, and an individualized approach appeared to be useful, particularly when communication to physicians was on a one-to-one basis or in small groups.[37] Physician-to-physician communication has been particularly effective.[36,38] Conversely, there has been little success with programs in which the physician has been a passive consumer of information. For example, strategies in which the physician has been sent unsolicited print materials in the mail have not proven very fruitful in facilitating new practices.[37,39]

## Critique of the Literature

The literature on adoption of innovation is plentiful and diverse, and has focused on most, if not all, medical disciplines. Unfortunately, a review of the literature reveals little building on the findings of previous studies in other clinical disciplines, such as nursing. Similar questions have been asked; similar results have been produced.

Christensen and Wertheimer,[40] for example, examined the prescribing of medications, as have Manning and Denson,[7] Lockyer et al,[17] and Peay and Peay.[41] Each of these investigators has described similar findings with respect to the resources which physicians use in the adoption process and their data bear marked resemblance to the landmark study conducted by Coleman et al.[1] Moreover, studies that have looked for evidence that physicians have adopted an innovation following a seminal study or report have demonstrated how slow physicians have often been to adopt innovations despite the quality of the research.[22,29,42-44]

For the most part, adoption studies have been of a relatively limited scope and based on small groupings of physicians working in narrowly defined geographic regions.[16,21,40] The studies have typically relied on one methodology, for example, a phone or mail survey, network analysis, or chart review. In only a few instances have researchers attempted to use more than one approach to examine and verify adoption patterns.[21,44] The study by McMillan et al[21] was a small-scale pilot project, and therefore its replicability in other settings is uncertain.

Several hypotheses related to the adoption of innovation by physicians have been put forward,[3,6,45] but these require testing to see if, how, and when they apply. Research that has been done in this area has not drawn on work in related fields. For example, recent work in the area of physician commitment to change shows that physicians who make an *a priori* commitment are more likely to change practices.[46,47] While this work complements the adoption of innovation literature, interventional studies should begin to integrate a level of physician commitment into their design. Likewise, little research has been done examining the synergistic effect of work involving multiple professional disciplines and the lay public. Recent investigations in preventive medicine, particularly in public health strategies related to "heart health,"[48] may suggest new models and strategies for intervention.

Work is also needed to advance theoretical models of change and adoption of innovation. For the most part, such models assume a fairly static stage-by-stage process of change. As de Ven and Rogers[49] have pointed out, researchers should instead be moving to a dynamic, continuous conception of the process by which innovation variables are sequenced and analyzed over time. They conclude that a theory of such change should explain how structure and purposive action are linked at the micro and macro levels of analysis, how innovation is produced both by the internal functioning of organization structure and by the external purposive actions of individuals, and how the process becomes stable or unstable over time.

# Implications for CME Research

This analysis of the literature suggests a number of directions that CME researchers can take to improve the understanding and working knowledge about physician adoption of innovation.

First, continued effort is needed to improve research methodologies. Since data collection is generally limited to one method, triangulation of information sources (for example, the use of multiple methods) would be productive, particularly in those studies which rely on self-report. Some work has already been done in this area by Lomas et al[44] and Curry and Purkis[47] to verify and strengthen the results of research. Multiple data collection methods would also help to achieve more dependable data and allow researchers to learn more about the relative validity, reliability, and usefulness of each method. Similarly, techniques (such as focus groups, clinical recall interviews, and ethnographic techniques) could be useful in pursuing and broadening the qualitative information about barriers to adoption and allowing clinicians to elaborate on their rationales and decision making.[21]

Second, models of the adoption of innovation need to be tested and refined and new models developed. Meta-analysis of studies done to date could prove beneficial in this area.

Third, there is a need for future studies in complementary areas. These might include studies of manipulative, coercive, and "top-down" approaches to change. Preliminary work by Fox et al[18] suggested that physicians resist adoption of innovations presented in this manner, although there may be circumstances involving costly investigations and procedures of uncertain benefit in which this approach could be justified. Similarly, research needs to be conducted to assess the relationship between planned interventions and the natural process of change. Do physicians make such changes without sophisticated interventions? Preliminary work has been done to examine the role that commitment to change makes in the change process[46,50]; it should continue. Interviews with early adopters and laggards, or with exemplary and remedial physicians, and with novice and expert MDs, could also illuminate the process of adoption.[51]

Interventional studies, (ie, those studies which attempt to accelerate the process of adoption) hold promise.[21,29,37] Research needs to build on the theoretical foundations established by Fox et al[18] and Nowlen.[6] Further, studies need to decrease their reliance on information dissemination as the primary method of facilitating change. This singular approach often ignores other important factors such as practitioner motivation to change, the context in which clinical decisions are made, how information is presented,[52] the clinical reasoning process itself,[53] and the environment in which physicians work.[6] Not surprisingly, approaches limited solely to the dissemination of information have limited degrees of success[35,54] (see chapter 12).

In each of these endeavors, researchers must proceed with caution. There are at least two ethical issues that deserve consideration. First, one must be sure that the relevant medical science warrants the adoption of an innovation before designing a study to accelerate the process. Second, thoughtful consideration must be given to approaches to encourage change in the physician with suboptimal management techniques.

# Implications for CME Providers

Studying how physicians adopt change can help direct the provision of CME. It is important to determine the point at which it is logical to intervene in the adoption process. There are times, for example, when a program or workshop in a new surgical procedure would be highly marketable within a community and times when it would be premature or too late. Another intervention involves physicians who are respected by their peers (described as "educational influentials"); Stross and his colleagues[55] have defined their role as those physicians who provide the necessary leadership in a clinical area to facilitate the adoption of innovations. Continued study of adoption will contribute to the delineation of appropriate windows of opportunity for other, similar interventions.

The CME provider and the learner form a dynamic partnership. While CME providers need to focus attention on the individualized needs of the learner, learners need to be encouraged to reflect on and describe changes they have made in the past, and how those changes have been incorporated in their practices. Both strategies may facilitate more efficient adoption of new ideas in the future. Skills in lifelong learning, including the ability to reflect on educational needs and practice changes, need to be introduced to novice physicians in undergraduate and post-graduate training. In the future, CME needs to be targeted towards individuals as much as it has traditionally been aimed at groups (see chapter 10).

Partnerships should be created between CME providers and other health care providers to maximize diffusion of innovation. Work in the field of "heart health" has demonstrated that interventions targeted to both community and professional levels have an additive and synergistic effect. For this reason, CME providers need to look at ways to ensure that the education of physicians, nurses, other professionals, patients, and the community occur in a systematic or synchronous fashion so that the impact of an adoption program is enhanced.

Finally, providers should facilitate the use of information systems developed to provide information to physicians about their own practices (and how these practices compare with those of their peers) and about ideal standards of practice. These systems become important as physicians increasingly work in group, corporate, and managed health care settings. Computerized reminder systems and flow charts show promise in this regard,[56-58] as do systems that couple individualized feedback with peer comparison data.[34,59] Expert systems, such as *Iliad*, also display promise in assisting physicians with their diagnosis investigations, and management of patients.[60,61]

The process by which physicians adopt innovation is worthy of continued study. As CME has emerged as a discipline, its professionals have expended resources examining more efficient ways to disseminate and test the diffusion of innovation. Work must continue in this field.

At the same time, it is important to note that progress has been made in delineating the circumstances under which change occurs within a medical community by individual physicians. Local support is necessary for adoption.[24] For individual physicians, it is important to be aware that change takes time, personal commitment, and multiple sources of information.[18]

CME programmers can assist this process by becoming more interactive, targeted, and integrated with other local initiatives aimed at improving patient care. For particularly complex changes—those which consume expensive resources yet pay high dividends in the reduction of morbidity—comprehensive CME strategies with different delivery methods and with the support of local leaders will achieve the common goal of teaching and reinforcing appropriate behaviors.

*The authors gratefully acknowledge the contributions, in group discussion, of Bart Galle and Michael Gannon.*

## References

1.  Coleman JS, Katz E, Menzel H. *Medical Innovation: A Diffusion Study.* Indianapolis, Ind: The Bobbs-Merrill Co, Inc; 1966.

2.  Rogers EM. *Diffusion of Innovation.* 3rd ed. New York, NY: The Free Press; 1983.

3.  Geertsma RH, Parker RC Jr, Whitbourne SK. How physicians view the process of change in their practice behavior. *J Med Educ.* 1982;57(pt 1):752-761.

4.  Fennell ML, Warnecke RB. *The Diffusion of Medical Innovations.* New York, NY: Plenum Press; 1988.

5.  Ford L, Kaluzny AD, Sondik E. Diffusion and adoption of state-of-the-art therapy. *Semin Oncol.* 1990;17:485-494.

6.  Nowlen PM. *A New Approach to Continuing Education for Business and the Professions,* New York, NY: Macmillan Publishing Co; 1988.

7.  Manning PR, Denson TA. How internists learned about cimetidine. *Ann Intern Med.* 1980;92:690-692.

8.  Grilli R, Apolone G, Marsoni S, et al. The impact of patient management guidelines on the care of breast, colorectal, and ovarian cancer patients in Italy. *Med Care.* 1991;29:50-63.

9.  Battista RN, Williams JI, MacFarlane LA. Determinants of preventive practices in fee-for-service primary care. *Am J Prev Med.* 1990;6:6-11.

10. O'Connor GT, Plume SK, Olmstead EM, et al. A regional prospective study of in-hospital mortality associated with coronary artery bypass grafting. *JAMA.* 1991;266:803-809.

11. Anderson GM, Lomas J. Monitoring the diffusion of a technology: coronary artery bypass surgery in Ontario. *Am J Public Health.* 1988;78:251-254.

12. Anderson JG, Jay SJ. Computers and clinical judgment: the role of physician networks. *Soc Sci Med.* 1985;20:969-979.

13. Anderson JG, Jay SJ, Schweer HM, Anderson MM. Physician utilization of computers in medical practice: policy implications based on a structural model. *Soc Sci Med.* 1986;23:259-267.

14. Freiman MP. The rate of adoption of new procedures among physicians: the impact of specialty and practice characteristics. *Med Care.* 1985;23:939-945.

15. Fuhrer MJ, Grabois M. Information sources that influence psychiatrists' adoption of new clinical practices. *Arch Phys Med Rehabil.* 1988;(69 pt 1):167-169.

16. Abelson J, Lomas J. Do health service organizations and community health centers have higher disease prevention and health promotion levels than fee-for-service practices? *Can Med Assoc J.* 1990;142:575-81.

17. Lockyer JM, Parboosingh IJ, McDougall G, Chugh U. How physicians integrate advances into clinical practices. *Mobius.* 1985;5:5-12.

18. Fox RD, Mazmanian PE, Putnam RW. *Changing and Learning in the Lives of Physicians.* New York, NY: Praeger Publishers; 1989.

19. Hillman BJ, Joseph CA, Mabry MR, Sunshine JH, Kennedy SD, Noether M. Frequency and costs of diagnostic imaging in office practice—a comparison of self-referring and radiologist-referring physicians. *N Engl J Med.* 1990;323:1604-1608.

20. Chassin MR, Brook RH, Park RE, et al. Variations in the use of medical and surgical services by the Medicare population. *N Engl J Med.* 1986;314:285-290.

21. McMillan DD, Lockyer JM, Magnan L, Akierman A, Parboosingh JT. Effect of educational program and interview on adoption of guidelines for the management of neonatal hyperbilirubinemia. *Can Med Assoc J.* 1991;144:707-712.

22. Kosecoff J, Kanouse DE, Rogers WH, McCloskey L, Winslow CM, Brook RH. Effects of the National Institutes of Health Consensus Development Program on physician practice. *JAMA.* 1987;258:2708-2713.

23. Manning PR, Denson TA. How cardiologists learn about echocardiography: a reminder for medical educators and legislators. *Ann Intern Med.* 1979;91:469-471.

24. Greer AL. The state of the art versus the state of the science: the diffusion of new medical technologies into practice. *Int J Technol Assess Health Care.* 1988;4:5-26.

25. Weiss R, Charney E, Baumgardner RA, et al. Changing patient management: what influences the practicing pediatrician? *Pediatrics.* 1990;85:791-795.

26. Means RP. How family physicians use information sources: implications for new approaches. In: Green JS, Grosswald SJ, Suter EM, Walthall DB, eds. *Continuing Education for the Health Professions.* San Francisco, Calif: Jossey-Bass Publishers; 1984:72-86.

27. Williamson JW, German PS, Weiss R, Skinner EA, Bowes F III. Health science information management and continuing education of physicians: a survey of US primary care practitioners and their opinion leaders. *Ann Intern Med.* 1989;110:151-160.

28. Jordan HS, Burke JF, Fineberg H, Hanley JA. Diffusion of innovations in burn care: selected findings. *Burns.* 1983;9:271-279.

29. Lomas J, Enkin M, Anderson GM, Hannah WJ, Vayda E, Singer J. Opinion leaders vs audit and feedback to implement practice guidelines: delivery after previous cesarean section. *JAMA.* 1991;265:2202-2207.

30. Stross JK. Relationships between knowledge and experience in the use of disease-modifying antirheumatic agents: a study of primary care practitioners. *JAMA.* 1989;262:2721-2723.

31. Schwartz JS, Lewis CE, Clancy C, Kinosian MS, Radany MH, Koplan JP. Internists' practices in health promotion and disease prevention: a survey. *Ann Intern Med.* 1991;114:46-53.

32. Peddecord KM, Janon EA, Robins JM. Substitution of magnetic resonance imaging for computed tomography: an exploratory study. *Int J Technol Assess Health Care.* 1988;4:573-591.

33. Sloan FA, Valvona J, Perrin JM, Adamache KW. Diffusion of surgical technology: an exploratory study. *J Health Econ.* 1986;5:31-61.

34. Keller RB, Soule DN, Wennberg JE, Hanley DF. Dealing with geographic variations in the use of hospitals: the experience of the Maine Medical Assessment Foundation Orthopaedic Study Group. *J Bone Joint Surg Am.* 1990;72:1286-1293.

35. Lomas J. Words without action? The production, dissemination, and impact of consensus recommendations. *Annu Rev Public Health.* 1991;12:41-65.

36. Ray WA, Schaffner W, Federspiel CF. Persistence of improvement in antibiotic prescribing in office practice. *JAMA.* 1985;253:1774-1776.

37. Soumerai SB, Avorn J. Predictors of physician prescribing change in an educational experiment to improve medication use. *Med Care.* 1987;25:210-221.

38. Schaffner W, Ray WA, Federspiel CF, Miller WO. Improving antibiotic prescribing in office practice: a controlled trial of three educational methods. *JAMA.* 1983;250:1728-1732.

39. Sibley JC, Sackett DL, Neufeld V, Gerard B, Rudnick KV, Fraser W. A randomized trial of continuing medical education. *N Engl J Med.* 1982;306:511-515.

40. Christensen DB, Wertheimer AI. Sources of information and influence on new drug prescribing among physicians in an HMO. *Soc Sci Med.* 1979;13:313-322.

41. Peay MY, Peay ER. The role of commercial sources in the adoption of a new drug. *Soc Sci Med.* 1988;26:1183-1189.

42. Stross JK, Harlan WR. The dissemination of new medical information. *JAMA.* 1979;241:2622-2624.

43. Dunn DRF. Dissemination of the published results of an important clinical trial: an analysis of the citing literature. *Bull Med Libr Assoc.* 1981;69:301-306.

44. Lomas J, Anderson GM, Domnick PK, Vayda E, Enkin MW, Hannah WJ. Do practice guidelines guide practice? The effect of a consensus statement on the practice of physicians. *N Engl J Med.* 1989;321:1306-1311.

45. Greer AL. Medical technology and professional dominance theory. *Soc Sci Med.* 1984;18:809-817.

46. Parker FW III, Mazmanian PE. Commitment, learning contracts, and seminars in hospital based CME: change in knowledge and behavior. *J Cont Ed Health Prof.* 1992;12:49-63.

47. Curry L, Purkis IA. Validity of self-reports of behavior changes by participants after a CME course. *J Med Educ.* 1986;61:579-584.

48. Mittelmark MB, Jacobs DR, Bracht NF, et al. Community-wide prevention of cardiovascular disease: education strategies of the Minnesota heart health program. *Prev Med.* 1986;15:1-17.

49. Van de Ven AH, Rogers EM. Innovations and organizations: critical perspectives. *Communication Research.* 1988;15:632-651.

50. Martin KK, Mazmanian PE. Anticipated and encountered barriers to change in CME: tools for planning and evaluation. *J Contin Ed Health Prof.* 1991;11:301-318.

51. Manning PR, DeBakey L. *Medicine: Preserving the Passion.* New York, NY: Springer-Verlag; 1987.

52. Kanouse DE, Jacoby I. When does information change practitioners' behavior? *Int J Technol Assess Health Care.* 1988;4:27-33.

53. Schmidt HG, Norman GR, Boshuizen HP. A cognitive perspective on medical expertise: theory and implication. *Acad Med.* 1990;65:611-621.

54. Hill MN, Levine DM, Whelton PK. Awareness, use, and impact of the 1984 Joint National Committee consensus report on high blood pressure. *Am J Public Health.* 1988;78:1190-1194.

55. Stross JK, Hiss RG, Watts CM, Davis WK, Macdonald R. Continuing education in pulmonary disease for primary-care physicians. *Am Rev Respir Dis.* 1983;127:739-746.

56. McPhee SJ, Bird JA. Implementation of cancer prevention guidelines in clinical practice. *J Gen Intern Med.* 1990;5:116s-122s.

57. Lawrence RS. Diffusion of the US Preventive Services Task Force recommendations into practice. *J Gen Intern Med.* 1990;5:99s-103s.

58. Dickinson JC, Warshaw GA, Gehlbach SH, Bobula JA, Muhlbaier LH, Parkerson GR Jr. Improving hypertension control: impact of computer feedback and physician education. *Med Care.* 1981;19:843-854.

59. Berwick DM, Coltin KL. Feedback reduces test use in a health maintenance organization. *JAMA.* 1986;255:1450-1454.

60. Lincoln MJ, Turner CW, Haug PJ, et al. Illiad training enhances medical students' diagnostic skills. *J Med Syst.* 1991;15:93-110.

61. Clayton PD, Evans RS, Pryor T, et al. Bringing HELP to the clinical laboratory: use of an expert system to provide automatic interpretation of laboratory data. *Ann Clin Biochem.* 1987;24:5-11.

**Chapter 3**

# The Characteristics of Self-directed Learning

*Penny Jennett*
*Deborah Jones*
*Terrill Mast*
*Kathleen Egan*
*Martyn Hotvedt*

# The Characteristics of Self-directed Learning

*"An individual who has achieved final formal certification for entering practice is assumed to be prepared to guide all of his or her further continuing education. Many (most) do so. For others however, the assumption that the practitioner has both the inclinations and the learning skills to maintain professional vitality is not accurate."*[1]

Continuing professional education learning needs are best met by attending and responding to the ongoing, changing needs of a profession, as well as to the real and perceived day-to-day needs of the individual practitioner.[2,3] Practitioner-initiated self-directed learning activities and planned formal CME programs form the core of how physicians keep up-to-date. In medicine, the half-life of knowledge, the information explosion, new diseases, innovative diagnostic technology, advanced treatment methods, changing societal expectations and practice patterns, and the specific needs of individual practices necessitate this broadened perspective.[4-7] Continued learning by professionals is incremental and complex, requiring both formal and informal approaches.[8,9]

Self-directed learning is a primary mode of learning for adult practitioners to meet professional needs. It is a legitimate, essential form of learning critical to the ongoing maintenance of competence and quality practice. Indeed, it has become an intrinsic way of life for professionals who wish to maintain the currency of their knowledge and skills.[10-14] It is therefore critical that CME providers better understand and define the concept of self-directed learning, its strengths and limitations as a format for learning, and the skills and motivation required to pursue it. In addition, familiarity with the research findings and studies that address this core learning format is central.

The contents of this chapter attempt to help continuing professional agencies, professional associations, and individual practitioners provide the needed support for self-directed learning. Initially, definitions and characteristics for self-directed learning are presented, three types of self-directed learning are described in detail, and self-directed learning, as it applies to medical practice, is discussed. The chapter then turns to research issues. Past self-directed learning research activities are reviewed and future directions posed. Relevant research methods and questions are summarized. Finally, implications that evolve from current views of self-directed learning are offered for the medical profession, the practitioner, and medical educators. The specific role motivation plays in self-directed learning is addressed in chapter 4.

# Definitions, Characteristics, and Types of Physician Self-directed Learning

The commonly accepted and frequently cited definition proposed by Knowles[12(p18)] has worn well through the years:

> *. . . a process in which individuals take the initiative, with or without the help of others, in diagnosing their learning needs, formulating goals, identifying human and material resources for learning, choosing and implementing appropriate learning strategies, and evaluating learning outcomes.*

A definition proposed more recently by Hammond and Collins[15(p17)] draws heavily from Knowles, adding social awareness, reflection, and critical analysis to the process:

> *. . . a process in which learners take the initiative, with the support and collaboration of others, for increasing self- and social awareness; critically analyzing and reflecting on their situations; diagnosing their learning needs with specific reference to competencies they have helped identify; formulating socially and personally relevant learning goals; identifying human and material resources for learning; choosing and implementing appropriate learning strategies; and reflecting on and evaluating their learning.*

Types and characteristics of physician self-directed learning share many of the qualities discussed by adult education theorists. Adult and self-directed learning activities have been characterized variously in the adult and general learning literature and are seen to contain four elements constituting common denominators. First, adult learning activities tend to be deliberate, systematic, and sustained.[11,12,16] Tough[11] found that adult learning activities generally consisted of a series of related episodes totaling at least 7 hours over a period of 6 months. The purposes of these learning activities varied, from obtaining new information and developing new skills to reexamining attitudes and/or beliefs. A second characteristic common to adult learning activities is that they are self-initiated.[17-19] Individuals often recognize a need to learn and take responsibility for their own learning.[19] Penland[17] found that 76% of individuals over the age of 18 were involved in self-initiated learning projects. Third, adult learning activities tend to be learner dominated and managed, with the learner taking an active role in the development of the learning program[20] and controlling the process.[15] In discussing adult learning activities, Knowles[12,19] noted that a prerequisite to self-directed learning is the desire and capability of an individual to plan and manage his or her own learning. Individuals engaging in self-directed learning have a self-concept amenable to holding themselves responsible for their own learning. The final characteristic common to adult learning activities is the specialization of the context.[19,21] Knowles[19] noted that adults not only know how the proposed learning will benefit them, but also are most ready to learn those things that will contribute to their own performance of life tasks. The motivation for engaging in adult learning activities typically comes from an immediate prob-lem, task, or decision that demands certain knowledge or skill[2,11] or arises from personal interest, pleasure, or curiosity.[11]

In describing the lifelong learner, several characteristics reappear in the literature. The individual is aware of the relationship between learning and "real life" and recognizes the need to be a lifelong learner; is motivated to engage in sustained learning activities; enjoys a self-concept that favors responsibility for self and self-determination in learning; and possesses the skills necessary to set realistic objectives, bring appropriate prior experience to bear, identify and access relevant resources, analyze and integrate material from disparate areas, and use a variety of learning strategies.[19,21,22]

## Self-directed Learning in Medicine

The concepts set forth in the adult learning literature apply readily to self-directed learning in medical practice. In medicine, control by the practitioner is the critical distinguishing characteristic of the self-directed learning experiences of physicians. Richards[23] described a continuum of control to characterize learning activities in medicine. In this view, traditional CME is completely faculty controlled and at one end of the continuum. Activities such as hospital-based CME and home-study or self-assessment programs fall at intermediate points. With the exception of the most teacher-dominated situation (in which the teacher fully determines content and method), the individual physician exerts varying degrees of control and assumes varying degrees of responsibility for the learning activity. Fox[24] takes this issue further conceptually, noting that "the pattern of formal and informal resources is what the learner controls, not necessarily the teaching or the learning experience." Self-direction may be viewed as an individual's control over the exercise of intentions, decisions, and actions in a given situation. In fact, self-directed learning has long been a staple of physician educational experiences.[25] A proposed typology regarding three specific types of self-directed learning follows.

## Types of Self-directed Learning Activities

Physician self-directed learning may take a variety of forms, ranging from informal and unstructured activities to intentional formal educational activities based on identified needs. For purposes of this discussion, three distinct forms of physician self-directed learning have been identified: 1) informal, ongoing, habitual activities directed to the maintenance of competence; 2) semi-structured learning experiences that typically have their basis in immediate patient problems; and 3) formal, intentional, planned activities.

### Informal self-directed learning

Considered by many physicians to be part of their "activities of daily learning," habitual self-directed learning is the most informal. It is undertaken on a routine basis as a matter of course without the assistance of others. The physician does not develop specific objectives to meet self-perceived needs, but rather engages in the activity to keep abreast of recent developments, much as CME professionals attend annual meetings.

Geertsma et al[26] have characterized this type of learning as "focusing," the process by which physicians become aware of new therapies, practices, or technologies, and thus set the stage for additional learning. Alternatively, in the face of rigorously controlled studies of educational effectiveness, Goldfinger[27] has referred to this form of learning as "contamination." Richards[23] simply describes these learning activities as "random learning." Types of activities that fall into this category include journal reading,[23,28-30] ad hoc conversations with colleagues or recognized experts (such as "educational influentials"),[30-34] interaction with pharmaceutical or equipment representatives,[33] attendance at regular CME events (such as grand rounds),[28,33] preparation for lecturing or writing,[35] and even attendance at traditional CME courses.[31] Informal physician self-directed learning tends to constitute routine, habitual, ongoing activities[23] that are used to maintain currency in the field or to satisfy intellectual curiosity.[36] These activities may or may not be based on documented learning needs, and the outcomes may or may not be formally evaluated by the learner. Rather, these activities are based on self-initiated scans of the physician's practice environment and are rapidly accessed, and their execution (ie, the selection of the topic or material and conduct of the activity) is solely the responsibility of the learner.[23,24]

### Semi-structured self-directed learning

A more structured form of physician self-directed learning is that learning associated with immediate patient problems.[6,7,37-39] In these instances, physicians have specific learning needs and objectives related to current patient care decisions. This type of self-directed learning may take the form of consultations with colleagues[37,40] or contact with educational influentials,[41,42] literature searches and medical informatics,[38] or reading.[29,30,37,43] As with informal self-directed learning activities, semi-structured learning is undertaken by the physician without assistance from others. Typically, semi-structured self-directed learning activities are practice-generated, with learning embedded in daily work.[39,43-45] Due to the problem- or disease-orientation of this activity and the acute need for information,[39,45] the methods must be convenient and efficient. While this type of learning activity is focused, it is also reactive to a unique set of circumstances and thus cannot be planned. Medical informatics assumes increasing importance as a tool in this category of self-directed learning.

## Formal self-directed learning

The most structured forms of physician self-directed learning are those intentional efforts to learn about specific problems or issues.[9,11,46] Penland[17] identified a hierarchy of formal, intentional, planned projects that is useful for describing formal self-directed learning activities of physicians. Four categories of formal projects are described: self-planned projects, and those employing a nonhuman planner, human planner, or group planner.

Self-planned projects of physicians were considered by Richards[44] to be a "frontier area for CME." The study of Geertsma et al[26] laid the groundwork for the study of change in physician practice behavior, and further work has focused on physician self-planned learning projects.[9,30,47]

In CME, learning resources in print and other media (eg, programmed instruction, TV, and printed material with a learning blueprint) most often serve the needs of self-instruction and self-study.[42,48,49] The use of patient management problems with annotations that provide discussion of important points is a further example of the use of nonhuman planners in CME.[50] These methods are often combined in voluntary self-assessment programs such as those offered in the American College of Physicians Medical Knowledge Self-Assessment Program, which combines a syllabus, references, and multiple-choice questions,[51] and the American College of Surgeons Surgical Education Self-Assessment Program. These types of self-directed learning resources offer the learner flexibility, efficiency, and accessibility.

The use of human planners (such as mentors or CME facilitators in face-to-face interaction) has been a popular format for self-directed CME, as evidenced by the use of learning contracts,[52] formal traineeships,[53] informal traineeships,[54] specifically tailored experiences,[44,55] and educational consultants.[55] Manning et al[52] have reported the effectiveness of combining learning contracts, information brokering, and colleague discussion groups into a self-directed learning project.

Group planners may also play a role in physician self-directed learning. While activities provided by group planners often refer to events such as workshops, CME courses, and specialty society meetings (ie, the traditional lecture courses), planned group activities are able to incorporate self-directed learning experiences. One example is the Opportunity for Self-assessment CME (OSCME)[46] in which participants rotated through different stations. In one station, participants audited their own charts and scored themselves; in another they employed critical incidents from their own practices to fuel discussion. Another example is the group practice intervention described by Premi,[56] in which practitioners met in a group to discuss their own practice problems. Specific issues were identified and educational strategies formulated for use by the group, including sharing literature searches and inviting consultants to join the group to address various issues.

In each of these formal projects, goals and objectives are specified,[52] and the learner takes major responsibility for self-assessment, for planning of objectives and resources to access, for conducting the learning experience, and for evaluating the outcomes.[57] In all types of formally planned projects, the learner is an active participant.

### Common ground

Despite their many differences, informal, semi-structured, and formal self-directed learning activities share a variety of features. Self-assessment plays a critical role in physician self-directed learning, whether the need is identified directly by the physician[45] or by techniques or programs such as computerized home evaluation,[58] the Individual Physician Profile,[55] or the Practice Integrated Learning Sequence.[59] The recognition of the need for the learner to take responsibility for his or her own learning pervades all forms of physician self-directed learning.[60,61] Learners are thus actively involved,[34,44,46,52,56,59] and typically draw on multiple resources, both human and print, in the conduct of their self-directed learning.[9,26,28,29,34,43,47,52,62-64] With the exception of those projects undertaken for pleasure or interest,[35,65] self-directed learning projects tend to be problem-based and related directly to patient care.[30,34,35,43,56,59] The perception of the discrepancy between actual and ideal performance, and thus acknowledgment of the need to know more, gives rise to cognitive dissonance.[9,22,24,65] CME credit is not an issue.[31,35,54] Rather, immediate problems, tasks, or decisions operate as key motivating forces.[35,37,65]

The growing understanding of definitions, concepts, and characteristics associated with these different types of self-directed learning is evident when one examines how research in that area has evolved and unfolded.

# Research Directions and Implications

This section reviews past self-directed learning research activities from the perspectives of focus, research questions, and approach. It outlines a shift in research emphasis and offers directions, questions, and methods appropriate for future attention. This subject is broad and catholic: the study of physician self-directed learning is actually a study of all of the learning done by physicians, since all of their (or any other professionals') learning is ultimately self-directed. In the 1960s, 1970s, and 1980s, physicians reported that they kept up with new developments in medicine primarily through self-directed efforts—reading, contact with colleagues, self-assessment programs,[51] and self-selected CME courses.[63,66,67]

The evaluation of formal CME activity, including workshops, has occupied much of CME research. Assessment by a "happiness index," as well as studies of short- and long-term impact, have evolved.[9,48,68,69] In contrast, self-reports of "informal" self-directed learning were accepted initially on their face value and were not studied in depth. Early studies of self-directed learning focused on the learning method and comprised descriptive studies of how physicians learned or how physicians directed their own studies. For example, Curry and Putnam[29] surveyed Canadian maritime physicians about how they spent their learning time, how they preferred to learn, and what methods they found effective. Further, Ferguson and Caplan[34] surveyed physicians' preferred learning methods and sources of information, as did Stinson and Mueller.[63] Northup et al[43] and Geertsma et al[26] focused on physicians' clinical information needs. These studies all depended on self-reported data, garnered via survey or interview, and generated quantifiable results: ratings, rankings, and frequency or hours of use of specific methods (eg, reading, colleagues, or short courses). A few studies, not based on self-report (but rather on audits of use of library information systems), complemented the self-report data. They focused on specific self-directed learning methods and how to increase their use.[38,45,70]

Research questions posed in these self-directed learning studies centered on issues such as "What kinds of self-directed learning do physicians pursue and prefer?", "How much of their learning was self-directed?", "Is self-directed learning related to self assessment?", "What clinical problems trigger self-directed learning?", and "Does successful self-directed learning promote the increased use of self-directed learning?"

Findings from these types of self-directed learning studies, not surprisingly, suggest that this distinct and central form of learning is much more complicated than at first glance. Observational studies have contradicted self-reports in some respects.[6,37,71] For example, increasing difficulty with using reading as an effective vehicle for "keeping up" due to the size and increasing complexity of the literature has been noted. In addition, problems have been uncovered with the skills needed for critical reading and interpretation of the literature. Thus, reading, by itself, has not been found necessarily to be a direct path to new knowledge.[43,72] Lastly, it has proven possible to measure differences among physicians' access to colleagues and literature for self-directed learning, and these differences appear to be greatest along specialty and practice setting lines.[73]

As researchers began to look at self-directed learning more critically, a shift in research methods, foci, and conceptual approaches evolved. Earlier research methods, almost all of which had been descriptive, moved from quantifiable approaches to those of a more exploratory and qualitative nature. Studies which gathered quantifiable data gave way to studies which collected qualitative data— data less easy to categorize and count. The study of Fox et al,[9] using in-depth interviews relating self-reported changes made in practice to causes of changes and learning, was a prime example of this redirection. In addition, the research focus moved from studying self-directed learning methods to studying practice changes that were presumed to result from using self-directed learning. The research questions included: "How does self-directed learning lead to changes in practice?" and "How does a desire to change practice lead to self-directed learning?" Also, new conceptual self-directed learning models were offered.[14,23,32,74,75]

# What Methods Should be Used in Future Research?

Desirable methods in self-directed learning research are those that provide the most power for answering those research questions being asked. For some questions, a qualitative, ethnographic case study may be the most powerful. For others, quasi-experimental, multivariate analysis, or randomized controlled trials may be more appropriate. There is an ongoing need for descriptive studies of self-directed learning that yield testable hypotheses and lead to hypothesis-testing, experimental studies. In addition, careful consideration must be given to longitudinal, multi-disciplinary or interdisciplinary, and/or collaborative perspectives when these are appropriate to answer the questions being posed. Studies using multiple methodologies (such as that by Williamson et al[6]) also provide attractive and pursuable research models.

Future directions in self-directed learning research activities are tied to appreciating both past research findings and documented research shifts. Central to moving forward is a reflection on which core research questions need to be studied and in what order of priority, as well as which research methodology is most appropriate given the research questions. Because self-directed learning practices occur at the level of the individual, because learning is difficult to measure, and because some self-directed learning will always be random learning[44] or "contamination,"[27] continuing the focus on the outcome (eg, a change in practice) rather than on the means (ie, self-directed learning methods), will, in general, be more successful. Noting both first-order and second-order outcomes will also be important, as will the quality of research (from the planning [design] phase to the reporting stage), buttressed by appropriate standards to ensure excellence.[5,24,76-78]

# What Questions Need to be Studied?

Questions that warrant study in the future can be categorized into five areas: (1) the nature of self-directed learning; (2) the self-directed learner; (3) the relationship between self-directed learning and self-assessment; (4) the interface between self-directed learning, CME, and practice; and (5) the interface between self-directed learning research, CME research, and practice research.

## (1) The nature of self-directed learning

The theoretical perspectives of Knowles[2] and Schön[79] serve as two key perspectives for the concept of self-directed learning as applied to the individual and informal learning activities of physicians. Knowles is widely recognized as having best portrayed the characteristics of adult learners that distinguish them from children as learners. Schön has described the self-reflective process employed by professionals to refine and improve their practices. To the extent that physicians share in the characteristics of all adults and all professionals as learners, it is appropriate to generalize from these theoretical frameworks. As we work to further develop the construct of self-directed learning in medicine, however, one task will be to discover what additional theoretical frameworks are needed. The fields of cognitive, organizational, and professional science, for example, all have perspectives to consider. New reflections on concepts of self-directed learning and their association with lifelong learning need in-depth study.[14]

Questions that link theory and self-directed learning (for example, "What can the sciences of cognition, organizational theory, and professionalism tell us about self-directed learning?" and "Can the social, psychological, and educational dimensions across the three types of self-directed learning [informal, semi-structured, and formal] be defined and measured?") require further investigation. In addition, explorations into how self-directed learning fits with the natural patterns of learning are needed. Such questions as, "Is self-directed learning multi-faceted?", "Is self-directed learning more suitable for some content than others?", "What is a self-directed learning curriculum?", "How cost-effective is self-directed learning?", "Are self-directed learning skills learnable?", "Do self-directed learning activities yield better retention and application than other learning methods?", and "How does past CME impact on, and facilitate, self-directed learning?" come to mind.

## (2) The self-directed learner

As noted, several publications outline the characteristics of self-directed learners and self-directed learning activities.[11,14,15,19-21] The reasons individuals engage in learning are also documented.[9,31,80-82] Further work in the area of physicians' self-directed learning, however, is appropriate—for example, "What characterizes the more self-directed learner physician from the less self-directed?", "What are the relationships between age and stage of career to self-directed learning?", "Why are some physicians (teachers and learners) attached to the passive learner mode of traditional CME?", "Do different types of physicians differ in their learning style needs?", and "Are internists more likely to be self-directed learners than surgeons?".

## (3) The relationship between self-directed learning and self-assessment

The relationship between self-directed learning and self-assessment provides another area for research attention. Schön[13] emphasizes the importance of reflection, in which self-evaluation is critical component. Reflection may also serve as a trigger for change.[9,26] If self-directed learning results from physicians' self-assessment, how accurate are their self-assessments?

Another area for query is how frequently self-directed learning is used to fill a gap identified by self-assessment.[22,83] Do gaps in knowledge or skills always lead to self-directed learning? Which gaps do and which do not? How self-assessment fits with motivation and leads to self-directed learning is also important.[9,84]

Self-directed learning and self-assessment are key features in maintaining competence—a major reason for physicians deciding to change and engage in learning.[9,31] Here, two questions are: "What is the impact of self-assessment programs that are now in place?" (eg, the American College of Physicians Medical Knowledge Self-Assessment Program) and "Should CME providers use traditional CME modes to provide physicians more opportunities to learn how to assess their learning needs?" Furthermore, questions such as "How should these assessment opportunities be provided?" are addressed in section II.

### (4) The interface between self-directed learning and practice

Work on change, learning, and organizational theory promoted by Fox et al,[9] Schön,[13] Lewin,[83] Vroom,[84] and Knox[22] form the basis of this work supported by research addressing stages of learning.[9,13,85-87] Several questions serve as examples in this area: "How are practice experience and self-directed learning intertwined?", "What is the role of the practice environment (context) in learning?", "How does the offering of self-directed learning activities interact with the social, political, and economic contingencies within the practice world?", "Do the three types of self-directed activities (ie, informal, semistructured, and formal) differ regarding their impact on physicians' competence, performance, and patient care?", "How do models of change, learning and organizational theory interrelate with self-directed learning within practice?", "How do variables such as practice site, patients within a practice, and colleagues affect the three types of self-directed learning?", and "How does self-directed learning specific to a selected clinical disease or procedure 'fit' with how physicians change and learn in practice?"

### (5) The interface between self-directed learning research, CME research, and practice research

The importance of sharing concepts, approaches, and findings among areas of research is critical to ensure efficient forward movement. Two questions currently presented for inquiry are: "Does self-directed learning research meld with CME and/or practice research? If so, how, when, and where?," and "What characteristics (design, approach, and implications) of self-directed learning research can be applied to CME and/or practice research, and vice versa?"

Findings from current research have implications for CME planners, medical educators, the medical profession, and the practitioner. We need to ask "Are some CME organizations better at facilitating self-directed learning? If so, why?," "What products and services can CME organizations offer that will support physicians in productive and effective self-directed learning?", and "What changes are needed in the structure and organization of CME providers to enable them to offer products and services that are effective in supporting excellent self-directed learning?" Further comments related to new directions for reflection by the medical profession, medical practitioners, CME providers, and academics with interest in this field are outlined in the section to follow.

# New Directions

Adequately understanding and accurately describing the mosaic of self-directed learning, along with its role in medical practice, raises many challenges for the medical profession, for the medical practitioner, for CME providers, and for academics in the field. However, in-depth knowledge of self-directed learning is critical if optimal approaches are to be designed to support this type of learning, and if its impact on clinical practice and patient outcome is to be positive.

# The Medical Profession and Medical Practitioners

Central to every profession, including medicine, is its exclusive ownership of an expert body of knowledge, skills, and values. This expertise must be responsive to the ongoing, changing needs of society, its clients, and the discipline itself. In order to preserve this identity, practitioners within a profession, collectively and individually, must value the need to continuously self-initiate, plan, participate in, and evaluate both learning and change. Medicine, among the most sophisticated applied sciences, is strongly anchored in this belief. As such, for medical practitioners, the readiness to recognize both perceived and real learning needs, manage information, seek out resources, and participate in continuous improvement, (as well as in self and peer assessment) is central.[6,13,88] The habits and methods needed to accomplish these goals must be fostered by the profession.

A number of specialty societies (eg, the American College of Physicians, the American Academy of Dermatology, the American College of Obstetrics and Gynecology, the American College of Chest Physicians, and the College of Family Physicians of Canada, among others) increasingly offer to their members and subscribers self-study tools, materials, and enhanced access to the literature in print and computerized form. Professional medical associations in North America have begun to follow this path (for instance, the American Medical Association and the Royal College of Physicians and Surgeons of Canada). These integrated policies, procedures, and opportunities acknowledge and reward the essentials of self-directed learning. Leaders and role models within medicine must continually foster, reward, and model such new directions. To do so they must have a deep commitment and responsibility to understanding the principles and concepts that relate to self-directed learning and lifelong learning. A select few must devote specific energies to helping their profession grasp the importance of this for its members and for the profession itself.

# Medical Schools

Learning climates and activities that reflect a learner-directed and problem-linked focus must be designed and offered on an ongoing basis throughout the training program. The skills and habits associated with self direction and information management must be observed, practiced, and fostered by the practitioners of tomorrow until such skills are highly refined and the behaviors are habitual. Opportunities for these habits to develop must be provided within the professional training period.  In addition, remedial self-directed mechanisms must be available to respond to feedback from self and peer evaluation activities.  The importance of these approaches to learning and evaluation by a practitioner, to practice-linked learning, to the maintenance of competence, and to the profession itself, should be articulated and shared.

Medical school staff increasingly include professionals who possess expertise in how to design and provide self-directed learning and student-directed learning opportunities and who network with other faculty members who can provide guidance in this area.  Knowledge of the types and characteristics of various self-directed learning activities is critical in order to ensure that adequate and appropriate resources are available for student learning.  Learning documentation and activities currently in place should be reviewed to determine the degree of learner responsibility that is being fostered.  Student and faculty development seminars addressing different approaches to learning (teacher-directed and student-directed) may be required to implement these ideas.

Members of medical faculties must continue to research both theoretical[2,12,19] and practical[13] self-directed learning perspectives.  Their research must employ clear definitions, pose central questions, and choose sound and appropriate methodologies.  In addition to providing annotated bibliographies and reviews, they must disseminate findings for their colleagues in the field.[6]  Acting and modeling on a day-to-day basis the skills and habits of self-directed learning and "continuous improvement"[85] in a responsible and professional fashion, are central to faculty members who continuously interact with tomorrow's physicians.

## CME Providers

Providers, within and outside of medical schools, must advocate and practice learner-directed and teacher-facilitated approaches to CME.  They must foster sensitivity to the application of learning to practice.[2,9,44]  Recognizing that both formal and practical self-directed learning activities are critical to responding to practitioners' needs[8] is central to the operation of CME offices and programs.  Recognizing that much learning and change take place in the practice context (and is therefore influenced by political, social, and environmental factors associated with physicians, patients, and significant others) is also important.[9,89]

Today's CME providers facilitate networking between practitioners, literature retrieval sources, expert resources, and teachers.  Such providers are now familiar with, or have access to, the technology that will permit practitioners to carry this out individually or collectively as needed.[90]  Multiple initiatives have already been undertaken to make the medical literature more accessible in terms of availability and format.[63,70,91,92]  Competent CME providers differentiate between group and individual learning needs, access resources as needed by their client group, and reward participation appropriately.

Their challenge is to design, promote, conduct, and evaluate cost-effective self-directed learning activities that are shown to meet the learning needs of their clients, impact practice, and have the potential to improve patient health. Those learning activities must also be attractive enough to win the participation and financial investment of physicians. To be successful in the long term and fulfill their mission, all CME organizers will need to shift a growing portion of their resources to self-directed activities.

If the medical profession, the practitioners within that profession, medical schools and faculty members, and CME providers grasp the current concepts, characteristics, and applications of self-directed learning discussed in this chapter and integrate them into practice, then will collectively increase future chances that self-directed learning will contribute more powerfully to physician excellence in practice and to improved patients outcomes.

*The authors gratefully acknowledge the contribution of Kenneth Warren in group discussion.*

## References

1.  Mawby RG. Lifelong learning and the professional. *Mobius.* 1986;6:35-39.

2.  Knowles MS. *The Adult Learner: A Neglected Species.* 4th ed. Houston, Tex: Gulf; 1990.

3.  Houle CO. *Continuing Learning in the Professions.* San Francisco, Calif: Jossey Bass; 1980.

4.  Catley-Carlson M. Global considerations affecting the health agenda of the 1990s. *Acad Med.* 1992;67:419-424.

5.  Davis D. Meta-analyses and metaphors in CME literature. *J Contin Ed Health Prof.* 1991;11:85-86.

6.  Williamson JW, German PS, Weiss R, Skinner EA, Bowes F III. Health science information management and continuing education of physicians: a survey of US primary care practitioners and their opinion leaders. *Ann Intern Med.* 1989;110:151-160.

7.  Manning PR. Continuing medical education: the next step. *JAMA.* 1983;249:1042-1045.

8.  Cervero RM. The importance of practical knowledge and implications for continuing education. *J Contin Ed Health Prof.* 1990;10:85-94.

9.  Fox RD, Mazmanian PE, Putnam RW, ed. *Changing and Learning in the Lives of Physicians.* New York, NY: Praeger; 1989.

10. Osler W. *Aequanimitas with Other Addresses to Medical Students, Nurses, and Practitioners of Medicine.* 2nd ed. Philadelphia, Pa: Blakiston; 1906.

11. Tough A. *The Adult Learning Projects: A Fresh Approach to Theory and Practice in Adult Learning.* Toronto, Canada: Ontario Institute for Studies in Education; 1971.

12. Knowles MS. *Self-Directed Learning: A Guide for Learners and Teachers.* New York, NY: Association Press; 1975.

13. Schön DA. *Educating the Reflective Practitioner.* San Francisco, Calif: Jossey Bass; 1987.

14. Candy PC. *Self-Direction for Lifelong Learning: A Comprehensive Guide to Theory and Practice.* San Francisco, Calif: Jossey Bass; 1991.

15. Hammond M, Collins R. *Self-Directed Learning: Critical Practice.* New York, NY: Nichols/GP Publishing; 1991.

16. Szczypkowski R. In: Knox A, ed. *Developing, Administering, and Evaluating Adult Education.* Washington, DC: Adult Education Association of the USA; 1980.

17. Penland P. Self-initiated learning. *Adult Educ.* 1979;29:170-179.

18. Hiemstra R. The older adult's learning projects. In: Lumsden DB, ed. *The Older Adult as Learner.* Washington, DC: Hemisphere Publishing Corporation; 1985.

19. Knowles MS. *Using Learning Contracts: Approaches to Individualizing and Structuring Learning.* San Francisco, Calif: Jossey Bass; 1986.

20. Knox AB, ed. Approach. *Developing, Administering, and Evaluating Adult Education.* Washington, DC: Adult Education Association of the USA; 1980.

21. Knapper CK, Cropley AJ. *Lifelong Learning and Higher Education.* London, England: Croom Helm; 1985.

22. Knox AB. Influences on participation in continuing education. *J Contin Ed Health Prof.* 1990;10:261-274.

23. Richards RK. Physicians' self-directed learning: a new perspective for continuing medical education. I: Reading. *Mobius.* 1986;6:1-13.

24. Fox RD. New research agendas for CME: organizing principles for the study of self-directed curricula for change. *J Contin Ed Health Prof.* 1991;11:155-167.

25. Miller GE. Continuing education for what? *J Med Educ.* 1967;42:320-326.

26. Geertsma RH, Parker RC Jr, Whitbourne SK. How physicians view the process of change in their practice behavior. *J Med Educ.* 1982;57:752-776.

27. Goldfinger SE. Continuing medical education: the case for contamination. *N Eng J Med.* 1982; 306:540-541.

28. Manning PR, Denson TA. How cardiologists learn about echocardiography: a reminder for medical educators and legislators. *Ann Intern Med.* 1979;91:469-471.

29. Curry L, Putnam WR. Continuing medical education in maritime Canada: the methods physicians use, would prefer, and find most effective. *Can Med Assoc J.* 1981;124:563-566.

30. Blanchard D, Fox RD. A profile of nonurban physicians from the study of changing and learning in the lives of physicians. *J Contin Ed Health Prof.* 1990;10:329-338.

31. Richards RK, Cohen RM. Why physicians attend traditional CME programs. *J Med Educ.* 1980;55:479-485.

32. Richards RK. Physicians' self-directed learning: a new perspective for continuing medical education—learning from colleagues. *Mobius.* 1986;6:1-7.

33. Stross JK, Harlan WR. Mandatory continuing medical education revisited. *Mobius.* 1987;7:22-27.

34. Ferguson K, Caplan RM. Physicians' preferred learning methods and sources of information. *Mobius.* 1987;7:1-9.

35. Hummel LJ. An investigation of physician self-directed learning activities. In: *Proceedings of the 24th Annual Conference on Research in Medical Education*; Washington, DC. 1985;24:213-218.

36. Crandall SJ. The role of continuing medical education in changing and learning. *J Cont Ed Health Prof.* 1990;10:339-348.

37. Covell DG, Uman GC, Manning PR. Information needs in office practice: are they being met? *Ann Int Med.* 1985;103:596-599.

38. Jennett PA, Parboosingh IJT, Maes WR, Lockyer JM. The management of medical knowledge and information overload in rural practice: can a medical information system help? In: *Proceedings of the Annual Conference on Research in Medical Education;* 1989; Washington, DC. 1989;28:63-68.

39. Haynes RB, Mulrow CD, Huth EJ, et al. More informative abstracts revisited. *Ann Intern Med.* 1990;113:69-76.

40. Lockyer J, Parboosingh J. The role of the consultation process in physician learning. In: *Proceedings of the 25th Annual Conference on Research in Medical Education;* Washington, DC. 1986;25:151-156.

41. Stross JK, Hiss RG, Watts CM, Davis WK, MacDonald R. Continuing education in pulmonary disease for primary care physicians. *Am Rev Respir Dis.* 1983;127:739-746.

42. Stross JK, Bole GG. Evaluation of an education program for primary care practitioners on the management of osteoarthritis. *Arthritis Rheum.* 1985;28:108-111.

43. Northup DE, Moore-West M, Skipper B, Teaf SR. Characteristics of clinical information-searching: investigation using critical incident technique. *J Med Educ.* 1983;58:873-881.

44. Richards RK. Physician learning and individualized CME. *Mobius.* 1984;4:165-170.

45. Jennett PA, Lockyer JM, Maes W, Parboosingh J, Lawson D. Providing relevant information to rural practitioners: a study of a medical information system. *Teach Learn Med.* 1990;4:200-204.

46. Craig JL. The OSCME (opportunity for self-assessment CME). *J Contin Health Prof.* 1991;11:87-94.

47. Jones DL. Viability of the commitment for change evaluation strategy. *Acad Med.* 1990;65:s37-s38.

48. Sibley JC, Sackett DL, Neufeld V, Gerrard B, Rudnick KV, Fraser W. A randomized trial of continuing medical education. *N Eng J Med.* 1982;306:511-515.

49. Manning PR, Lee PV, Clintworth WA, Denson TA, Oppenheimer PR, Gilman NJ. Changing prescribing practices through individual continuing education. *JAMA.* 1986;256:230-232.

50. Jones E, Jones JV, Putnam W, Sowden S. A self-directed learning package in rheumatology for family physicians. *Med Teacher.* 1987;9:433-437.

51. Davidoff F. The American College of Physicians and the Medical Knowledge Self-Assessment Program paradigm. *J Contin Health Ed Prof.* 1989;9:233-238.

52. Manning PR, Clintworth WA, Sinopoli LM, et al. A method of self-directed learning in continuing medical education with implications for recertification. *Ann Intern Med.* 1987;107:909-913.

53. Kantrowitz M, Konis CN, Rezler AG. A personalized mini-residency program at the University of New Mexico School of Medicine: a seven-year perspective. *J Contin Ed Health Prof.* 1991;11:197-204.

54. Goldfinger SE, Bennett NL. Sub-rosa continuing medical education. *Mobius.* 1983;3:7-9.

55. Sivertson SE, Meyer TC, Hansen R, Schoenenberger A. Individual physician profile: continuing education related to medical practice. *J Med Educ.* 1973;48:1006-1012.

56. Premi JN. Problem-based, self-directed, continuing medical education in a group of practicing family physicians. *J Med Educ.* 1988;63:484-486.

57. Suter E, Green JS, Lawrence K, Walthall DB. Continuing education of health professionals: proposal for a definition of quality. *J Med Educ.* 1981;56:687-707.

58. Marshall JG, Banner S, Chouinard JL. *Physicians On-Line: Final Report of the CMA iNet Trial.* Ottawa, Canada: Canadian Medical Association: 1986.

59. Lanzilotti SS, Finestone A, Sobel E, Marks A. The practice integrated learning sequence: linking education with the practice of medicine. *Adult Educ Q.* 1986;37:38-47.

60. Osler W. The importance of postgraduate study. *Lancet.* 1900;2:73-75.

61. Association of American Medical Colleges. *Physicians for the Twenty-first Century: The GPEP Report. Report of the Panel on the General Professional Education of the Physician and College Preparation for Medicine.* Washington, DC. Association of American Medical Colleges; 1984.

62. Mason JL, Kappelman. *Continuing Medical Education: Utilization and Preferences of Primary Care Physicians.* Baltimore, Md: University of Maryland School of Medicine; 1979.

63. Stinson ER, Mueller DA. A survey of health professionals' information habits and needs. *JAMA.* 1980;243:140-143.

64. Lockyer J, McMillan DD, Magnan L, Akierman A, Parboosingh JT. Stimulated case recall interviews applied to a national protocol for hyperbilirubinemia. *J Contin Ed Health Prof.* 1990;11:129-138.

65. Means RP. *Information-seeking Behaviors of Michigan Family Physicians.* Urbana, Ill: University of Illinois, 1979.

66. Riddle JW. Report of the Council on Medical Education. *Cont Med Ed News.* 1981;10:2-20.

67. Rothenberg E, Wolk M, Scheidt S, Schwartz M, Aarons B, Pierson RN. Continuing medical education in New York County: physician attitudes and practices. *J Med Educ.* 1980;57:541-549.

68. Stein LS. The effectiveness of continuing medical education: eight research reports. *J Med Educ.* 1981; 56:103-110.

69. Lloyd JS, Abrahamson S. Effectiveness of continuing medical education: a review of the evidence. *Eval Health Prof.* 1979;2:251-280.

70. Haynes RB, McKibbon KA, Walker CJ, Ryan N, Fitzgerald D, Ramsden MF. On-line access to MEDLINE in clinical settings. *Ann Intern Med.* 1990;112:78-84.

71. Brody BL, Stokes J. Use of professional time by internists and general practitioners in group and solo practice. *Ann Intern Med.* 1970;73:741-749.

72. Bergman DA, Pentel RH. The impact of reading a clinical study on the treatment decisions of physicians and residents. *J Med Educ.* 1986;61:380-386.

73. Egan K. Practicing physician access to biomedical knowledge. In: *Proceedings of the 25th Annual Conference on Research in Medical Education*; Washington DC. 1987;26:209-213.

74. Tough A. *Learning Without a Teacher.* Toronto, Canada: Ontario Institute for Studies in Education; 1967.

75. Jennett PA. Lifelong self-directed learning: a critical ingredient of medicine as a profession. In: *Learning in Medicine: The Oslo Conference.* London, England: Oxford University Press; 1993:8-180.

76. Fox RD. New horizons for research in continuing medical education. *Acad Med.* 1990;65:550-555.

77. Escovitz GH, Davis D. A bi-national perspective on continuing medical education. *Acad Med.* 1990;65:545-550.

78. Yonke AM, Foley RP. Overview of recent literature on undergraduate ambulatory care education and a framework for future planning. *Acad Med.* 1991;66:750-755.

79. Schön DA. *The Reflective Practitioner.* New York, NY: Basic Books; 1983.

80. Houle CO. *The Inquiring Mind.* Madison, Wis: The University of Wisconsin Press; 1961.

81. Cross KP. *Adults as Learners: Increasing Participation and Facilitating Learning.* San Francisco, Calif: Jossey Bass; 1981.

82. Scanlon CS, Darkenwald G. Identifying deterrents to participation in continuing education. *Adult Educ Q.* 1984;34:155-156.

83. Lewin K. *Field Theory in Social Science.* New York, NY: Harper and Row; 1951.

84. Vroom VH. *Work and Motivation.* New York, NY: Wiley & Sons, Inc; 1964.

85. Putnam RW, Campbell D. The desire for competence. In: Fox RD, Mazmanian PE, Putnam RW, eds. *Changing and Learning in the Lives of Physicians.* New York, NY: Praeger; 1989.

86. Rogers CR. *Freedom to Learn.* Columbus, Ohio: Merrill; 1983.

87. Bennett NL. Theories of adult development for continuing education. *J Contin Ed Health Prof.* 1990;10:167-175.

88. Berwick DM. Continuous improvement as an ideal in health care. *N Eng J Med.* 1989;320:53-57.

89. Nowlen PM. A New Approach to Continuing Education for Business and the Professions. New York, NY: MacMillan Publishing Co; 1988.

90. Manning PR, Petit DW. The past, present, and future of continuing medical education: achievements and opportunities, computers, and recertification. *JAMA.* 1987;258:3542-3546.

91. Jennett PA, Parboosingh IJ, Maes WR, Lockyer JM, Lawson D. A medical information networking system between practitioners and academia: its role in the maintenance of competence. *J Contin Ed Health Prof.* 1990;10:20-24.

92. Haynes RB. The origin and aspirations of the ACP Journal Club: editorial. *Ann Intern Med.* 1991;114(suppl 1):A18.

**Chapter 4**

# The Role of Motivation in Self-directed Learning

*Karen Mann*
*Judith Ribble*

# The Role of Motivation in Self-directed Learning

*The physician, it is repeatedly stated, must be a continuous, lifelong learner. It is clear, however, that motivation to engage in self-directed learning is neither universal nor simple. The degree to which physicians actually direct their learning varies both across and within physicians; many factors affect this motivation and they may interact in multiple ways.*

Motivation in learning has been an important theme of learning theorists since the early behaviorists,[1] and the search for an underlying motivational structure to explain participation in adult learning has spanned the last three decades.[1] The purpose of this chapter is to identify possible motivators, and to develop a framework for thinking about motivation in self-directed learning. Using that framework, specific factors that have been associated with motivation, either conceptually or empirically, will be explored. These include factors within the individual, within the environment, or within the learning process itself. Following the exploration of these factors, an analysis of current research, including the strengths and weaknesses of the literature and our understandings to date will be reviewed. Remaining research questions will be considered. Finally, implications for the provider and the practice of CME will be discussed.

## Definition of Self-directed Learning

As noted by others,[2,3] confusion and debate have characterized the definition of self-directed learning. Debate has arisen concerning whether self-directed learning includes only those types of learning that are outside the bounds of the formal learning processes and structures, or whether it includes the use of many modes of learning, both formal and informal, wherein the ultimate control of the learning process lies with the learner. The former type of learning has been labeled autodidaxy by Candy,[2] to distinguish it from the latter, more inclusive approach to self-directed learning. A second debate has concerned whether self-directed learning is a process, or set of activities, or whether self-directedness is a personal attribute or combination of attributes within the learner. For the purposes of this chapter, this definition is used:

*"A program of learning activities, the structure, planning, implementation and evaluation of which are in the control of the learner."*

This definition permits examination of all aspects of motivation, including both the learner and the learning activities.

# A Conceptual Approach to Motivation and Self-directed Learning

The theoretical framework selected to guide this discussion is that of *social learning theory*, described by Bandura in 1977.[4] This theory has subsequently been written and enlarged upon by Bandura, who relabelled it *social cognitive theory* (1986).[5] Its relevance lies in the concept of reciprocal dynamic interaction, and in its fundamental tenets. Reciprocal determinism is described by Bandura[4,5] as the continuing, reciprocal, dynamic interaction among three elements: the individual, behavior, and the environment. The attributes, attitudes, and values of the individual continually interact with the individual's behavior. Similar interactions occur between the individual's behavior and the environment and the individual and the environment. These interactions are shown in Figure 4.1.

## Figure 4.1

## Interactions in social learning theory

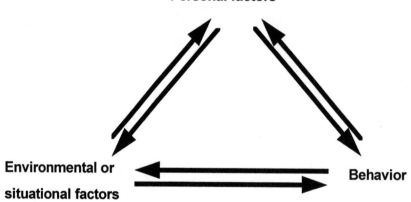

Social learning theory attributes several abilities to individuals. These include: symbolic (ability to store information and events in memory), vicarious (ability to learn through the observation of others), self-reflective and self-regulatory capabilities, and the potential for forethought. As a result of the capability to be inherently self-regulating, individuals are able to visualize desired goals and outcomes in the future, to set goals for themselves, to monitor progress toward those goals, and to reward themselves accordingly when they are achieved. The capacity to self-evaluate (to reflect on one's own behavior and make evaluative judgments accordingly) is critical to self-assessment. The ability to set goals makes self-directed learning a natural or inherent process.

This view of the individual as interacting with the environment is also held or implied by other learning theorists. Knox's[6] proficiency theory described a series of factors within the individual and the life situation that affects decisions to participate. In Knox's view, decisions to participate will have as their goal the achievement of a desired level of proficiency, either in personal or professional arenas.[7]

In 1983, Schon[8] described professionals' self-directed learning as an interaction with the environment in a reflective process, which he calls *"reflection-in-action."* In this process, the learner becomes aware of a learning need when a discrepancy or "surprise" is encountered as the professional conducts his or her tasks through a process called *"knowing-in-action."* Knowing-in-action is the automatic, embedded knowledge and skill that make up most of the practices of physicians.[9] When surprise is encountered, a deviation from routine practice or expectation, the individual is caused to reflect on this occurrence and on the previous actions in a process of reflection-in-action. This reflection may lead to the learner's selection of a solution or alternative action. The outcome of that action will provide the opportunity for the last link in the process—*"reflection-on-action."* It is in this final step that the learning that has occurred is incorporated into the individual's repertoire and becomes part of a "new" knowing-in-action.

Cross[10] also described learning as an interactive process, commencing with the individual's self-evaluation, and based in his or her set of attitudes toward education. These combine with the individual's estimate of the importance of the goals of learning and their likelihood of success should the learning be undertaken. In this construct, the importance of goals is affected by the unique circumstances in the individual's life, including barriers and opportunities to learning. Each of these interactions affects motivation to participate.

Fox et al[11] proposed a theory of learning and change that involves an interactive process among forces for change, the learning process, and subsequent changes. Key forces for change include professional, social, and personal forces impelling learning. Professional forces include the desire for enhanced competence or the pressures in the clinical environment. Personal forces (such as personal well-being) are sometimes mixed with professional goals or, less frequently, operate as the main motivating force. Finally, social forces act alone or in concert with professional forces (for example, collegial relationships) to motivate change.

Nowlen[12] described the individual's ongoing learning and function as the result of two separate, but intertwined strands of influence. These are the cultural strand (which carries, among other things, cultural meaning, expectations, norms) and the individual strand (which carries all the individual's past experience, growth, and cultural interactions). It is the continuous interaction of these two that helps to explain performance.

These theorists share a view of individuals as inherently self-regulating, capable of setting goals for themselves, working toward them, and rewarding themselves on their achievement. In addition, they acknowledge that the individual is unique and that the results of his or her interaction with the environment will also be unique. Within that framework, there are some specific factors that may motivate or enhance participation in self-directed learning and are supported by both theory and practice. As relatively few studies are reported about self-directed learning in CME, evidence from both theory and practice from many related fields, including behavioral medicine, health education, psychology, and education, has shaped this chapter's findings.

# Factors Within the Individual

In this section are presented factors residing within the individual that support or are associated with motivation to participate in self-directed learning.

## Forethought capability

Forethought capability is the capacity to hold events symbolically in the future, where they can act as an incentive or a desired outcome. Bandura[5] describes this as one of the most fundamental of cognitive and learning abilities. An important factor in the model proposed by Fox et al[11] is the individual's image of change, which may facilitate the process. This is consistent with the ability to visualize a desired outcome, which then acts as a motivating force.

## Goal-setting capability

Related to the ability to visualize future outcomes is the individual's inherent aptitude to set personal goals. The effectiveness of goals in human activity has been studied extensively, both in the context of social learning theory and by proponents of goal theory.[13,14] Goal-setting becomes a motivational force as it directs energy and effort, mobilizes attention and action, and generates strategies for the achievement of goals. Goals appear to be most effective as motivators when they are of average difficulty, ie, neither too difficult nor too easy. This inherent capability in all individuals to visualize the future, combined with an image of desired outcomes, is thus a potent motivator, and is particularly relevant for self-directed learning. Vroom[15] has also outlined a model of assessment of goals according to their value (valence) and the likelihood of achieving them (expectancy). He has termed this the *"path-goal model."* In fact, the valence-expectancy model of describing human behavior encompasses many approaches to the explaining of behavior and motivation, including social learning theory.

## Perception of a gap or need

A third element within the individual is the ability to perceive a gap between desired performance and perceived current performance. This may be viewed as an integral part of the goal-setting process or, as viewed by Knox,[7] as a desire for proficiency. The essence of this as a motivator is the desire to close the gap, and to meet the goal of desired performance. Clearly, this gap may be perceived in relation to a single, discrete skill (eg, a new technique) or to a larger area of expertise of personal or professional development (eg, enhanced involvement in health promotion or geriatrics).

## Self-efficacy

An important construct in social learning theory is self-efficacy, defined as the individual's view of his or her ability to execute a specific task.[4] This is separate from locus-of-control, in that it is generally task-specific (eg, pelvic examinations, dealing with dying patients) and amenable to change through intervention. Self-efficacy is believed by Bandura[16] to be the major determinant of the goals an individual will set and of the energy, effort, and perseverance that will be dedicated to their achievement.

## Previous success with self-directed learning

Self-efficacy may arise or develop from several sources. In order of their effectiveness, these sources are: personal experience (practice or achievement), vicarious experience (observation of others), persuasion (exhortation), and physiological feedback (racing pulse or anxiety).[4] As experience is the most effective enhancer of self-efficacy, previous successful experience with self-directed learning is likely to lead to higher perceived self-efficacy, which in turn will result in higher motivation for further involvement in self-directed learning experiences.

## Locus of control

Locus-of-control refers to the individual's perception concerning the source of control over events and outcomes.[17] Persons with an internal locus of control believe their actions to have an effect on the world around them; those with an external locus-of-control regard the control of events to be in the hands of powerful others or due to fate. Although they are two separate factors, the individual's locus-of-control may be linked to the perception of self-efficacy. Individuals with a high degree of self-efficacy toward a particular task (eg, counseling regarding smoking) may nevertheless fail to be motivated if they also perceive that, even if the task is successfully executed, it will have no effect on final outcomes. The presence of an internal locus-of-control has been linked to increased satisfaction with self-directed learning in undergraduate college students.[18] In contrast to self-efficacy, locus-of-control is generally viewed as a relatively stable trait, not easily amenable to change. However, where an internal locus-of-control is present, it may be a motivating force toward participation in self-directed learning. Although locus-of-control may not have been directly addressed, Penland's[19] findings (that a major reason for participation in self-directed learning activities was the ability to retain individual control) are consistent with that notion.

## Achievement

Achievement motivation has been widely studied in many contexts. A recent study[16] found that persons who selected self-directed learning activities were also likely to have a strong motivation to achieve when compared with those who selected more traditional forms of study.

## Curiosity

Curiosity motivates individuals to participate in learning for the interest the subject holds, for the purpose of gaining a broader understanding, and for the purpose of continually learning. It is generally associated with an openness to change. Fox et al[11] found that of 10 identified forces for change (encompassing personal, professional, and social forces), curiosity accounted for 4% of reported changes. Although the proportion is small, the changes associated with curiosity motivation were frequently significant, and some required extensive commitment in terms of time and persistence. Hummel,[20] in her investigation of family physicians and general surgeons, found intellectual curiosity motivated 18% of projects, second only to the motivation to solve patient problems. Personal interest motivated another 18% of projects cited. Woolf[21] found that personal interest was the main motivation for self-reported learning needs of physicians in semirural practice in Ontario. Curiosity may also act together with other forces, or may have a catalyzing, or mediating effect.[22]

## Professionalism

Professionalism was identified by Fox et al[11] as an important factor in learning and change. The majority of the changes the physicians in their study described were motivated by professional forces, including the desire to enhance and maintain competence and the desire for career development. These authors described professionalism as the internalization of societal and other external expectations, which has occurred throughout the process of professional socialization, and which involves the interacting of external expectations with the individual's personal experience, expectations, values, and other factors. Frequently, individuals do not make the distinction between the two (external and internal factors) and they become a potent internal motivator. As such, their motivational effects are not limited to self-directed learning. However, the changes recorded frequently involved self-directed learning as a central thread, suggesting that professionalism and self-direction are strongly linked.

## Attitudes toward and readiness for self-directed learning

Candy[2] has compiled a composite list of more than 100 competencies, grouped together based on qualitative similarities, which have been linked with successful independent learning. The general categories included are that the learner (1) is methodical and disciplined; (2) is logical and analytical; (3) is reflective and self-aware; (4) demonstrates curiosity, openness, and motivation; (5) is flexible; (6) is interdependently and interpersonally competent; (7) is responsible; (8) is venture-some and creative; (9) shows confidence and has a positive self-concept; (10) is independent and self-sufficient; (11) has information-seeking and retrieval skills; and (12) has knowledge and skill about learning processes and can develop and use criteria for evaluation. For each category, individual studies are identified.

The factors identified above do not represent an exhaustive analysis of all factors within the individual that affect motivation to participate in self-directed learning. Students of self-directed learning have attempted to measure self-directed learning "readiness" to identify whether high scores on specifically developed scales predict involvement in this type of learning activity. The Self-Directed Learning Readiness Scale (SDLRS) developed by Guglielmino[23] has been used most widely, although not without debate about the validity of its conceptual base. Also developed was the Oddi Continuing Learning Inventory (OCLI) to identify personality dimensions of self-directed learners.[24] The difficulties of the measurement scales are discussed later in this chapter in the section critiquing current research.

The question of attributes or attitudes that are associated with self-directed learning reflects the assumption that attitudes predispose individuals to act in certain ways toward their environment and toward the objects, events, and persons within it. If positive attitudes exist toward self-directed learning, the individual may be more likely to become involved in such learning activities than if those attitudes are absent. It has been shown frequently, however, that attitudinal predispositions are insufficient on their own to effect behavior or behavior change. Frequently, skills and an enabling environment are also necessary to bring about change.

## Factors Within the Environment

While environment for self-directed learning is clearly not subject to distinct boundaries, it may be helpful to think of the physician's environment as having several components. First, there is the practice environment, including the immedi-ate environment of the physician and his or her patients. Patients are an important factor in the physician's practice environment and they have a potent effect on physician behavior. In Hummel's study,[20] fully 21% of physicians were stimulated by the desire to solve a specific patient problem. Second, the environment also includes a larger involvement with physician colleagues in the practice and the community. Finally, there is a community from which both patients and physicians come, which exerts its own set of expectations.

The environmental factors that motivate self-directed learning may be grouped in any of several ways. For this discussion, they are categorized by their impact on three stages of the self-directed learning process: (1) asking the question, (2) finding the answer, and (3) integration of the new information or skill into practice. Clearly, there is some overlap of factors, and the distinction is somewhat artificial.

## (1) Asking the question

Asking the question refers to the process of identifying a learning need.  The factors discussed in this section are seen as positive factors that motivate self-directed learning activities.  In this case, they may also, in their absence, be viewed as barriers to participation in self-directed learning.

### Time to reflect

Schon's[25] description of the reflective practitioner is especially helpful at this point.  Reflection on one's action happens both deliberately and as a result of a "surprise" encountered in the course of practice.  The surprise that presents itself when a particular way of acting results in other than the expected outcome naturally causes reflection on the discrepancy.  The solution of the problem requires reflection on the unexpected event and self-reflection by the physician on his or her action.  That reflection may give rise to a need to learn (or a "question") about additional knowledge, attitude, or skill, which may effect a desired outcome.  This is the first, critical step in self-directed learning.  On a more deliberate level, physicians may wish to evaluate (as do all professionals) their practice (knowledge, information, and skill) periodically, to determine the presence of learning needs.  This reflection or self-assessment may also act as the first step in initiated self-directed learning.  Whether serendipitously or deliberately, the availability of time for reflection is essential for learning.  Frequently, work and patient obligations within the practice are such that either no formal reflection can occur, or questions raised in practice are not acknowledged or go unanswered.

### Availability of information systems

Information systems, either in print or an electronic medium, are necessary to assist the physician in asking questions and seeking solutions.  A recent needs assessment of practicing family physicians and specialists[26] revealed that although many physicians have access to such systems, (ie, there were computers in their practice), they frequently did not possess the skills to utilize them.  The question of availability then also includes accessibility as a function of physician skills.

### Interaction with colleagues

The most basic premise of social learning theory is that one learns from others and from interaction with the environment.  Physicians are influenced by the expectations of the environment, as expressed by colleagues, about keeping up-to-date.  They are also exposed, in an environment with other colleagues, to potent role models in self-directed learning.  Observational learning is driven in a powerful fashion by observing the actions of others and the consequences (ie, rewards or censure) of their behavior.  The behavior modeled by others (in terms of information, values, attitudes, and skills) can also provide a standard against which to assess one's own performance.  Discrepancies can be perceived as gaps to be filled to achieve desired levels of proficiency, and may serve as specific goals for attainment.  The absence of collegial interaction may exert a negative effect on the pursuit of self-directed learning. Physicians who are in solo practice appear more likely, over time, to experience difficulty in maintaining professional competence. Their risk appears to substantially exceed that of the physician member of a practice group.[27,28] In reviewing the literature on physicians' self-directed learning projects, Richards[29] observed that self-directed learning projects generally involved greater contact with others than did other-directed, primarily formal CME.

### Community expectations

Just as important as the interaction with colleagues are the implicit or explicit expectations about ongoing learning and maintenance of professional growth and competence. These expectations are powerful incentives. Of comparable importance are those interactions with the community—with the individual community member as a patient or as a member of a larger community of individuals. Increasingly sophisticated and well-informed patients have expectations of their physicians regarding ongoing learning, understanding, and awareness of current advances. There is also the expectation, not always successfully met, that physicians will be able to address emerging issues of psychosocial, socioeconomic, and other dimensions, which significantly affect health. These abilities, however, are not systematically addressed during most physicians' undergraduate medical education. Therefore, general expectations (and expectations regarding specifically emerging skills) act as powerful incentives toward self-directed learning. Hummel's[20] study found that 10% of self-directed learning projects undertaken were impelled by professional motivation to improve the profession, community, or society.[20]

### Mechanisms to identify needs

Several facets of identification of needs have been mentioned—reflecting on interactions with patients and patient problems, observing other colleagues in practice, and responding to expectations of colleagues, patients, and the community. These methods and opportunities are informal rather than formal. Where further assessments of a formal nature are required, the physician needs to seek assistance with such procedures as practice audit, or self-administered formal tests of knowledge and skill, explored in section II. The awareness of a gap or a need, or identification of a desired level of skill may be most helpful if the areas of need or standards of current performance can be defined. Feedback on one's current level of performance is essential to learning; in addition, goals are more often successfully attained (and at higher levels of achievement) if the learner has feedback on current performance.[15] In whatever way feedback is obtained, it can be powerfully motivating.

## (2) Finding the answer

There is no shortage of questions raised in practice.[30] In contrast, there appears to be a dearth of immediately available, efficient, and effective learning resources and of training for physicians in ways to pursue the needed answer. The process of self-directed learning requires that an answer be sought. Three factors are proposed that may motivate the physician to successfully complete the process: (1) assistance with focusing the question, (2) assistance with locating resources, and (3) access to those resources.

All three aspects have been addressed in a project reported by Jennett et al.[31] The objective of the Medical Information System at the University of Calgary, Alberta, Canada, is described as assisting individual physicians in clarifying their clinical questions. Physicians telephoned questions raised by patient problems to trained librarians and specialist physicians who identified and screened appropriate resources. Over the course of the 12-month pilot project, physician use was such that a subscription service for physicians was established. Successful solutions to information needs would be expected to reinforce the physician's use of the service and would also promote the development of more refined questions. Access to resources on the part of these physicians was not simply a question of obtaining the appropriate source, or a question of reasonable geographic proximity, since physicians have reported low use of both the university library and their local library.[26] Conversely (at least for family physicians and specialists in the same study), problems encountered in practice were most frequently addressed through the use of resources that existed in the physician's office (for example, personal texts). This behavior probably reflects learning patterns established early in one's education and embedded thoroughly in the process of conventional undergraduate medical curricula, where the emphasis is frequently on committing to memory thousands of facts from convenient teacher-prepared handouts, a survival tactic that allows little time or incentive for finding personal resourses.

## (3) Integration into practice

Learning is complete when new information, skills, or attitudes are integrated into practice. Schon[8] described this as the final step in the reflection-in-action process, in which what is learned becomes part of a new "knowing in action." Factors integral to this step also motivate further self-directed learning. Personal factors play a role in integration, as the successful integration increases satisfaction with personal goals attained or performance improved and also increases personal perceptions of self-efficacy. Heightened self-efficacy, in turn, increases motivation.

The important factors in the environment may be termed "reinforcing factors" in that their effect is to determine whether the new learning is continued.[32] Just as patient and colleague expectations may have a motivating effect, feedback from these sources may also be motivating. Colleagues' approval and respect (and patients' satisfaction and improved health outcomes) are important reinforcing factors.

# CME credits

The awarding of CME credits for participation in educational activities has been alternately lauded and criticized since the American Medical Association initiated the Physician's Recognition Award in 1968. The record-keeping and extensive paperwork required of accredited sponsors has added to the cost of CME activities, and the benefits of accumulating credits based on simply attending a CME seminar have been difficult to document. CME credits have traditionally been assigned a relatively unimportant role in encouraging physicians to participate in self-directed learning activities.[29-33]

A recent study,[34] however, has thrown new light on the subject. In a survey of 645 physicians who responded to a mailed questionnaire, a study commissioned by the Accreditation Council on Continuing Medical Education (ACCME) found that the single most important factor in choosing to attend a CME activity concerned the availability of CME credits. Category 1 credits carry the approval of an accredited organization and provide official assurance of an educationally sound program that has been developed independent of commercial influence. This sanction may serve as a powerful incentive for physicians who are looking for a way to recognize credible programs among the thousands of CME activities presented each year.

## Factors Inherent in the Learning Process That Motivate Self-directed Learning

As discussed in the previous section, factors emanating from personal needs and from the environment in which the physician works are linked to primary concerns in the hierarchy of issues that motivate self-directed learning. The flexibility of arranging study time and location to suit a busy schedule carries a strong appeal. After these factors have brought the physician to the table, however, other forces inherent in the learning process need to be present in order to motivate continued effort.

Formal CME activities impose external motivations that oblige the learner to complete the process of experiencing the program, even if it turns out to be boring, irrelevant, or counterproductive. National and regional seminars require advance planning for travel, lodging, and practice coverage, and the complexities and expense of these arrangements act as a deterrent to leaving early and discontinuing the seminar. Attendees may be too embarrassed to walk out of a lecture hall. Peer pressure or respect for eminent lecturers can keep the seats filled even if the minds wander. In contrast, in self-directed learning projects, the learner must be encouraged to persevere in the absence of the traditional enforcement mechanisms. Program developers need to build in incentives that will retain the attention of the solitary learner. The following mechanisms are illustrative of factors that may be intrinsic to successful educational programs that allow the learner to select the time, place, and topic of choice.

### Control of learning experience

The printed text of a self-assessment program can be soporific; care must be taken to avoid unrelieved pages of text by interspersing text with diagrams, graphs, bullet points, and illustrations. Computer-based programs that resemble printed materials offer little or no advantage over printed texts.[35] In fact, unadorned computer screens may deprive the learner of informative and relevant photographs and illustrations that cannot be keyed into the computer program. In order to reap the benefits available from this technology, educational designers need to develop programs that utilize computer-specific strengths, including branching logic, random access of cross-referenced information, and offering a variety of learning options tailored to the individual physician's learning style.[36]

Self-directed learning places the control of the curriculum in the hands of the learner and allows specific questions to be researched for immediate clinical use. Multimedia applications of computer programming can gather a myriad of learning tools at one electronic workstation, where the learner can call up appropriate modules that use text, graphics, audiotapes, and videotapes to answer questions as they arise in practice situations.

## Coaching/corrective feedback

Telephone hotlines that put physicians in contact with content experts provide access to a source of personal coaching in areas of expressed need. The Medical Information Services by Telephone (MIST) offered by the University of Alabama School of Medicine, Birmingham, engages specialists to return calls received by a toll-free number; callers can request written materials for further study or make referrals to the consulting physician.

In addition, self-assessment programs can confront learners with information in a manner that identifies weaknesses and challenges them to search for correct answers. Many medical speciality societies publish extensive self-assessment programs that are revised or rewritten periodically by groups of clinicians. These programs are designed to lead the learner through a structured curriculum by providing a syllabus, asking questions that are deemed important for the practitioner, supplying answers and critiques as feedback mechanisms, and adding bibliographic materials to encourage further reading.

## Effect of past experience

Adult education researchers emphasize the importance of accumulated knowledge based on prior learning experiences.[36] Material that can be related to what an individual already knows appears to be easier to remember and builds confidence incrementally. New studies on the effects of aging on the brain question traditional assumptions about the decay of learning abilities in the age cohort that includes many practicing physicians. The impact of prior knowledge on current learning suggests that experts and novices may think in different ways.[37] A wealth of knowledge in one area may enable a senior physician to skim over one section of a flexible curriculum while spending a great deal of time on another topic that younger colleagues with more recent diplomas would find elementary.

## Social interaction

Positive effects of social interaction can be stimulated by the formation of study groups and mentoring opportunities with influential peers. A study among primary care physicians reported improvement in cancer control performance as a result of an educational program that used interactive discussion groups, influential peers, and self-formulated contracts.[38]

Group dynamics can also create a disincentive to learning in certain instances. The implications of asking a question that might reveal a gap in essential knowledge and the competitiveness of some group members can be inhibiting to the acquisition of that knowledge. Self-study eliminates this barrier and allows physicians to take as much time as needed to acquire and practice new ways of thinking and acting, and to better past performance records.

## Educational components and strategies

Physician preferences regarding beneficial educational activities have been studied in various settings, but across-the-board comparisons are difficult to justify. The quality of the activities under scrutiny differ widely in different settings. If respondents are asked to rate a checklist of strategies, the items often differ among studies and confound any comparison of preferences. For example, a study involving 160 family physicians in Oregon found that "hotline consults" (telephone consultations), one-day regional workshops, and written protocols were preferable to methods that relied on electronic technologies held to be more frustrating to learn and operate.[39] In an Australian study, rural general practitioners who participated in a 2-year study reported a preference for individual, experiential study programs over formal CME programs.[40]

Reading printed material continues to be the quickest and most flexible way to assimilate knowledge.[41] Listening to audiotapes and watching television or videotapes expands the use of the senses and reinforces knowledge, but presents information in a linear fashion that does not allow random access to bits and pieces of related topics. The strength of self-directed study lies in the ability to access a sufficient number of options, so that the learner can find the method that suits the need of the moment today; and if desired, find a different method tomorrow.

## Enjoyment

Video games are considered to be entertainment, but the elements of fun and excitement that motivate teenagers to stand for hours in dimly lighted arcades can also be adapted for more serious subject matter. A study of learning outcomes at nine universities found that graduate students in degree-granting programs learned better by videotape than by live delivery of similar material.[42] The results, statistically significant in this study, suggest that lively, animated material designed to hold the viewer's attention enhances both the acceptance and the outcome of certain self-study programs.

### Achievement of a goal

The rewards that await the physician who submits to the discipline of self-directed study are many—the bridging of a knowledge gap; the comparison of self-assessment test scores against national norms and confirming an area of competence; and the satisfaction of having completed a rigorous, long-term study program. One author suggests that teaching individual physicians to do on-line literature searching has the potential for blurring the traditional "town/gown" distinction that works against private practitioners lacking access to medical librarians in academic medical centers.[41]

Manning et al[43] described a project that employed motivational factors in all three categories—personal factors, environmental factors, and factors within the learning process. Contract learning (self-formulated learning objectives), information brokering (linking physicians with consultants and community resources), and collegial networking (discussion groups) were integrated to assist physicians with speciality-board retraining through self-directed learning. Although the project did not study motivation to participate directly, 50% of participating physicians were successful in completing their learning plans, suggesting a high level of satisfaction.

The values inherent in the process of self-directed learning take many forms and provide multiple motivations for the physician to persevere with an individualized approach to CME. Flexner[44] emphasized that, if students were solidly grounded in a few subjects, they would be well prepared to continue in a lifelong search for new knowledge using the methods they had learned initially. Written in 1910, Flexner's words have currency today:

> *The actual value of these conceptions of [study of the sciences] and of the habits grounded on them depends less on the extent of his [sic] acquisitions than on his sense of their reality. Didactic information, like mere hearsay, leaves this sense pale and ineffective; a first-hand experience, be it ever so fragmentary, renders it vivid.*

## The Current Literature on Self-directed Learning: A Critique

### Definition

As noted earlier, the study of self-directed learning has been impeded by debate and disagreement concerning its nature and meaning. It has been studied both as a process and as a constellation of attributes of the learner. It has also been considered by some to include only those activities that fall outside the domain of formal organization, while others have included activities of all kinds, provided the control of the process lies with the learner.

## Difficulties in Interpretation

Studies of self-directed learning have, for the most part, followed Tough's[45] model of data gathering. While many populations of persons have been studied, socioeconomic status and ethnicity have not generally been reported. Merriam and Caffarella[3] have reviewed and summarized the literature on self-directed learning, addressing the deficits in published studies. They have also discerned three types of studies: verification research (confirming the existence of self-directed learning as a form of study), the learning process itself, and the styles and attributes of self-directed learners. First, serious concerns about verification studies have related to the populations studied and the methods of data collection employed. While most studies have been conducted on middle-class samples, thus limiting their general applicability, this sampling does not likely reduce the usefulness of the literature in applying it to physicians and other professionals. Similarly, regarding data collection, interview techniques allow for probing and reflection, but may generate results contaminated by the interviewer or those marred by difficulties attendant upon the use of retrospective measures. Brookfield[46] has added to these methodological criticisms, flagging the literature's emphasis on individual dimensions of self-direction at the expense of social or contextual dimensions.

Studies of the self-directed learning process, the second area of literature described by Marriam and Caffarella,[3] explore how the individual actually conducts the process and are the most likely to provide insight into the role and determinants of motivation. Most studies since Knowles[47] have assumed self-directed learning to be a linear process, planned well in advance. In fact, some exploratory studies have suggested that this is not always the case; rather, interactions with the environment and among variables within that environment may be involved.[48] This is certainly consistent with any dynamic learning theory serving as an underlying conceptual base. Other approaches to self-directed learning as primarily a means of solving problems have also been suggested.[49] These are congruent with Schon's theory of reflection-in-action[25] in which the situation, or a trigger, cue, problem, or surprise, becomes the motivation to learn. A final approach to the process of self-directed learning relates to the use of resources. Although it appears that a basic understanding of the resources used by self-directed learners exists, more clarification of the usefulness of each resource is required. Furthermore, the process by which educators can assist learners in finding and using those resources needs clarification.

The literature on the third type of study of self-directed learning, relating to self-directedness as a attribute, is smaller than that on the existence and nature of the process. This literature aims to better understand these learners, their personality characteristics, cognitive styles, and perceptions, and their motivation to learn in this manner. Oddi[50] has suggested this as an appropriate focus to facilitate studies of self-directed learning.

It is in this area that measurement and methodological difficulties have been rife. Guglielmino[23] has operationalized self-directed learning, as a series of characteristics indicating readiness to engage in this type of study. These characteristics

(openness to learning, self-concept as an effective learner, initiative and independence in learning, informed acceptance of responsibility, love of learning, creativity,
future orientation, and the ability to use basic study and problem-solving skills)
underlie the Self-Directed Learning Readiness Scale (SDLRS) that has been used in
numerous studies. Some controversy surrounds the use of this scale. A second
scale, the Oddi Continuing Learning Inventory (OCLI),[24] may also assist in measuring the existence of this characteristic. One aspect of these qualities is clearly
motivational. However, more information on this and other attributes is needed.

A major factor that affects all analyses of self-directed learning is the lack of a
unifying conceptual base, although some models have been proposed. These
models by Long,[51] Brockett and Hiemstra,[52] and Grow[53] assume the existence of
motivation to self-directed learning; however, specific motivational factors have not
been explored.

Candy[2] has criticized the largely positivist approach to the study of self-directed
learning and has proposed an interpretive approach to explore: (1) the learner's
views of learning in general, (2) the learner's intentions or purposes in the learning
situation, (3) attitudes toward direction or assistance, and (4) views of independent
learning and the development of personal autonomy. While, for Candy and others,
the learner is the central point of study for self-directed learning, the context of
learning is critical and it is necessary to operationalize and describe the reaction
between both learner and context.

It is possible, however, that the search for a unifying theoretical base may be an
impossible task, given the multiplicity of interacting factors and the unique nature
of each individual learner. Rather, the study of self-directed learning might profit-
ably continue within the broad framework of social learning theory. This theory
recognizes the dynamic, changing, interactive, and individual nature of human
functioning and learning. The process of learning can be studied effectively within
it by utilizing models and consistent theoretical approaches thoughtfully and eclecti-
cally. In addition, by enhancing the interpretive phenomenological study of the
process, further inductive insights can be gained.

Finally, for those studying self-directed learning in relation to professional development, in the field of CME, it is important to recognize that the information that
exists is found in several fields of study, including education, adult education, and
psychology (among others). The synthesis of all these research directions is ultimately necessary to complete an understanding of self-directed learning and of
motivation within it.

## Questions Remaining to be Answered

A review of possible motivational factors (and of the current status of research)
highlight several remaining research questions. Those that apply to self-directed
learning for all types of learners have been discussed above. They include: (1)
more inquiry into the nature and usefulness of resources used by self-directed

learners, (2) attempts to identify and describe personal attributes associated with participation in self-directed learning and to clarify their developments, (3) the effect of interventions on the development of self-directed learning, and (4) the predictive value of measurement scales. These questions apply equally to the self-directed physician learner, as do many others relative to the field of CME. Here an improved understanding of potential barriers to and facilitators of self-directed learning is critical prior to the development of studies to determine whether interventions may benefit physicians in their self-directed learning pursuits. A greater understanding of the skills of self-directed learning, their acquisition and development, and their related motivational elements, is essential for the continuum of medical education.

## Implications

Although much remains to be understood, the current state of knowledge has important implications for the practice and providers of CME:

(1) There is a need to create a system for access to useful learning resources. While some examples of this exist, the creation of a system of such resources needs to be more widespread. Further, training will be required to help individuals effectively select and access the resources they need.

(2) Increased participation in self-directed learning will increase the need for effective information-management systems. Such systems will be an important aspect of asking questions and finding answers. Physicians will need assistance in formulating their questions and in utilizing the systems effectively.

(3) CME providers and practicing physicians will need to better understand and operationalize the interaction between formal and self-directed learning activities. Resources may need to be shifted from formal activities to the development of resources for self-directed learning, including the need to provide opportunities for physicians to practice and acquire needed self-learning skills.

(4) Improved systems whereby self-directed learning can be documented will need to be developed and marketed. Better documentation of activities will allow better exploration of their nature and the role of motivation. Further, there will be a concurrent need to study documented self-directed learning activities to assist learning needs assessment, and to raise physician awareness of their own self-directed learning activities.

(5) Increased involvement in self-directed learning will necessitate change in expertise and new collaborative relationships in CME offices, eg librarians, distance learning, and informatics specialists.

(6) A new role may be added to the educational influential—that of acting as a role model for self-directed learning. These individuals need to be identified and assisted to provide such examples.

(7) Finally, recognizing the importance of the continuum of medical education, CME providers must promote the importance of acquiring skills in self-directed learning in undergraduate curricula and residency training. If these skills are successfully acquired early in the individual's medical career, they are likely to become an embedded source of motivation.

*The contributions of John Parboosingh, Dennis Wentz, Murray Kopelow, and Elizabeth Lindsay, to the discussions that formed the basis for this chapter, are gratefully acknowledged.*

## References

1.   Houle CO. *The Inquiring Mind.* 2nd ed. Madison, Wis: University of Wisconsin Press; 1988.

2.   Candy PC. *Self-Direction for Lifelong Learning: A Comprehensive Guide to Theory and Practice.* San Francisco, Calif: Jossey-Bass; 1991.

3.   Merriam SB, Caffarella RS. *Learning in Adulthood.* San Francisco, Calif: Jossey-Bass; 1991.

4.   Bandura A. *Social Learning Theory.* Englewood-Cliffs, NJ: Prentice-Hall; 1977.

5.   Bandura A. *Social Foundations of Thought and Action: A Social Cognitive Theory.* Englewood-Cliffs, NJ: Prentice-Hall; 1986.

6.   Knox AB. Proficiency theory of adult learning. *Contemp Educ Psychol.* 1980;5:378-404.

7.   Knox AB. Influences on participation in continuing education. *J Contin Ed Health Prof.* 1990;10:261-274.

8.   Schon DA. *The Reflective Practitioner.* New York, NY: Basic Books; 1983.

9.   Fox RD. New research agendas for CME: organizing principles for the study of self-directed curricula for change. *J Cont Ed Health Prof.* 1991;11:155-167.

10.  Cross KP. *Adults as Learners: Increasing Participation and Facilitating Learning.* San Francisco, Calif: Jossey Bass; 1981.

11.  Fox RD, Mazmanian PE, Putnam RW. *Change and Learning in The Lives of Physicians.* New York: Praeger Publishers; 1989.

12.  Nowlen PM. *A New Approach to Continuing Education for Business and the Professions.* New York, NY: MacMillan; 1988.

13.  Locke EA, Shaw KN, Saari LM, Latham GP. Goal-setting and task performance: 1969-1980. *Psychol Bull.* 1981;90:125-152.

14.  Locke EA. Motivational effects of knowledge of results: knowledge or goal-setting. *J Appl Psychol.* 1967;51:324-329.

15.  Vroom VH. *Work and Motivation.* New York, NY: John Wiley & Sons, Inc; 1964.

16.  Bandura, A. Self-efficacy mechanism in human agency. *Am Psychol.* 1982;37:122-147.

17.  Rotter JB. *Social Learning and Clinical Psychology.* Englewood-Cliffs, NJ: Prentice-Hall; 1954.

18. Grabinger RS, Jonassen DH. Independent study: cognitive and descriptive predictors. In: Proceedings of selected research papers of the annual meeting of the Association for Educational Communications and Technology; January 14-18, 1988; New Orleans, La.

19. Penland P. Self-initiated learning. *Adult Ed Q.* 1979;29:170-179.

20. Hummel LJ. An investigation of physician self-directed learning activities. *Proc Ann Conf. Washington, DC: Res Med Ed.* 1986;25:213-218.

21. Woolf CR. Personal continuing education (PECE) plan: stage 2, a model to supply physicians' perceived needs. *J Cont Ed Health Prof.* 1990;10:321-328.

22. Lanzilotti S. Curiosity. In: Fox RD, Mazmanian PE, Putnam RW, eds. *Changing and Learning in the Lives of Physicians.* New York, NY: Praeger; 1989:29-43.

23. Guglielmino LM. *Development of the Self-Directed Learning Readiness Scale.* Athens, Ga: University of Georgia; 1977. Thesis.

24. Oddi LF. Development and validation of an instrument to identify self-directed continuing learners. *Adult Ed Q.* 1986;36:97-107.

25. Schon DA. *Educating the Reflective Practitioner.* San Francisco, Calif: Jossey-Bass; 1987.

26. Mann KV, Chaytor K. Help, is anyone listening? An assessment of learning needs of practicing physicians. *Acad Med.* 1992;67:4s-6s.

27. McAuley RG, Henderson HW. Results of the peer assessment program of the College of Physicians and Surgeons of Ontario. *Can Med Assoc J.* 1984;131:557-561.

28. McAuley RG, Paul WM, Morrison GH, Beckett RF, Goldsmith CH. Five-year results of the peer-assessment program of the College of Physicians and Surgeons of Ontario. *Can Med Assoc J.* 1990;143:1193-1199.

29. Richards R. Physicians' self-directed learning: a new perspective for continuing medical education—the physician and self-directed learning projects. *Mobius.* 1986;6:1-14.

30. Covell DG, Uman GC, Manning PR. Information needs in office practice: are they being met? *Ann Intern Med.* 1985;103:596-599.

31. Jennett PA, Lockyer JM, Maes W, Parboosingh J, Lawson D. Providing relevant information to rural practitioners: a study of a medical information system. *Teach Learn Med.* 1990;4:200-204.

32. Green L, Eriksen MP, Schor E. Preventive practices by physicians: behavioral determinants and potential interventions. *Am J Prev Med.* 1988;4(suppl 4):101-107.

33. Goldfinger SE, Bennett NL. Sub-rosa continuing medical education. *Mobius.* 1983;3:7-9.

34. Slotnick HB, Raszkowski RR, Jensen CE, Wentz DK, Christman TA. A new study of physician preferences in CME: insights into education vs. promotion. Presented at the Third National Conference on Provider-Industry Collaboration in CME; October 8-9, 1992; Chicago, Ill.

35. Kramer JB. Computers and medical practice: an auspicious union. In: Nash DB, ed. *Future Practice Alternatives in Medicine.* New York, NY: Igaku-Shoin; 1987:303-341.

36. Chao J. Continuing medical education software: a comparative review. *J Fam Pract.* 1992;34:598-604.

37. Caffarella RS, Loehr L, Hosnick J. Cognition in adulthood: current research trends. In: Proceedings of the Adult Educational Research Conference. 1989; Madison, Wis.

38. Dietrich AJ, Barrett J, Levy D, Carney-Gersten P. Impact of an education program on physician cancer control knowledge and activites. *Am J Prev Med.* 1990;6:342-352.

39. Darr MS, Sinclair AE. HIV disease: educational needs of Oregon family physicians. *Fam Med.* 1992;24:21-23.

40. Davies PG, Davies JM. Continuing medical education undertaken by general practitioners using the rural registrar scheme. *Med J Aust.* 1991;155:157-159.

41. Douma A. The future of continuing medical education. In: Nash DB, ed. *Future Practice Alternatives in Medicine.* New York, NY: Igaku-Shoin; 1987:343-367.

42. Stone HR. *A Comparative Analysis of Interactive and Non-Interactive Video Delivery of Off-Campus Graduate Engineering Education.* Washington, DC: American Society for Engineering Education, Division of Continuing Professional Education; 1990.

43. Manning PR, Clintworth WA, Sinopoli LM, et al. A method of self-directed learning in continuing medical education with implications for recertification. *Ann Intern Med.* 1987;107:909-913.

44. Flexner A. *Medical Education in the United States and Canada.* New York, NY: Heritage Press; 1973.

45. Tough A. *The Adult's Learning Projects: A Fresh Approach to Theory and Practice in Adult Learning.* Toronto, Canada: Ontario Institute for Studies in Education; 1971.

46. Brookfield S. Self-directed adult learning: a critical paradigm. *Adult Ed Q.* 1984;35:59-71.

47. Knowles MS. *The Modern Practice of Adult Education: From Pedagogy to Andragogy.* 2nd ed. New York, NY; Cambridge Books; 1980.

48. Spear GE. Beyond the organizing circumstance: a search for methodology for the study of self-directed learning. In: Long HB, ed. *Self-Directed Learning: Application and Theory.* Athens, Ga: University of Georgia Press; 1988:199-221.

49. Peters JM, Lazzara PJ. A knowledge acquisition model for building expert systems: studying adult reasoning and thinking. In: Adult Education Research Conference. 1988; Calgary, Canada.

50. Oddi LF. Perspectives on self-directed learning. *Adult Ed Q.* 1987;38:21-31.

51. Long HB, ed. *Self-Directed Learning: Emerging Theory and Practice.* Norman, Okla: University of Oklahoma; 1989.

52. Brockett RG, Hiemstra R. *Self-Direction in Adult Learnig: Perspectives on Theory, Research, and Practice.* New York, NY: Routledge and Kegan Paul; 1991.

53. Grow GO. Teaching learners to be self-directed. *Adult Ed Q.* 1991;41:125-149.

**Chapter 5**

# Developmental Perspectives in Learning

*Nancy Bennett*

# Developmental Perspectives in Learning

*"Advanced age seems almost always to be associated with lower levels of performance, [but] we cannot tell how much difference between the young and the old is due to a failure of the latter to acquire new knowledge or skill and how much is the result of a loss of knowledge or skill originally possessed."[1]*

This statement strikes directly at the concern for providing appropriate CME, clearly focuses on the need to understand professional development, and directs us to learn more about factors which contribute to lower levels of performance. However, if age is a critical element in assessing clinical competence, why has it received so little attention in the literature?

The continued professional development of physicians is a central theme of CME, in which experience, performance, and age are all interwoven. Assuming a simple connection between age and competence, however, ignores the complexity of the experiences that shape any physician's performance throughout a career. Age itself is not an indicator that answers many of the important questions about the quality of practice performance. We must reframe the question to understand the professional development of physicians and define factors important to that development. A look beyond age links learning experiences and events to patterns of practice.

Physicians learn how to practice medicine in less than 10 years, but use the results of that effort for many decades. Understanding how that knowledge base is adapted, enhanced, and used over time is limited. It is unclear what parts of the knowledge base are most important, how individual parts contribute to the whole, whether old knowledge is dropped in favor of new ideas, or when and how shortcuts are developed as the result of expertise. The goal of this chapter is to define what is known about the parts of professional development that are linked to age and experience and to understand their impact on the ways physicians practice medicine.

## Relationships Between Age and Physician Attributes

While understanding professional development contributes to the way we clarify how physicians change their thinking about managing patients, the literature that links age to performance and experience in medicine is not readily available. There are, however, examples of clinical behavior studies that use age or years of experience as one physician characteristic. One way to organize these studies is to separate the traditional elements of knowledge, skills, or attitudes of physicians as linked to age.

## Linking Knowledge and Age

In this chapter, eight studies are reviewed, linking knowledge and age.[1-8]  In one of these, physicians in three hospitals in a large northeastern city were surveyed about their use of blood products.  Older attending physicians routinely scored lower on knowledge tests compared to younger residents, yet their scores for confidence in using blood products were higher.  The authors equated age with experience to show a shift from novice to expert, and argued that expert status is linked to a knowledge base that is readily accessible and which increases physicians' confidence in their ability to solve medical problems.  Confidence may be misplaced, however.  New information inconsistent with current beliefs is not readily accepted or adapted.[2]

An Illinois study of family physicians reflects the contrast between the relative ease of incorporating new information in undergraduate medical education and the problems inherent in disseminating knowledge to practicing physicians.  In this study, younger physicians were found to enter practice with a better recall of the causes of dementia but little opportunity to become comfortable with the knowledge because of the smaller geriatric population in their practice.  On the other hand, older physicians were better able to evaluate their diagnostic abilities in geriatrics.[3]

Knowledge gaps and amount of learning relative to age were the focus of a Minnesota study on knowledge of cancer pain management in older, middle-aged, and younger physicians.  The authors found that older physicians reported learning more from CME than younger physicians and that older and middle-aged practitioners learned more from consultants than their younger colleagues.  Of the three age groups, younger physicians felt most strongly that staff conferences were the preferred place to learn.  Finally, the study indicated that younger and middle-aged physicians preferred to use literature as a learning resource to a greater extent than older physicians.[4]

Clarifying factors which link knowledge and age, Donabedian[1] proposes an epidemiology of quality.  He indicates that the key attributes influencing physician performance are training, experience, and specialization.  Further, the author defines experience in terms of years in practice and volume of similar cases treated, and suggests that while the effect of experience is additive over years of practice, it becomes shaded by obsolescence of knowledge.

Supporting Donabedian's findings, a study of internists with the American Board of Internal Medicine concluded that there was an inverse correlation between test scores and the number of years since certification.  In this study, knowledge declined sharply within 15 years of certification and procedure-oriented subspecialists scored less well than other internists when asked about general medical knowledge.[5]  Similarly, Day and colleagues[6] found that success on recertifying examinations declined with age or time since completion of training.  In this study, questions were categorized by the degree to which they probed stable, changing, or new knowledge.  Scores for new or changing knowledge decreased with age, suggesting that, while older physicians may experience more difficulty with the examination format, the decline in performance with age may be related to the way in which physicians update and expand their expertise rather than to the loss of the original knowledge base.

Lockyer et al[7] confirm that the use of formal CME is somewhat different for different ages. In a study of family physicians, they indicated that frequent attendance at CME courses was more common among younger physicians, and that year of graduation and certification status were strongly associated. In a further analysis of learning patterns, Lockyer and colleagues[8] provided evidence that younger physicians were more apt to consider the advice of colleagues when making changes while older physicians were more prone to use CME courses.

## Linking Skills and Performance With Age

Five studies are discussed that analyzed the link between skills and age.[9-13] In this instance, "skills" also covers studies of performance or behavior. A 5-year peer assessment program in Ontario[9] found that 35% of physicians 75 years of age or older were of serious concern to examiners, based on failure to meet minimal standards of documentation and patient care. This was compared with 9% of those 50 years of age or younger and 16% of those from 50 to 74 years old.

Physician characteristics, including age, were thought to be a factor in cesarean birthrates in New York City.[10] Older, more experienced physicians performed fewer cesarean sections and more forceps deliveries and breech extractions. The authors found a high correlation between age and type of experience, including differences in management based on techniques acquired in training. Gender and practice setting were not found to be associated with the operative delivery rates.[10]

A study of obstetricians and gynecologists found that younger physicians in "nonsolo" practices were involved in more birth-related activities.[11] The authors hypothesized that energy levels may be higher for younger physicians or that there is a life cycle pattern in the doctor/patient relationship with pregnancy as an entry point. Specialization declined and generalized practice increased with age, with older physicians spending less time on pregnancy and birth. It may be that, with age, there is a decrease in the degree of concentration on delivery and related care, along with an increase in the range of diseases treated—and a subsequent reallocation of time and energy.[11]

Roos and colleagues[12] found that surgical experience accounted for a large part of the probability of complications following cholecystectomy and, marginally, following hysterectomy. In this study, experience appears to be defined primarily by continued high numbers of procedures in a given year rather than by expertise acknowledged in other ways.

Finally, Freiman[13] surveyed the number of new procedures adopted by a group of 484 physicians during a 1-year period.  He found that, up to about 50 years of age, there were continued increases in the number of new procedures adopted, achieving a maximum of procedures at this mid-life stage.

## Linking Attitudes and Age

Among five studies using physician attitude and age as factors for exploration, experience influenced the ways physicians thought about making treatment decisions in a Michigan study about willingness to proceed with treatment.[14]  Four clinical case vignettes were used to differentiate between case-related clinical experience and general experience.  The role of case content was found to be significant in decision making, indicating that more experience with a problem led to a greater willingness to proceed with treatment without additional information.  For cases involving arthritis, a fever of undetermined origin, or *cor pulmonale*, usually one or two encounters provided enough experience to treat without additional information.  Younger physicians, when compared to older colleagues who had more experience, were more willing to treat patients without seeking additional information and preferred to maintain full responsibility for patient care.  The authors concluded that experience does not alter the strategies for accessing information but allows a physician to delay in seeking it.  They also suggested that attitudes or perceptions about problem-solving ability are important in assessing the value of even a single clinical problem.[14]

Reuben and Robertson[15] compared physicians aged 35 to 54 years to those older than 65 years.  Elderly physicians devoted a larger proportion of their practice to elderly patients.  They tested less often for mental status and vision and less frequently assessed the need for physical therapy.  On the other hand, they provided more counseling, performed more general examinations and Pap smears, and spent more time on each office visit.  The authors hypothesized that attitudes directed toward these behaviors may be due to training in different eras, having a greater body of clinical experience, knowing patients well, or failing to keep up-to-date.

A Canadian author[16] found that those who graduated before 1969 differed significantly in their understanding and beliefs about contraception than did those who graduated after 1969.  When asked about beliefs, younger and older physicians differed in responses about attributes of women, contraceptive devices, adverse effects of contraception, and problems created for physicians by contraceptive issues.  Three methods of contraception were included in the study.  The authors questioned the existence of regional, gender, and age differences that affect family practitioners in Canada, producing variations in the perceptions of efficacy, adverse effects, and suitability of contraceptive methods.[16]

A Massachusetts study[17] about cost containment found age to be a significant factor in attitudes about the importance of major technologies, inappropriate ordering of diagnostic tests, excessive utilization of radiographs, and the therapeutic effect of test ordering.  Physicians 60 years of age and older reported their perception of major technologies as "very important" compared to perceptions of lesser importance reported by those under 60 years. The older physicians also noted that inappropriate ordering of diagnostic tests was very important in influencing health-care costs. The authors concluded that education about cost containment must allow for physicians' ages.[17]

A final study[18] relating attitudes to age described life satisfaction among practicing internists, and analyzed characteristics of work, health, and life styles. An important factor was age: older physicians reported greater satisfaction with life. A number of other coping and health habits were explored, many of which were also significant.

While age can clearly be important in looking at performance, all of these references provide glimpses into the role of age and experience when performance is defined within very specific parameters. For a broader base of understanding professional development, it is helpful to look at literature in other areas. Adult development, life span, career development, cognition theory, and performance theories each contribute some useful ideas, models, and constructs.

## Adult Development Theory

One adult development theory is illustrated by a study defining seasons of life that change with time. Levinson et al[19] outlined age ranges during which usual tasks of development take place. The authors used intensive interviews with a group of 40 men to describe adult life as ten stages grouped in three eras. An era was defined as a period of stability interrupted by times of adjustment and transition; issues that emerge must be resolved during each period in order to build a strategy for resolution of new issues in the next period. The process of resolving issues may be lengthy, with each period lasting about 5 years. Three major eras are charted, beginning with early adulthood based on childhood and adolescence. This first era focuses on entering the adult world, through the age-30 transition, and ends with "settling down." The second era, the midlife transition, proceeds through middle adulthood, through the age-50 transition, and ends with middle adulthood, and the commencement of the third era, late adulthood.

Early adulthood tasks usually include moving away from one's childhood family to create an independent home and find work. People often marry and may begin having children during early adulthood. During the early stages of adulthood, physicians are involved in intense full-time schooling and training that may force postponement of many other parts of their lives. As school ends, many physicians seem to have a sense of needing to catch up; a greater focus on one's personal life may compete with the need to start a practice and open an office or to begin other full-time work in medicine.

Near age 30, many men make new choices or affirm old choices in defining their personal views of adulthood. This leads to the second era in adulthood that often places a high value on work, attaining seniority, or achieving ambitions. Although responsibilities and pressure increase, there may also be some expanding sense of expertise based on clinical experience that provides new definition for practice goals. Practice life may be more stable, with an income and schedule that are more predictable. Some physicians shift to devote more time to parenting or community concerns, while others branch into new styles of medical practice such as limiting patients to a specific type of problem or a specific setting. Some practitioners devote all their energy to their chosen field, while others apportion time quite differently to include personal growth, family, or community.

The second era of adult life, middle adulthood, provides the opportunity to question and search for meaning in life. There may be a series of changes or crucial marker events such as a major job change, a serious illness, a divorce, or a move. Resolution of these questions and issues can result in a sense of creativity and fullness in the life cycle; lack of resolution may signal the beginning of decline.

Physicians rarely change jobs in the corporate sense. Some may move into administrative or educational positions, leaving behind clinical practice, or relinquish other activities to focus on patient care. As more physicians work in health maintenance organizations (HMOs) or other large groups, this may change, but, for now, advancement is often seen in a subtle fashion. Informal consultations with colleagues or networks used for problems may readily provide a clear sense of those designated as "experts." Experts may also be found by reviewing the literature for those writing opinions in prestigious journals or noting those individuals invited to teach CME courses. Given the range of positions in health care, few physicians drop out of medicine even when they do not maintain a clinical practice.

Because of the delayed introduction to full-time professional life, there may be some unevenness in the development of a physician's personal and professional lives. That may become apparent by choices made during middle adulthood. Active participation in professional organizations or community activities may become more important. A focus on parenting may result in fewer hours at work. Interest in hobbies, religion, friends, or community service may become more central. Some physicians may decide to devote all their energy to medicine.

The later periods of adulthood require further refinement of adult life with appropriate changes to match professional and personal goals with what has been achieved to date for a satisfactory life structure. A sense of crisis occurs for many people when it is obvious that the dreams from earlier periods require reshaping.

These refinements and reorientations lead to the third era, late adulthood, during which older physicians often receive mixed messages about their role in medicine. Some patients do not want to begin a relationship with a physician who will soon retire. On the other hand, some older physicians are recognized as elder statespersons providing wisdom and compassion about difficult medical decisions. This era is marked by several issues: concerns about being sued when income is declining; being viewed as not up-to-date; poorly defined roles for most retired physicians to continue contributing in ways that fill gaps in society; and, finally, difficulty in leaving medicine as a central role in all aspects of physicians' lives. Retirement requires much advance planning to break off relationships and relinquish responsibilities.

# Life-span Theory

Life-span theory assumes that many of the tasks of adulthood are completed about the same time for most people. While not tied to age in the same way as adult development theory, life-span theory assumes that sequential changes provide a framework for an understanding of adult life, while recognizing that each person is shaped by the forces in the environment. Three major types of events contribute to the form of adult life. First, life events may be age related. A first job, marriage, and retirement are examples set by social norms and biology. Second, life events may be related to historical events, such as wars, recessions or depressions, or political changes. That impact may be linked to age. Third, events like illness, death of a family member, loss of a job, or a career change may be a great force in an individual's history.[20-22]

Life-span development accounts for the ways in which an event may have different meanings to different people. An event may be more stressful if it is perceived as being "off schedule" for an individual. A "late" marriage or start of parenting, an "early" retirement, or a "late" start in training are reported to be stressful. A downswing in the economy may block career development or force other choices based on available resources or ability to find an income. One of the classic examples of a powerful historical event was the death of the late President John Kennedy, which was experienced differently according to one's age.

Life-span theory also includes the professional and personal development of physicians as adults. Long years of training with little income may be a source of stress in the perception of being off schedule. Shifts in the role of a physician in the community, changes in health-care costs, and uncertainty in social norms may be stressful for physicians practicing medicine in a changing world. Several examples illustrate these shifts. First, cutbacks in insurance, coupled with more options within HMOs and clinics provide more salaried positions. Second, the needs of underserved populations and populations of new immigrants without health insurance create societal demands that physicians are asked to help solve. Third, the increasing numbers of geriatric patients and of children with few resources compel physicians to help make choices within limited resources.

# Career Development Theory

Several theories exist in the literature that help to explain the ways in which careers develop. Nowlen[23] uses a double helix to describe the relationship between the values, expectations, and missions of a culture, intertwined with an individual's attributes, experiences, and limitations. Culture gives meaning to work and to an individual's history. The theory helps to clarify the need to address the context of work within the experience of the individual; neither can be addressed without appreciating the impact of the other. Even in private practice, physicians operate within the health care system. Thus, using CME to change the way some problems are handled cannot be separated from how our society views that problem and what is expected of the physician. AIDS, abortion, and child abuse are all obvious medical problems closely coupled to complicated social and political agendas. Similar issues include organ transplantation, geriatric care, and aggressive therapy for the terminally ill, each of which extend life and demand enhanced clinical skills in the face of limited resources and unclear societal values.

Houle[24] envisages a career as a lengthened line of learning beyond schooling. The first stage (about 5 years) of professional life demands that professionals extend their proficiency in practical techniques within their domain of practice. The next 5 years often shifts that need to one of improved basic theoretical understanding. The third phase of a career (years 10 through 15) often reflects promotions into new positions that require more administration or management of relationships with coworkers and subordinates than was learned in school. The next stage for many is a push to understand one's own work in the greater context of history, society, and the economy, and, after 20 years, many professionals ask for a broader orientation to all knowledge. Houle[24] describes the shifts in the ways these professionals, including physicians, view their work. Moving from a narrow understanding of the clinical care to a broader, administrative view, for example, demands new skills and new ways of solving problems. Similarly, mastering technical issues often extends thinking about ways that address some of the societal issues involved in caring for people. This theory provides an interesting view of the limitations of initial training in which the knowledge base must expand to meet new demands that come with the development of professional expertise.

Super[25] identifies five stages of a career, beginning with *childhood. Exploration* generally occurs between 15 and 24 years old, during which early work activities and a full-time job are used as a testing ground. *Establishment* occurs from 25 to 44 years old, with the development of a permanent place in the work world, and the need for stability and security. This period may be a very creative time for many people. From 45 to 64 years old, Super describes a *maintenance* phase that consolidates a position or situation, following which he envisages stage five *decline* for those 65 years of age and older, with erosion of physical and mental power and the end of a major occupational role. The career stages are age based, and assume work within a traditional setting. Created within the context of the business world, they provide examples of the assumptions of age and work effort that are common in society.

Schein[26] proposes a theory of career anchors based on the motivations, attitudes, and values that are formed early in each person's career. These anchors are seen as shaping what individuals look for in life and how they interpret their experiences. Schein's study identified five such anchors—managerial competence, technical-functional competence, security, creativity, and autonomy and independence:

1) *Those professionals using the managerial anchor are motivated by a desire to be competent in the activities thought of as management, such as the ability to influence, supervise, lead, manipulate, and control people to achieve organizational goals. There is a desire to rise in the organization with greater levels of responsibility.*

2) *A focus on the challenge of the actual content of work defines the technical or functional anchor. Individuals in this group prefer to stay within their area of practical expertise rather than be promoted just to supervise.*

3) *One group of people tie a career to a given setting or organization for a sense of security. Some people who fit within the security anchor change jobs, but generally stay within the same type of company position, preferring stability to autonomy.*

4) *The creativity anchor fits those individuals who need to create something, perhaps as an entrepreneur, inventor, or developer of a new product or service. Independence allows the development of new ideas rather than requiring a response to corporate goals.*

5) *Those anchored by autonomy and independence often find organizational life too restrictive because their primary concern is for a sense of freedom without the restrictive aspects of organizational life.*

Schein's constructs are instructive and helpful in understanding how a basic orientation toward a career may shape how it unfolds. A preference for creativity, for example, may push one physician to structure clinical practice quite differently from one who has a preference for technical-functional competence. The creative physician may develop an innovative system for follow-up, new ways to help patients stop smoking, or patient educational materials describing treatment options. For the technically oriented physicians, a computer system might track diagnosis and treatment for specific diseases within the practice, while those who push for managerial competence may build or make better use of interdisciplinary teams. The concept of anchors may be helpful for an individual sorting out career and learning options, or, conversely, for members of a health-care organization to think about ways that professionals function as they move forward in their careers.

Defining career stages is one way to look at the changes that physicians experience as they continue in medicine. Bennett and Hotvedt[27] divide physicians' careers in medicine into the following three stages. (1) The first stage, *breaking in*, is the period during which a physician sets up practice and begins to perform the roles of a physician. At this stage, physicians perceive few options for the way they practice experience and many demands to conform to local standards. Their learning is more apt to be at the local level, driven by an interest in understanding the local practices and meeting influential colleagues. (2) The second stage, *fitting in*, is the time during which physicians refine a place in medicine consistent with professional and personal goals. Intense questioning about how medicine fits with all the other adult roles in life may occur. Some physicians may specialize, or shift the focus of a practice; others may limit work in favor of parenting, community involvement, or time to pursue other activities; and some may devote all their energy to medicine. Learning may take place away from home more often since physicians at this stage have more money and control of time to allow travel. Further, they may have special interests which demand expertise found only in selected settings, often outside their own locale. (3) *Getting out* is the third stage. Physicians report changes in physical status, professional standing, their view of the world, and the world's view of the older physician. The informal and formal processes of withdrawing from a practice often take many years. Learning may move back to the local level in response to the need for others in the medical community to recognize these physicians as competent and actively engaged in the practice of medicine.

## Cognition Theory

Another tack to take in thinking about professional development has been to look for places where enhanced performance or learning takes place—called *situated cognition*. Brown and colleagues[28] argue that conceptual knowledge cannot be abstracted from learning situations. Knowledge is only one part of the whole activity of learning, dependent on the culture of a learning environment which determines or predicts what will be learned. Situated cognition may be helpful in looking at knowledge gains and adaptation to change, relative to the environment in which learning and change take place. For example, differing cultures of care in hospitals and ambulatory clinics require different practice and subsequent learning strategies. Thus, providing education in more settings, including hospitals, clinics, and community-based sites, may extend the ways that physicians see similar problems and encourage the formulation of a greater variety of practice setting-specific solutions. Situated cognition is linked to age in several ways, the most obvious of which is that shifts in curriculum may provide very different learning situations for different training eras.

Another way to extend learning that makes use of specific settings is the notion of *cognitive apprenticeships*. Cognitive apprenticeships lay out a progression of skills leading to expertise, guided by a master or expert who helps the learner by modeling expert strategies in the context of a problem. A key component of this model is effective self-critique that leads to independence in learning.

Cognitive performance has been directly measured in the psychological literature. Salthouse[29] reviewed studies that compared age and experience, and concluded that, given limitations in methodology, it is not possible to determine whether experience minimizes cognitive differences. Despite this critique, cognitive performance literature is one of the underutilized sources from which CME professionals could borrow to expand their thinking.

Another way to look at the role of experience and age is to consider how a physician moves from *novice to expert*. The definition of expert implies use of experience that expands the knowledge base. Schmidt et al[30] found that, rather than superior reasoning skills, expertise is based on cognitive structures they called "illness scripts." Novice physicians are apt to use pathophysiology (ie, principles) in their reasoning when new problems arise. Intermediate physicians move away from an active use of pathophysiology to more elaborate information systems. Experts collect information in an abbreviated form from a patient, and use it to compare and match this problem with available illness scripts in their experience base. Thus, different knowledge structures are used at each stage. Further, rather than losing earlier knowledge, physicians store and retrieve it when necessary in the form of clinical information that has been effective in defining specific illnesses.

# Performance

One of the central goals of professional development is enhanced performance. Schon[31] uses experience as the critical piece of performance to understand how a professional's knowledge changes with what he terms a "reflective practice." Professionals use a specific knowledge base to formulate and generate their professional work. Experience allows that knowledge base to expand in ways that are not the same as learning from traditional teaching methods. Technical rationality says that professionals are technicians who select optimal solutions for a given problem, and that increased technical expertise widens the range of problems that can be solved. In contrast, reflective practice proposes that real problems are often not well defined or clear, and that indeterminate situations, those difficult to clearly define, are the usual rather than the unusual. While increased technical expertise may not clarify such problems, past performance, experience, and reflection allow some professionals to create innovative or new solutions to problems that are not simple or clear.

Professionals look for problems they can solve. A problem is understood or framed by possible answers, determined by discipline, training, background, and interests. The complexity or indeterminacy of many problems is partly due to the lack of ready solutions available to the professional and may result in different views of the problem, with different actions by different professionals. Many problems do not have a single or correct response but can be approached in a variety of ways;  a good solution matches the expectations of both the health professional and the patient.

Examples of how to learn problem framing are common in the education of professionals, often made clear by the terminology we use to describe learning. Medical interns and residents treat patients with the guidance of senior physicians. Student professionals perform or execute productive practice that is demonstrable to professionals acting as teachers. In Schon's model,[31] learning is directed by performance problems, and teaching is seen as guiding or coaching performance rather than a more distant traditional telling of facts and theory. Students learn by working on specific professional problems, standing next to a professional as teacher/coach in the field.  Schon[31] also describes the "right kind of telling" that takes place when students work closely with faculty to learn how to frame questions and to respond as professionals do.

Another way to look at performance was offered by Stross and Bole,[32] who identified "educational influentials."  They hypothesized that primary care physicians rely on informal and personal methods of education frequently influenced by opinion leaders within their community.  For the greatest impact, academic centers can teach those physicians designated by their peers as influential, who then function as both formal and informal consultants to others in the community, and as disseminators of new information.  While educational influentials were not grouped by age in this study, the study does provoke questions about the relationship between career stages and position as an influential professional.

## Figure 5.1

### Developmental perspectives on age and stage of career

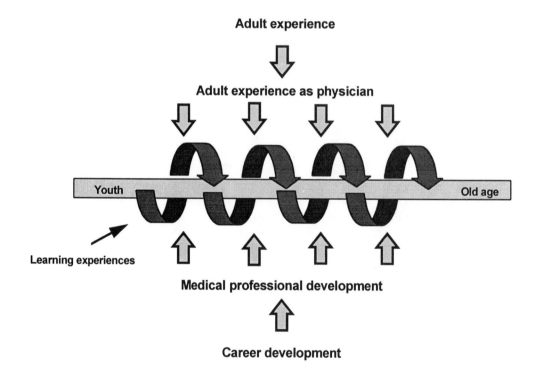

# Consensus

Age and experience contribute to the quality of performance, but they are not primary factors, and their relative place with other factors is less easily defined. Age becomes important as part of the pattern of development when linked (for example) to the number of years in practice, the volume and variety of cases seen, and relative expertise. Age and age-related factors affect but do not predict competence. Professional development is shaped by many factors such as motivation to learn, desire and ability to be a self-directed learner, interest in clinical competence, ability to assess learning needs, and systematic participation in a well developed, individualized CME program. These factors combine to provide a look at the important reasons physicians learn, make changes, and become experts. Neither age nor years of experience are the centerpiece of a model for professional development, however professional development is tightly tied together by age and range of experiences. Enhanced performance based on experience gathered over time *is* professional development.

The perception of age in our society, as in medicine, is tied to societal norms. The patient's perception of his doctor's stage of career and expertise is shaped outside of medicine. The health care system has not addressed how it wants to involve physicians at different stages of their careers and the impact of age. That impact varies widely. If a physician follows the local guidelines for commonly ordered tests during the first phase of his career, then shifts to tests recommended by a given professional society, and finally orders a large number of tests to protect himself from legal action at the end of his career, the dollar variation may be tremendous, and both the style of care and its rationale shifts.

There is no provision to consider the use of retired physicians in selected ways or in positions that are not funded. Older physicians face conflicting issues and messages. For example, while there are age limitations for physicians to admit patients to hospitals, there are usually none for treating patients in private practice. In addition, on the one hand we see the wise older physician using his experience to define a strategy for difficult problem, while on the other hand we hear anecdotes about incompetence stemming from older physicians' out-of-date information or skills.

Medical schools seek ways to provide optimal teaching in a short period of time. One of the current shifts in undergraduate education has been to provide more attention to the ways students learn and how that essential function will be used in the practice of medicine. Extending that thinking into shifts in teaching patterns for CME is under discussion and of interest to many. A model of small groups of physicians using real problems as forums for discussion, however, creates a crisis for the current CME system since the financial base for most programs is from large enrollments. While there is a consensus that age and experience make a difference in what physicians need and want, CME providers rarely put into practice programs and strategies to address questions of professional development. The development of a continuum of learning from medical school through an entire career appears to be an achievable and desirable goal.

One of the ways to think about age in relation to professional development is in terms of the way that age ties together the parallel continua of life and career development. Learning activities respond to needs and interests from a variety of sources, and may, in turn, generate more learning activities. Intense concentration in one area may demand learning focused primarily on professional issues, for example. Age ties together the concurrent streams of development, for both the personal and professional life of a physicians. All adults deal with general life events and experiences with variable outcomes. At the same time, physicians manage general career issues as well as issues specific to the practice of medicine.

# Next Steps: Implications for Research and Practice

The research agenda is exciting and complicated: the questions are both subtle and pervasive with potential, significant impact on the health care system and on CME. There are three major areas of questions around understanding career stage, developing expertise, and defining the role of CME in professional development.

First, while some early ideas exist about the shape of a career, details are lacking that may be helpful to both individuals and CME experts. Can stage theory be confirmed? What happens to learning at transition points? Although some things are known about shifts in physicians' attitudes toward health care that appear with age, what are the details of the impact on the kind of care received by individual patients and the costs of time and money involved? How is age linked to professional identity? When physicians are treated by colleagues as "old," remaining up-to-date is somewhat more difficult because informal opportunities are not offered as often or there is a perception of negative feedback from colleagues. Do we help older physicians move toward the periphery by informal attitudes? What are appropriate roles for older physicians in a system that has limited resources and uneven distribution of physicians?

The second group of questions focuses on how physicians move from novice to expert. What defines an expert and how does a physician reach that point? What is the role of experience and learning in expert behavior? How does experience contribute to the knowledge base? Can CME provide experiences that will support that transition? What are intermediate points along the way? What is the impact on health care of those physicians who do not become experts?

The third group of questions concerns the role of CME in professional development. Can skills be taught so that each physician has a system to assess specific learning needs using reviews of real cases? How do physicians link assessment of their own competence with learning needs? What are the details of the motivations for physicians to remain competent at each stage of their career? Or, conversely, what are the factors that predict when physicians will stop adding to their clinical expertise? What parts of expertise remain constant over a career, and what parts change?

What is the role of training in determining who becomes expert? When do physicians learn to be competent self-directed learners? Does CME have a role in that process?

CME providers can use the research agenda to create program options that respond to understandings of physician development. Programs can designate the necessary levels of expertise to work fully with the content. We may be able to have experts display their lines of reasoning, talk about how patterns are seen, and amplify how solutions are framed. An expert-level course could display ways to extend the number of available solutions for complicated problems. Programs could also be designed to address age-related needs. The market could be segmented with special workshops to address new concepts in a given area contrasted with protocols that are becoming out of date. Older physicians might wish to learn more about what is no longer acceptable or optimal treatment, and details about alternative treatments. Programs could offer tutorials, apprenticeships, or variations in setting to address problems for which the learning context is important.

Age is important in understanding performance. Of even more importance is a better understanding of how we can translate the impact of age on professional development and on CME. To create and elaborate understandings of how physicians change and learn, we must be able to explain the ways that life and career events push professional development. These snapshots from available work shape the beginning of a CME practice and research agenda centered on revealing a more sophisticated view of the connections between the interwoven strains of age, experience, and performance.

## References

1. Donabedian A. The epidemiology of quality. *Inquiry*. 1985;22:282-292.
2. Salem-Schatz SR, Avorn J, Soumerai SB. Influence of clinical knowledge, organizational context, and practice style on transfusion decision making. *JAMA*. 1990;264(4):476-483.
3. Rubin SM, Glasser ML, Werckle MA. The examination of physicians' awareness of dementing disorders. *J Am Geri Soc*. 1987;35(12):1051-1058.
4. Elliott TE, Elliott BA. Physician acquisition of cancer pain management knowledge. *J of Pain and Symptom Mgt*. 1991;6(4):224-229.
5. Ramsey PG, Carline JD, Inui TS, et al. Changes over time in the knowledge base of practicing internists. *JAMA*. 1991;266(8):1103-1107.
6. Day SC, Norcini JJ, Webster GD, Viner ED, Chirico AM. The effect of changes in medical knowledge on examination performance at the time of recertification. *Res Med Educ*. 1988;27:139-144.
7. Lockyer JM, Jennett P, Parboosingh JT, McDougall GM, Bryan GL. Family physician registration at locally produced short courses. *Can Med Assoc J*. 1988;139:1153-1155.
8. Lockyer JM, Parboosingh JT, McDougall GM, Chugh U. How physicians integrate advances into clinical practices. *Mobius*. 1985;5(2):5-12.
9. McAuley RG, Paul WM, Morrison GH, Beckett RF, Goldsmith CH. Five-year results of the peer assessment program of the College of Physicians and Surgeons of Ontario. *Can Med Assoc J*. 1990;143(11):1193-1199.

10. Berkowitz GS, Fiarman GS, Mojica MA, Bauman J, deRegt RH. Effect of physician characteristics on the cesarean birth rate. *Am J Obstet Gynecol.* 1989;161(1):146-149.

11. Baumgardner JR, Marder WD. Specialization among obstetrician/gynecologists. *Med Care.* 1991;29(3):272-282.

12. Roos LL, Cageorge SM, Roos RP, Danzinger R. Centralization, certification, and monitoring. *Med Care.* 1986;24(11):1044-1066.

13. Freiman MP. The rate of adoption of new procedures among physicians. *Med Care.* 1985;23(8):939-945.

14. Gruppen LD, Wolf FM, Vorhees CV, Stross JK. The influence of general and case-related experience on primary care treatment decision making. *Arch Intern Med.* 1988;148:2657-2663.

15. Reuben DB, Robertson JB. The care of elderly patients by elderly physicians. *J Am Geri Soc.* 1987;35:623-628.

16. Russell ML, Love EJ. Contraceptive prescription: physician beliefs, attitudes, and sociodemographic characteristics. *Can J Public Health.* 1991;82(4):259-263.

17. Greene HL, Goldberg RF, Beattie H, Russo AR, Ellison RC, Dalen, JE. Physician attitudes toward cost containment. *Arch Intern Med.* 1989;149(9):1966-1968.

18. Linn LS, Yager J, Cope DW, Leake B. Factors associated with life satisfaction among practicing internists. *Med Care.* 1986;24(9):830-837.

19. Levinson DJ, Darrow CN, Klein EB, Levinson MH, McKee B. *The Seasons of a Man's Life.* New York, NY: Ballantine; 1978.

20. Fitzgerald JM. *Lifespan Human Development.* Belmont, Calif: Wadsworth; 1986.

21. Lerner RM, Hultsch DF. *Human Development: A Life-Span Perspective.* New York, NY: McGraw Hill; 1983.

22. Skolnick AS. *The Psychology of Human Development.* San Diego, Calif: HB & J; 1986.

23. Nowlen PM. *A New Approach to Continuing Education for Business and the Professions.* New York, NY: MacMillan; 1988.

24. Houle CO. The lengthened line. *Perspect in Biol Med.* 1967;11:37-51.

25. Super DE. *Career Education and the Meanings of Work.* Washington, DC: US Dept of Health, Education, and Welfare; 1976.

26. Schein EH. *Career Anchors.* San Diego, Calif: University Association; 1985.

27. Bennett NL, Hotvedt MO. Stage of career. In: Fox RD, Mazmanian PE, Putnam RW, eds. *Changing and Learning in the Lives of Physicians.* New York, NY: Praeger; 1989.

28. Brown JS, Collins A, Duguid P. Situated cognition and the culture of learning. *Ed Research.* 1989;18:32-42.

29. Salthouse T. Influence of experience on age differences in cognitive functioning. *Human Factors.* 1990;32:551-569.

30. Schmidt HG, Norman GR, Boshuizen HPA. A COGNITIVE PERSPECTIVE ON MEDICAL EXPERTISE. *Acad Med.* 1990;65:611-621.

31. Schon DA. *Educating the Reflective Practitioner.* San Francisco, Calif: Jossey-Bass; 1987.

32. Stross JK, Bole GG. Evaluation of a continuing education program on rheumatoid arthritis. *Arthritis Rheum.* 1980;23:846-849.

**Chapter 6**

# Future Directions in Research on Physicians as Learners

*Robert  Fox*
*Jennifer Craig*

# Future Directions in Research on Physicians as Learners

Although the four preceding chapters review and interpret research and theory related to physicians as learners, there are new ideas that hold promise but lack a substantial body of investigations. Two notions are particularly promising. The first grows out of the need to integrate ideas related to continuing education and learning to clinical performance, rather than focusing on traditional ideas about knowledge and skills or competency. The second (related) theory suggests that clinical experience is a learning laboratory. Both sets of ideas seek to bring learning and education closer to the work of medicine. Each deserves some attention for its potential to influence future research.

## Performance

There are times in the history of any discipline when the overall perspective of the investigators and practitioners shift from one viewpoint to another. The forces behind such transitions may be diverse and powerful. CME has experienced its share of frustrations in several areas that may have contributed to this impending shift.

First, learning and education for physicians has become increasingly expensive. This, along with an increase in pressures for accountability, have created a swell of interest in the cost-effectiveness and ultimate value of teacher-driven education. It has also raised the question about the notion that simply bringing doctors up-to-date in terms of their medical and scientific knowledge is inadequate. Second, pragmatic interests in demonstrating the clinical outcomes and advantages for patient care of physicians' behavior have shifted attention from the classroom to the practice. Third, the testimony of physicians that much, if not most, of their learning is woven into patient care has caused educationists to wonder if interest should shift to what doctors actually do rather than what they are competent to do. Finally, new research findings related to change and to self-directed learning and change in practices, suggest that what physicians do may be an organizing principle for their learning activities. Because of the weight of these forces and the logical arguments of scholars such as Nowlen[1] and Cervero,[2] the focus of attention in research on CME has begun to shift from questions related to the knowledge and skills of physicians to their actual performance in practice.

In 1988 Nowlen[1] described professional performance as the interaction of two strands of development. The first strand represents the personal and professional history of the professional. It includes such things as education and training (eg, college, university, medical education, and CME), important and memorable professional events (eg, critical incidents such as pointed clinical successes or failures), and personal life histories (eg, illness, marriage, or loss of a loved one). The second strand is the culture of the profession. Culture may be thought of as the fabric of meaning derived from special language, artifacts, roles, and circumstances associated with practicing medicine. Professional culture gives meaning to actions and events. It is based on experiences in the role of physician, especially as that role is perceived and reinforced by patients, other physicians, and other professionals. Together, culture and personal history form a "double helix," interacting with each other and predisposing the physician to act in a certain way as he or she performs the role of physician.

This perspective on performance offers several important considerations for those in CME research and practice. First, the process of developing or changing performance is affected by many other variables than participating in formal CME. Second, the planned changes that are sought by physicians and educators must account for some of these other factors. Third, CME (and learning associated with changing performance) must accept a place within this broader explanation of performance and must develop services that facilitate the process that may be beyond the traditional mission of formal CME organizations. Fourth, in order to be successful, efforts to educate physicians and efforts to understand learning must "fit" within the culture of medicine. Meaning must be matched to the meanings commonly held in this culture if success is to follow. This requires a significant reinterpretation of ideas drawn from education, psychology, and sociology to make these ideas useful for understanding and acting within the medical culture.

If performance replaces competency and the fund of knowledge of medicine as the most important object of CME practice and research, it may require a reassessment of the role of the educator and educational researcher in the practice of medicine. Certainly, acceptance of the idea of performance as the organizing concept for research will alter the makeup of the research community and the body of literature that will guide CME in the future. Epidemiologists, sociologists, medical anthropologists, economists, and clinical investigators will join educational researchers as those who contribute to the practice of CME. Studies related to what affects performance will be drawn from these areas for interpretation and for their implications for the practice of CME.

## Learning From Experience

Learning from experience refers to the characteristics of learning that are not based on teaching but on practicing medicine. Learning from experience in the clinical setting is a way of both solving a clinical dilemma and generating a means for altering practices in similar situations. It is self-teaching with the clinical encounter as a learning resource and reflection on practices as a primary method. It is also a skill that can be developed more fully.

Learning from experience involves five distinct stages through which a physician passes. Each stage affects the next, with the last stages cycling back to the zone of mastery. Schon's model describes these five stages in a model he terms "reflective practice."[3] These have been modified slightly to fit better with the research of CME and the situation of physicians.

The first stage of learning from experience is what Schon refers to as *"knowing-in-action."* Knowing-in-action incorporates the automatic and deeply imbedded knowledge and skill that make up most of the practices of physicians. This is consistent with some of the principles described in the literature of problem-based learning. Schon makes the assumption that practitioners cannot practice effectively if they do not have this embedded, action-oriented knowledge. In effect, knowing-in-action represents those practices that are routine and automatic, so deeply learned that they require little active reflection or effort. Recognition of the diagnosis within a commonly seen presentation of symptoms or signs is one example. The use of a set dosage of a particular medication when treating a specific condition may be another. The physician can recall the explanations and find the studies that justify these actions if necessary, but that knowledge has become embedded in his or her actions rather than actively reflected upon in the clinical encounter. It is at this level that practice is based on fact and science.

However, it is clear that many cases may not be managed competently by embedded knowledge and ensuing automatic action. Uniqueness, conflict, or ambiguity come into play and present physicians with *"surprises,"* forming the second stage of Schon's model. Surprises may take the form of an inconsistent finding in the history or examination, an odd laboratory finding, or some other inconsistency with what one should expect to find in a given patient encounter. For example, a history of heavy drinking may complicate the treatment of arthritis with nonsteroidal anti-inflammatory drugs. A history of anxiety may mask or complicate the presentation of depressive symptoms. Illiteracy may suggest possible problems with patient compliance with a complex dosing schedule.

Once surprised, physicians move to the third stage of the model, *"reflection-in-action."* Reflection-in-action occurs when physicians are surprised during patient care and must reconstruct the knowledge skills and events that brought them to understand the surprise and develop a way to resolve the uniqueness, conflict, or ambiguity it indicates. Reflection-in-action occurs during the patient-physician interaction. The physician reviews the practices, knowledge, and information gleaned from the patient in an attempt to delineate exactly what it is that is different about this particular case and what should be done next. It may take the form of an unusual answer to a usual question, followed by a reconstruction of facts and information related to that patient in light of the knowledge and skill of the physician. The objective of reflection-in-action is to develop a response that may be appropriate during the patient encounter.

The fourth stage of Schon's model is the *"experiment."* This does not imply that good doctors experiment on their patients and should not be interpreted as it usually is in medical research. Here, in the face of surprise and based upon their reflection-in-action, physicians decide to attempt something in an effort to gain more information or resolve some clinical dilemma. Experiments can be as simple as the rephrasing of a question or as complicated as the changing of medication dosages, surgical procedures, or therapeutic regimens. These experiments are ad hoc in nature. They reflect the ability of the physician to reconstruct the information, knowledge, and skills needed to accommodate the unusual features of the case.

The fifth stage of Schon's model occurs after the patient encounter is completed. The physician reflects back on what occurred in the patient-care episode. The purpose is to make sense of the surprise, the way he or she thought about that surprise (reflection-in-action), and the experimental attempt to resolve it. *"Reflections-on-actions"* have an impact on knowledge-in-action. In effect, reflection-on-action is the loop that brings learning from recent experience to bear on general procedures, and develops new frames of reference for future cases. Figure 6.1 depicts the relationships among the different components of the process of learning from experience. It is a representation of how physicians navigate in the swamp of conflict, ambiguity, and uniqueness that characterizes many cases. It is this process that encompasses the art of medicine and a principal means that physicians use to expand the zone of mastery.

## Figure 6.1

## Learning from experience
**(adapted from Schön, 1987)**

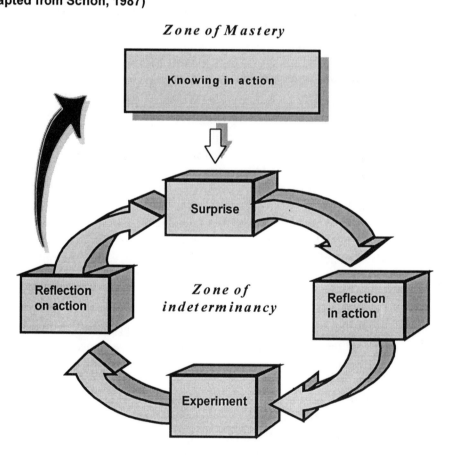

By providing a picture of the means by which learning from clinical experience occurs, the model has several implications for physicians as learners who are constantly working to expand their zone of mastery, and for physicians who are helping colleagues, residents, students, and other health professionals to learn from their experience. It provides a framework for organizing reflections-on-practices that may facilitate the process of more effectively incorporating new and better practices into the zone of mastery.

The research base underlying this powerful idea is yet to be developed, since the theoretical model was built from studies of professions other than medicine. It has only begun to be interpreted as a useful model for understanding important ways that physicians may learn and alter their practices. It does, however, provide a new perspective that needs research to link it to the existing literature of CME.

Ideas about physicians' performance as an organizing principle for CME and the important role experience plays in learning will require additional investigations before these ideas occupy a key role in the literature of CME. Important questions for future investigators are:

- *What are the variables that affect performance?*

- *How do critical incidents (past experiences) relate to patterns in performance?*

- *Can the negative effects of critical incidents on performance be counter acted or "unlearned"?*

- *What kinds of barriers to change are by-products of the culture of medicine?*

- *Are the stages of learning from experience accurate representations of how physicians learn from their clinical experience?*

- *Can physicians learn to learn from their experiences?*

- *How can new beliefs, values, and skills be introduced so that they are more compatible with the "culture of medicine"?*

- *How can learning from experience be incorporated into the design of CME?*

These questions represent only a few of the ways that researchers may test and apply these ideas to future research. Because these notions about performance as the basis of education and learning from experience were developed outside of medicine, they must first be analyzed for the extent to which they translate into useful models for understanding physicians' learning. Probably many of the initial investigations will be qualitative, in an effort to ground these ideas in empirical evidence. Methods of investigation may include case studies, observations, and case-stimulated recall interviews. Out of these first studies will come formal hypotheses that will guide subsequent investigations. With careful exploratory studies, the exact applications of these ideas will be known.

### References

1.  Nowlen PM. *A New Approach to Continuing Education for Business and the Professions: The Performance Model.* New York, NY: MacMillan; 1988.

2.  Cervero RM. *Effective Continuing Education for Professionals.* San Francisco, Calif: Jossey-Bass; 1988.

3.  Schon DA. *Educating the Reflective Practitioner: Toward a New Design for Teaching and Learning in the Professions.* San Francisco, Calif: Jossey-Bass; 1987.

# Section I

# Annotated Bibliography

**Anderson JG, Jay SJ, Schweer HM, Anderson MM.** Why doctors don't use computers: some empirical findings. *J R Soc Med.* 1986;79:142-144.

> This paper analyzes the attitudes of medical students, residents, and practicing physicians toward computer applications in medicine. While physicians recognize the potential of computers to improve patient care, they are concerned about the possibility of increased governmental and hospital control, threats to privacy and ethics, and legal problems. Attitudes appear to be somewhat independent of prior computer experience, and they significantly affect the extent to which physicians use clinical computer systems.

**Bandura A.** *Social Learning Theory.* Englewood Cliffs, NJ: Prentice-Hall; 1977.

> This book provides a clear and complete description of social learning theory as developed by this author. In particular, the role of cognitively based motivation and the concept of self-efficacy are explored.

**Brody EW.** *Managing Communication Processes.* New York, NY: Praeger Publishers; 1991.

> The communication process is seen as a variable to be managed, important to determining the success of an organization as it provides service to its many constituents. Partnerships with communications users are seen as key to successful organizational development.

**Brookfield S.** Self-directed adult learning: a critical paradigm. *Adult Educ Q.* 1984;35:59-71.

> This paper advances four criticisms regarding the current state of self-directed learning research, and offers suggestions for shifts in direction of the research paradigm commonly guiding the field. These include: (1) the emphasis on middle-class adults as the predominant sample studied; (2) the almost exclusive use of quantitative measures to document self-directed learning; (3) the emphasis on individual dimensions, to the exclusion of the social or contextual dimensions; and (4) the absence of discussion concerning the implications of these decisions for social and political change.

**Brookfield S.** Self-directed learning, political clarity, and the critical practice of adult education. *Adult Ed Q.* 1993;43:227-242.

> Two inherently political dimensions of self-directed learning include: (1) recognition that the intellectual heart of self-direction involves issues of power

and control; and (2) any authentic exercise of self-directedness requires certain political conditions to be in place.

**Budrys G.** 'Keeping the faith' and market realities: physician in an HMO. *Qual Health Res.* 1991;1:469-496.

To overcome negative attitudes toward prepaid practice plans, participating physicians constructed roles that exceeded their perceptions of traditional caregivers, emphasizing patient care and avoiding what they considered to be mundane administrative tasks. The study suggests that adherence to preconceived notions of traditional medical professionalism contributes to the loss of patients.

**Candy PC.** *Self-direction for Lifelong Learning: A Comprehensive Guide to Theory and Practice.* San Francisco, Calif: Jossey-Bass; 1991.

This book presents a comprehensive survey and an analysis of self-directed learning theory and practice. It also presents a new theoretical construct for self-directed learning.

**Coleman JS, Katz E, Menzel H.** *Medical Innovation: A Diffusion Study.* Indianapolis, Ind: Bobbs-Merrill; 1966.

This book discusses prescribing practices during the 16 months following the introduction of a new drug. While several channels of influence preceded the adoption of the drug, adoption was dependent on contact with a social intermediary (eg, detail person or colleague) rather than impersonal media (eg, journals).

**Collins A, Brown JS, Newman SE.** Cognitive apprenticeship: teaching the craft of reading, writing and mathematics. In: Resnick LB, ed. *Cognition and Instruction: Issues and Agendas.* Hillsdale, NJ: Lawrence Erlbaum Assoc.

This chapter deals with the construct of situated cognition, useful to the reader interested in residency training, CME traineeships, or innovative, problem-solving methods such as peer mentoring, chart-stimulated recall/review, or small group teaching. Important methods in the construct include modeling, coaching, scaffolding (providing resources or supports), articulation, reflection, and explanation.

**Crandall SJS, Volk RJ, Loemker V.** Medical students' attitudes toward providing care for the underserved. *JAMA.* 1993;269:2519-2523.

First-year and last-year medical students completed questionnaires concerning overall attitudes, perceived societal expectations, physician/student responsibility, personal efficacy, and provision of care. Final-year students were less favorably inclined toward caring for the medically indigent than first-year students. Such differences were apparent only for males.

**Curry L, Putnam WR.** Continuing medical education in maritime Canada: the methods physicians use, would prefer, and find most effective. *Can Med Assoc J.* 1981;249:563-566.

This survey finds that a majority of maritime Canadian physicians use individual learning methods (reading) to update knowledge, but that these activities get no support from universities or continuing medical educators. The authors believe that CME should supply physicians easy access to up-to-date information, train them in how to assist and tutor each other, and provide them with the resources to refresh their knowledge and skills at the universities.

**Deber RB, Baumann AD.** Clinical reasoning in medicine and nursing: decision making vs problem solving. *Teach Learn Med.* 1992;4:140-146.

The authors cite evidence to support their claim that the clinical reasoning process possesses two components—problem solving and decision making.

**Dunn DRF.** Dissemination of the published results of an important clinical trial: an analysis of the citing literature. *Bull Med Libr Assoc.* 1981;69:301-306.

The extent to which the results of a trial on photocoagulation in treating diabetic retinopathy were disseminated through the published literature is investigated by citation analysis. The results of this study suggest that a large number of citations to a clinically significant paper in the literature does not of itself ensure that the information reported will reach the appropriate practicing physician.

**Fennell ML, Warnecke RB.** *The Diffusion of Medical Innovations.* New York, NY: Plenum Press; 1988.

The book explores the emergence and development of the organizational network and its role in the diffusion of modern medical technology by analyzing data. Regional networks established to promote the diffusion of state-of-the-art treatment for head and neck cancer to community practitioners are studied. The author suggests that the classic innovation diffusion theory that describes the innovative physician as lone scientist and solo practitioner is inadequate for understanding innovation in the modern medical setting.

**Fox RD, Mazmanian PE, Putnam RW, eds.** *Changing and Learning in the Lives of Physicians.* New York, NY: Praeger Publishers; 1989.

This book is based on an analysis of interviews with 340 practicing physicians, and explores changes made and learning associated with those changes. Forces for change include those considered to be professional, personal, and social. Learning as process and as a response to change is explored. The interrelationship of these forces is affected by the physician's image of the consequences of the change. A model is proposed that describes the overall relationship between forces for change, learning, and types of change.

**Franks P, Clancy CM.** Physician gender bias in clinical decision making: screening for cancer in primary care. *Med Care.* 1993;31:213-218.

In this article, women who have a female physician as their usual provider (compared with those who have a male physician) were more likely to have tests and mammograms. There was a smaller, but nonsignificant, similar trend for breast examinations. No gender bias was evident for blood pressure checks. The results support the idea that physician gender bias exists in clinical decision making and represents an area for quality improvement.

**Freiman MP.** The rate of adoption of new procedures among physicians: the impact of specialty and practice characteristics. *Med Care.* 1985;23:939-945.

This article describes a survey of physicians on the number of new procedures they adopted during a 1-year period. A simultaneous statistical analysis of factors affecting the adoption of new procedures displays that age, board certification status, and solo practice all affect adoption.

**Geertsma RH, Parker RC Jr, Whitbourne SK.** How physicians view the process of change in their practice behavior. *J Med Educ.* 1982;57:752-761.

After constructing a hypothetical change model, the authors describe an interview of physicians dealing with the change process. A hypothetical model of this process is proposed: (1) priming—dissatisfaction is felt about some aspect of practice; (2) focusing—an awareness of alternatives is developed; (3) follow-up—further thinking about the change occurs; (4) rationalization—solutions are envisioned to practical problems associated with the potential change; and (5) triggering—the change is implemented after a clear communication regarding the desirability of the change.

**Goldfinger SE.** Continuing medical education: the case for contamination. *N Engl J Med.* 1982;306:540-546.

The author asserts that "contamination" (other sources that provide as educational message such as lectures or consultation) should not be treated as a hindrance to studies of CME, but should be recognized as an integral part of the learning process.

**Goldman G, Pineault R, Bilodeau H, Blais R.** Effects of patient, physician and hospital characteristics on the likelihood of vaginal birth after previous cesarean section in Quebec. *Can Med Assoc J.* 1990;143:1017-1024.

Although vaginal birth after a previous cesarean section is advocated in most cases, it has not yet been adopted as widespread policy. Charts of women in Quebec who underwent vaginal birth after a previous cesarean section were compared to the charts of women who had a repeat cesarean section in an attempt to identify factors that favored vaginal delivery. The authors describe physician characteristics relating to type of practice and the degree of hospital specialization as significant factors in predicting the type of delivery.

**Greer AL.** Medical technology and professional dominance theory. *Soc Sci Med.* 1984;18:809-817.

This paper examines the theoretical and empirical bases for hypotheses of professional dominance and the utility of these hypotheses in explaining hospital decisions to adopt new medical technologies. The analysis indicates that appropriate application of the concept requires specification of the type of physician exercising influence and of the hospital decision systems within which it is exercised.

**Grow GO.** Teaching learners to be self directed. *Adult Ed Q.* 1991;41:125-149.

Based on the situational leadership method of Hersey and Blanchard (*Management of Organizational Behaviour: Utilizing Human Resources.* 5th ed. Englewood Cliffs, NJ: Prentice-Hall; 1988), the author describes the staging of the staged self-directed learning skills, and that the teacher can help or hinder that progress. The article is helpful in discussing various teaching methodologies and their match to the learner's degree of readiness for self-direction.

**Habermas J.** *The Theory of Communicative Action.* Boston, Mass: Beacon Press; 1987.

The basic conceptual framework of normatively regulated and linguistically mediated interaction is examined. The author suggests that the development of society must itself give rise to problem situations that afford contemporaries privileged access to general structures.

**Hill MN, Levine DM, Whelton PK.** Awareness, use, and impact of the 1984 Joint National Committee consensus report on high blood pressure. *Am J Public Health.* 1988;78:1190-1194.

This is a survey of Maryland physicians following the dissemination of a consensus report on treatment of high blood pressure. One year after publication, 62% of physicians participating in both parts of the study were aware of the report. Although familiarity with the recommendations (81%) and the extent to which care was based on the guidelines (65%) were high, use of the report in practice (17%) and the amount of change in practice behavior required to adhere to the guidelines (18%) were low.

**Hillman BJ, Joseph CA, Mabry MR, Sunshie JH, Kennedy SD, Noether M.** Frequency and costs of diagnostic imaging in office practice: a comparison of self-referring and radiologist-referring physicians. *N Engl J Med.* 1990;323:1604-1608.

To assess possible differences in physicians' practices with respect to diagnostic imaging, the authors compared the frequency and costs of imaging examinations as performed by primary physicians who used imaging equipment in their offices (self-referring) with those ordered by physicians who always referred patients to radiologists (radiologist-referring), by using a large, private insurance-claims database. Physicians who did not refer their patients to radiologists for medical imaging used imaging examinations more frequently than did physicians who referred their patients to radiologists.

**Hummel LJ.** An investigation of physician self-directed learning activities. Proc Res in Med Educ. Washington, DC. *Assoc Am Med Coll.* 1986:213-218.

This study reports on the self-directed learning activities of physicians to determine the extent to which physicians engaged in this type of learning. Both family physicians and general surgeons were included. Tough's model (see last entry in this bibliography) of a learning project form the basis for the study. Interviews focusing on nine specific characteristics of self-directed learning revealed that less learning projects occur in family physicians compared to specialists, and that motivations related to solving clinical problems.

**Jordan HS, Burke JF, Fineberg H, Hanley JA.** Diffusion of innovations in burn care: selected findings. *Burns.* 1983;9:271-279.

This study examines the diffusion of innovations in burn treatment discussed at the US National Institutes of Health 1978 Consensus Development Conference on Supportive Therapy in Burn Care. The study traces the awareness and use of innovations in burn care, the source and timing of new information to physicians, and the ways in which characteristics of both innovations and physicians are related to the diffusion process. The three most important sources of information about the advances are staff conferences, journals, and medical schools.

**Knowles MS.** *The Adult Learner: A Neglected Species.* 4th ed. Houston, Tex: Gulf; 1990.

This book is a classic in the field of adult learning, human resource development, and adult education. It is one of the few resources that contains, in one volume, the wide range of research related to the field of adult learning.

**Knox AB.** Influences on participation in continuing education. *J Contin Ed Health Prof.* 1990;10:261-274.

This article provides an overview of the complex set of personal and situational influences on participation in what the author terms "systematic learning activities, which reflect discrepancies or gaps between a learner's current and desired proficiencies." A list of suggestions are included for providers to use when planning, conducting, and assessing effective learning activities.

**Levinson DJ, Darrow CN, Klein EB, Levinson MH, McKee B.** *The Seasons of a Man's Life.* New York, NY: Ballantine; 1978.

In-depth interviews with 40 men provide the data for the development of a theory of the stages through which most adult men pass. The interviews are used to create representative stories of four men that help the reader understand one of the classic sources of adult development theory.

**Liebes T.** On the convergence of theories of mass communication and literature regarding the role of the 'reader'. In: Dervin B, ed. *Progress in Communication Sciences.* Norwood, NJ: Ablex Publishing Corporation; 1991;10:123-143.

The meaning of a transmitted message is simultaneously constructed and interpreted by the receiver of the message. What influences that social construction and interpretation is an area deserving of further study.

**Lindberg DAB, Siegel ER, Rabb BA, Wallingford KT, Wilson Sr.** Use of MEDLINE by physicians for clinical problem solving. *JAMA.* 1993;269:3124-3129.

Critical incident technique was the method used in this study. MEDLINE searches were carried out by and for physicians to meet a wide diversity of clinical information needs. Physicians reported that literature via MEDLINE was at times critical to sound patient care and favorably influenced acquired patient outcomes.

**Lockyer JM, Parboosingh JT, McDougall G, Chugh U.** How physicians integrate advances into clinical practices. *Mobius.* 1985;5:5-12.

This paper reports on the sources of information family physicians and specialists use in the process of making changes in their clinical practices. An average of 3.08 sources of information are utilized for each change and more than 50 percent of the changes are complete in less than 1 year.

**Luria AR.** *Cognitive Development: Its Cultural and Social Foundations.* Cambridge, Mass: Harvard University Press; 1976.

Experiments with villagers of Uzbekistan support the concept that important manifestations of human consciousness are directly shaped by the basic practices of human activity and forms of culture.

**Lurie N, Slater J, McGovern P, Ekstrum J, Quam L, Margolis K.** Preventive care for women: does the sex of the physician matter? *N Engl J Med.* 1993;329:478-482.

Analyzing claims data for nearly 100 000 women, differences between male and female physicians were determined in the frequency of mammograms and Pap smears ordered. Women were more likely to have Pap smears and mammograms if they saw female rather than male physicians, particularly if the physician was an internist or family practitioner.

**Manning PR, DeBakey L.** *Medicine: Preserving the Passion.* New York, NY: Springer-Verlag; 1987.

Through interviews with exemplary physicians and surgeons, the authors identify the successful methods that physicians use to maintain their competence.

**Manning PR, Denson TA.** How internists learned about cimetidine. *Ann Intern Med.* 1980;92:690-692.

This survey of general internists explores how they first heard about, learned the clinical principles of usage of, and gained update information on cimetidine. Medical journals remain the single most popular source of information in all stages of learning; the next most common sources are CME programs and discussion with colleagues.

**Merriam SB, Caffarella RS.** *Learning in Adulthood.* San Francisco, Calif: Jossey-Bass; 1991.

This book explores research and theory-building efforts in self-directed learning. The studies are categorized to include those that address, (1) self-directed learning as a form of study, including the process of self-directed learning, and (2) self-directedness as a personal attribute. Major issues that researchers must address are reviewed.

**Norman GR, Schmidt HG.** The psychological basis of problem-based learning: a review of the evidence. *Acad Med.* 1992;67:557-565.

This extensive literature review finds evidence that problem-based learning in undergraduate medicine may foster self-directed learning, increase retention of knowledge, and enhance interest in clinical subject matter.

**Oddi LF.** Perspectives on self-directed learning. *Adult Ed Q.* 1987;38:21-31.

This paper reviews work on self-directed learning as a process. The author suggests that the understanding of self-directed learning could be improved if the process were studied as it relates to the learner's personality. The author suggests that an understanding of the characteristics of personality that lead an individual to initiate and persist in learning would provide a more comprehensive focus for the study of self-directed learning.

**Osherson DN, Smith EE.** *Thinking.* Cambridge, Mass: MIT Press; 1990.

Studies in the following areas are reviewed: (1) remembering, (2) categorization, (3) judgment, (4) choice, (5) problem solving, (6) cognitive development, and (7) rationality. Thinking is viewed in terms of evolution and cognitive science.

**Paisley W.** Information and work. In: Dervin B, Voigt MJ, eds. *Progress in Communication Sciences.* Norwood, NJ: Ablex Publishing Corporation; 1980.

Properties of information use are provided: quantity, quality, structure, function, and normative versus actual information use. Individual factors such as cognition, personality, and motivation are discussed in relation to social factors that affect information use. Social factors include work teams, employing organizations, formal professional groups, and informal groups of professionals working around the same issues.

**Parboosingh JT, Gondocz ST.** The maintenance of competence (MOCOMP) program: motivating specialists to critically appraise the quality of their continuing medical education activities. *Can J Surg.* 1993;36:29-32.

A credit system for personal CME participation is described. It is designed to facilitate recognition of high-quality CME, and to encourage specialists to compare their CME efforts with those of their colleagues. This is a carefully crafted attempt to encourage and evaluate self-directed CME activities by means of a diary.

**Parente R, Anderson-Parente JK.** Retraining memory: theory and application. *J Head Trauma Rehabil.* 1989;4:55-65.

Techniques are offered for retraining memory to enhance cognition. Research is presented implying that educators should consider neuropsychological variables in discerning educational needs.

**Penland P.** Self-initiated learning. *Adult Educ.* 1979;29:170-179.

The author uses a national probability study to verify some of Tough's work (see last entry in this bibliography) regarding self-initiated and self-planned learning. Reasons for undertaking lifelong or self-initiated projects include a wish to keep the learning strategy flexible and the desire to put one's own structure on a learning project.

**Renschler HE, Fuchs U.** Lifelong learning of physicians: contributions of different educational phases to practice performance. *Acad Med.* 1993;68:S57-S59.

This pilot study determines when in their education physicians thought they had acquired the competencies they used in their daily practices. Physicians were queried 5 years after completion of their formal training. Specialty education is believed to contribute most to the physician's daily practices, with a median contribution of 20%. Practice-based independent learning was found to be superior to formal continuing education.

**Rogers EM.** *Diffusion of Innovation.* 3rd ed. New York, NY: The Free Press; 1983.

This classic text provides an analysis of the common features of innovation diffusion from the perspective of the world's research on innovation adoption. It describes the process of adoption, characteristics of early vs late adopters, and factors that facilitate adoption.

**Schein EH.** *Career Anchors.*  San Diego, Calif: University Association; 1985.

Schein's work deviates from the traditional view of the stages of a career by explaining individual orientation in the context of work.  His model of career anchors describes ways that individuals interpret their career and their orientation to continuing education.

**Schmidt HG, Norman GR, Boshuizen HPA.**  A cognitive perspective on medical expertise. *Acad Med.* 1990;65:611-621.

The authors propose a new theory of the development of expertise in medicine. They outline assumptions that expertise does not necessarily imply superior reasoning skills, but rather is the result of using cognitive structures (or illness "scripts") that describe prototypes.  Novice physicians use pathophysiological causes of symptoms, while illness scripts provide the model to solve problems for experts.

**Slotnick HB, Raszkowski RR, Jensen CE, Wentz DK, Christman TA.**  A new study of physician preferences in CME: insights into education vs promotion.  Presented at the Third National Conference on Provider-Industry Collaboration in CME; October 8-9, 1992; Chicago, Ill.

This paper explains the results of an independent study funded by the Upjohn Company, US, exploring issues physicians consider in deciding which CME activities to attend.  It searches for evidence that doctors may confuse promotion with education.

**Super DE.** *Career Education and the Meanings of Work.*  Washington, DC: US Dept of Health, Education, and Welfare; 1976.

The traditional view of work life in business is represented as stages that occur over time.  The stages convey common traditional assumptions of age and work in our society.

**Tough A.** *The Adult Learning Projects: A Fresh Approach to Theory and Practice in Adult Learning.*  Toronto, Canada: Ontario Institute for Studies in Education; 1971.

This book describes the findings and implications of studies of adult learning projects that illuminate the entire range of deliberate adult learning, self-planned learning and private lessons, as well as courses and workshops.  Tough discusses what and why adults learn, how they learn, and what help they obtain in doing so.

# Section II

# The
# Assessment
# of
# Learning Needs

"The failure lies in the fact that continuing education activities have not been correlated with continuing competence, but rather with continuing education hours, as though that were the same as continuing competence."

Boisenneau R.
The Failure of Voluntary Continuing Education.
In: *Continuing Education in the Health Professions.*
Rockville, Maryland:
Aspen Pub;
1980.

# Introduction to Section II

This section is a bridge, linking section I, the world of the learner, to section III, the world of CME provision. It also moves us from a relatively passive, if instructive, consideration of the characteristics of the learner toward a more active role in ensuring clinical competence.

Why would we want to write a section on the assessment of physician competence and clinical performance? Shouldn't physicians, at least the vast majority of them (and at least the ones that we are interested in), know their own strengths and weaknesses? Isn't that a basic assumption of all CME? An illustration might help justify our consideration of this issue, derived from the Sibley study,[1] outlined in the introduction to section I.

> *To recap, Jack Sibley and co-workers determined that they would mail printed materials to community-based primary care docs on a variety of family medicine topics, those that the practitioners considered "high" and "low" priority. While the high priority items displayed no significant change in the charts of the physicians who received relevant CME materials, the low priority items did—a fact hidden in the mostly negative findings and subsequent press that the study received following its publication. What does such a finding imply?*

- First, that the physicians in this study may (knowing that their charts were going to be reviewed) have chosen topics that they felt proficient in as high priority.

- Second, that the doctors were not knowledgeable in some areas, and did not know, at least in these areas, what they did not know.

- Third, that doctors may need some gold standard in practice, some means by which they can gauge their competence—for example, the extent to which they used harmful, useless, or out-of-date practices.

It might be helpful if we put this consideration of self versus other assessment on a continuum, ranging from the perception of the learner (identifying so-called "perceived needs"), through those assessments accomplished in the test environment (competency assessments), to those which are derived from the practice setting (performance assessments). This continuum is not always seamless in the life of the physician, and frequently becomes compartmentalized, one section bearing little or no relation to another. We could represent this continuum by a line, in which subjective self-assessment of wants is placed at one end and objectively determined needs based in patient care data are at the other. An imaginary CME and learning problem might add a little flesh to these conceptual bones.

*A group of physicians in the Saltfleet Health Care Group (an HMO) has set aside travel money for years, allowing each partner to attend one major conference or convention a year. The newest member of the group indicates that, while she enjoyed her most recent conference on the menopause, she came away with no new knowledge, and has not changed her practice as a result of it. She asks if setting aside the travel expenses is a good expenditure of practice-generated income, especially in a time of cost restraint. She proposes that the group do monthly chart reviews, using the data to identify practice needs and develop practice-based programs.*

This HMO example gives us several insights, some similar to those gleaned by the Sibley study—physicians may choose CME topics in areas not directly related to practice or patient care needs, and may in fact already be practicing at optimal levels in those areas. They may also choose CME activities on the basis of nonpractice factors, such as the site of a conference or a desire to assure that they are keeping up with current practices (explored by Donald Moore and his colleagues in chapter 11). However, the newest member of the group has inserted the question of a gold standard (although she probably wouldn't use that phrase) into her colleagues' practice life. Two notions central to the assessment of learning needs can be found here—the standards or norms of her practice group, and the use of charts as a marker of performance and a stimulator of discussion and learning.

Here's another example:

*The AAPG, the American Academy of Pediatric Geriatricians (we assume they focus on the health of 19-year-olds), has for years based its Enhancement of Clinical Competence Program, (called ENCOMP) on an annual meeting and on a bimonthly self-assessment program of multiple-choice questions. Because of complaints regarding the self-assessment questions (members say they're too esoteric) and frankly, because of declining revenues from the annual meeting, the AAPG is considering a re-certification program. This process would include office simulations, computer-based programs, chart review with peers, and other measures.*

The AAPG example furnishes us with an illustration of several issues: the movement to a more objective means of determining (or enhancing) competence from one of self-assessment, and the use of multiple assessment measures to perform this function. There are several questions not raised by the AAPG model, however. These questions include the reliability and validity of these measures, the degree to which they test or don't test the specific capabilities of the competent pediatric geriatrician (we wouldn't presume to know what they are), and the acceptability of this program to the members of the AAPG. Does a computer-based program test clinical aptitudes or computer skills? What does it mean, for example, if a member "fails"?

This issue of failure (the other side of the objective assessment coin in many minds) is considered in the next and last vignette.

*The Joint Liaison Council of the Wesley Urban Faculty of Medicine and its
affiliated teaching hospitals recently met to discuss the issue of
incompetence.  Specifically, three primary care practitioners and one
general surgeon in the system have been found to be performing at
suboptimal levels.  The medical school, with its experience in setting tests
and determining the abilities of its residents and undergraduates, has been
asked to put forward a proposal at the next council meeting.  The proposal
is to include strategies to identify practitioners operating at such levels,
means by which specific deficiencies may be determined, and remedial or
corrective methods.*

This example allows us to tease apart several issues and to raise some questions.
First, the finding of suboptimal performance implies that someone or some group
has established optimal standards such as professional standard review organizations, or those set by quorum.  But what do these mean and how are they set?
Second, how would an organization begin to screen for physician performance?
Third, there are issues of testing or measuring the performance of the identified (and
maybe, down the road, other) physicians.  Fourth is the very important (and recur-
rent, it would appear) issue of incompetence, its relationship to practice, its negative
connotation, and the effectiveness of something called remedial education.

Attempts to answer these questions and explorations of these issues are offered in
this section.  Terrill Mast's chapter deals with the broad sweep of the definition and
meaning of competence, providing us with a brief taxonomy and theoretical construct.  It also deals with issues of self-assessment and the abilities of the physician
(as in the case of the HMO's newest member) to reflect on practice patterns, and
provides a cooperative framework on which more may be accomplished in research
and provision of service in this area.  Two examples of tools useful in the objective
assessment of competence are described in some detail in this section: the use of the
standardized patient is explored by Murray Kopelow; and a rich exploration of the
potential in record review as a performance measurement tool forms the content of
the concluding chapter of this section by Jocelyn Lockyer and Van Harrison.

## Reference

1.    Sibley JC, Sackett DL, Neufeld VR, et al.  A randomized controlled trial of continuing
      medical education.  *N Eng J Med.* 1982;306:511-515.

# Chapter 7

# Concepts
# of
# Competence

*Terrill Mast*
*David Davis*

# Concepts of Competence

*This last point is . . . the key to continued effectiveness as a clinician: learning how to decide when current diagnostic and management maneuvers are no longer good enough and need to be changed.[1]*

This chapter begins by distinguishing between competence and performance; presents various dimensions of, and methods to assess, physician competence and performance; and concludes by presenting the implications for research and practice in continuing physician education.

## Competence or Performance?

The phrase "the assessment of competence" is frequently used in medical education as is the word "performance." Both require clarification. The two terms are generally taken to refer to what one can do (competence), and what one does do (performance). This general understanding is found beyond CME, and even beyond education. In linguistics, for example, Chomsky[2] distinguished between linguistic competence as the speaker-hearer's knowledge of language, and linguistic performance as the actual use of language in concrete situations. Closer to home for continuing medical educators, Norman[3] defined competence as what a doctor is capable of doing, and performance as what a doctor actually does in day-to-day practice.

A helpful distinction between the terms performance and competence is employed by psychometricians, whether speaking of medical, linguistic, or any other domains. This distinction avoids the confusion inherent in these terms, and clarifies that competence is a theoretical construct, which is never observable, just as intelligence is a nonobservable construct. On the other hand, performance is behavior which can be observed, and from which competence can be inferred, just as it is an observable performance on so-called intelligence tests from which we infer a construct we call intelligence. Although this may seem like a semantic technicality, the distinctions are necessary for at least three reasons: (1) it is important to define the terms being used, and both terms (competence and performance) are being used frequently; (2) some authors and researchers treat competence and performance as qualitatively and quantitatively different things; and (3) some writers seem to treat competence and performance as the same thing, changing the terms only for stylistic variety.

Thinking of competence as a construct avoids the assumption that measurements of performance in a "controlled test setting" produce pure measures of competence. Performance in such testing environments is affected by different, perhaps fewer, variables (eg, time limitations, examinee expectations about observer standards, examination room logistics, or reluctance to perform invasive physical examinations) than performance in a busy clinical practice setting. Although performance in the controlled test setting may be closer to demonstrating true competence, it remains a measure of performance rather than a direct measure of competence.

In an address to the Research in Medical Education Conference on the assessment of clinical skills, Miller[4] offered his definitions of competence and performance in the context of a pyramid to describe the various assessment methods that might be used to provide data on "anything so complex as the delivery of professional services by a successful physician." That framework is worth reviewing here in some detail.

At the base of Miller's model is knowledge. Assessments of knowledge seek to measure what the learner knows. Rather than measure just anything an individual knows, assessment seeks to measure how much of a specific body of knowledge he or she possesses. Further, Miller asserts that our assessments must measure whether an examinee knows how to use his or her knowledge. Miller terms this "competence," and suggests it comprises these features: the skill of acquiring information from a variety of human and laboratory sources, the ability to analyze and interpret such data, and the ability to develop management plans. Patient management problems, methods based on human models, and complex computer-based simulations are all methods of assessing competence.

Miller calls the third step of his pyramid "performance." Assessments at this level are characterized by encounters with human subjects. For example, when physicians display how they diagnose and treat patients in clinical settings under observation, Miller would say their performance is being assessed. Evaluations of examinees' encounters with standardized patients appear to provide sufficient validity and to overcome the problem of standardization across examinees. Standardized patients are, for many, currently the method of choice for measuring performance. Their background and use are explored in greater detail in chapter 8. At the peak of Miller's assessment pyramid is "action." Here examiners must assure that physicians will perform specific functions in the practice setting rather than solely in the artificial test setting. So, for Miller, action depends on performance, which builds on competence, which builds on knowledge.

These four levels provide very useful distinctions, but it should be noted that Miller's concept of competence differs from the more commonly held view (eg, Norman's[3] and Senior's[5]) that competence is what a doctor is capable of doing, and that performance is what a physician actually does in day-to-day practice. This further demonstrates the need for commonly held definitions of terms.

Regardless of the terms used, the key operative distinction lies between assessment of behavior in the test setting and behavior in the natural setting. In the test setting, the doctor reports to and performs within a medical school's (or state's, province's, or professional society's) assessment framework, with the knowledge that he or she is being evaluated. Examples of these situations are commonplace, including recertification and licensing examinations, and certification activities such as advanced cardiac life support and advanced trauma life support. Regardless of the assessment method (eg, written questions, oral examinations, or standardized patients), this is an artificial situation. By contrast, a clinical practice forms a natural setting in which the examinee or doctor is primarily under the scrutiny of his or her own professional conscience, and is concerned primarily with the patient's well-being. The doctor may also be concerned with indirect observations and assessments by licensing bodies, members of the practice group, hospital quality assurance measures, or payer oversight systems, and most likely is aware of issues of malpractice.

In summary, it important to distinguish between competence and performance, and to think of competence as a theoretical construct of which performance is the observable and measurable manifestation. The conditions under which examinees perform, and even the conditions under which they are observed, must be considered in inferring the degree of competence underlying the performance. We can directly measure performance; we can only indirectly assess competence by making inferences from performance measurements.

# Dimensions of Competence

## Traditional Dimensions

Inasmuch as the subject of this text is physician learning, both the dimensions and domains of competence are clearly tied to the practice of medicine. Practical assessments of physician competence require narrower definitions, such as those provided by emergency medicine, ophthalmology, or hypertension, as well as dimensions of competence such as history taking. Listing the dimensions of competence permits a determination of its component parts. This process also guides the design of the assessments, allows an analysis of tasks, and provides assurance that all relevant aspects of competence are included in the list. A traditional broad cut at analysis might be this one, proposed by Norman[3]—knowledge (eg, of diseases, or management strategies), skills (such as interpersonal, communication, or clinical), and attitudes (such as motivation to learn, beliefs, or values).

Other groups have provided similar, though more detailed, schema. One is the American Board of Medical Specialties[6] framework, comprising three dimensions: the tasks of the physician (eg, history taking or use of tests), the clinical situations or subject matter of the discipline, and prerequisite abilities (eg, knowledge, problem-solving ability, and attitudes). Another is the competency structure of the American Board of Internal Medicine:[7] the relevant abilities of the physician (eg, knowledge, technical skills, and interpersonal skills); problem-solving tasks (eg, data gathering, diagnosis, and continuing care); the nature of the medical illness, including the problems encountered by the physician; and the social and psychological aspects of the patient's problem, especially those which relate to diagnosis and management. A third is the Cambridge Conference on Clinical Assessment[8] working classification of seven dimensions for assessing competence: (1) knowledge, (2) interviewing/interpersonal skills, (3) history taking, (4) physical examination and technical skills, (5) problem-solving (clinical reasoning and diagnosis), (6) decision-making (use of investigations and management), and (7) personal qualities (eg, responsibility and value).  Finally, as if seven dimensions aren't enough, Southern Illinois University requires all medical students to pass a clinical performance examination before graduating, which assesses 13 competencies.[9]

## Self-reflection and Self-learning: A New Dimension of Competence

The ability to learn from experience is undeniably necessary for any physician to keep up with changes in clinical practice.  This ability is implicitly portrayed only in the model of Southern Illinois University.  This process has been best described by Schön,[10,11] and is explored in chapter 6.  A brief restatement of the theory is included here, with reference to possible mechanisms by which the competency may be tested.

Briefly, Schön has drawn attention to the lack of regularity and routine in professional practice.  This phenomenon flows from several sources: ambiguity (derived from lack of information about the task, the problem, or its solution), conflict (arising from inherent differences in information, intended outcomes, and values inherent in the clinical problem), and finally, uniqueness (aspects specific to that particular problem or patient).  By undergraduate and graduate training and through clinical experiences, health professionals develop "flexible templates" of knowledge and skill which they apply to tasks, the so-called clinical algorithms or decision-making models of the practiced clinician.  In sensitive and well-trained physicians, these templates, described by Schön as "knowing-in-action," grow more sophisticated, richer, and more automatic as they are modified over time.[10]

"Surprises," by which Schön means the unexpected clinical problem or feature, must be recognized by the clinician in order to perform effectively in the immediate clinical context, and in order to develop abilities to perform optimally in further clinical efforts.  Thus, the ability to recognize the uniqueness, conflict, or ambiguity inherent in a clinical encounter is a key feature of the competent physician.  Following its recognition, the competent clinician conducts what Schön refers to as an experiment—a different, nonroutine approach to the problem—referred to as "reflection-in-action."  Such an approach generally requires no new knowledge, but rather a focusing on past experiences or information, to develop a different diagnostic or therapeutic strategy.  Occasionally, new information is required, and the information-seeking skills of the physician become important to the process.
Having applied the experimental element to the encounter (for example, by asking a different, nonroutine question in a patient interview), the competent physician is in a position in which he or she can assess the effectiveness of the experiment.  This later, evaluative phase is referred to by Schön as "reflection-on-action," referring to the physician's contemplation on the now-completed process.

This brief review of both traditional and recent models of competence leads to the conclusion that there is no "correct" set of dimensions of medical competence, just as there is no one "correct" way to cut up a chicken.  Rather, it is apparent that the dimension used for guiding assessment needs to reflect the purposes of the assessment. Any implicit dimensions which are considered essential, such as the ability to learn from experience, must be made explicit if they are to guide the design of assessment methods or systems.

# Measurement Methods and Applications

Prior to considering the entry of competency and performance assessment methods into everyday educational and clinical practice, it is necessary to discuss issues of limit setting, and the selection of appropriate measurements and instruments.

## Setting Standards: Identifying Incompetence

Not within the domain of most CME providers, many licensing bodies, peer review organizations, and other associations have demonstrated an increasing interest in the assessment of competence and its corollary, the detection of physicians of less-than-adequate competence. Detecting incompetence must involve some kind of measurement, since identifying incompetent physicians really means identifying physicians whose observable performance does not meet certain standards. The problem of setting standards in regard to any measures of performance in the medical setting is difficult, and various approaches have been taken. One approach is to set an arbitrary, norm-referenced cutoff, such as that employed by the National Board of Medical Examiners.[12] Regardless of absolute levels of performance, Part I examinees whose scores fall more than 1.2 standard deviations below the mean of a criterion group are considered to be incompetent, and do not pass the examination.

Setting criterion-referenced passing levels demonstrates another approach to standard setting. In this approach, all examinees need to perform well on important test items. "Performing well" is defined by some decision-making group, with regard to the specific tasks measured by the test. It is generally accepted by psychometricians that tests of medical performance should be criterion referenced and, further, that the cutoff score (that is, the score above which the physician is considered to be competent) be set through the judgement of experts in consideration of the specific items or tasks of the examination. Criterion-referenced standards, unlike those that are norm-referenced, are set by an analysis of the test items, rather than by an arbitrary process.

The following section describes: first—measurement instruments in the determination of physicians' abilities or competency assessment, and second—measures of performance assessment in the work or practice setting. Implications for the use of these tools, and the potential for the development of tools of use in the determination of internally set self-assessment activities, are explored in concluding paragraphs.

# Measuring Competence

## Multiple-choice questions

Multiple-choice questions are a frequently used measure of knowledge testing, their popularity stemming from their ease of application, their proven proficiency in testing recall and interpretation of factual knowledge, and their ability to sample a wide range of clinical areas.[13] Their use crosses the medical education continuum— from undergraduate examinations, to certification and fellowships examinations, to self-assessment programs and other uses in relicensure and recertification.  The experience of the National Board of Medical Examiners described by Hubbard[14] provides an example of an extensive system of competency assessment.  In addition, physician self-assessment programs, such as that described by Marshall,[15] have grown in sophistication and use.

The widespread use of multiple-choice questions exists in the face of moderate criticism of the method: the tendency to test esoteric, academic knowledge at the expense of relevant practical information, their ability to "cue" responses, and the failure to credit partial knowledge or to portray the broad range of clinical competencies.  Despite these criticisms, however, well-designed multiple-choice questions are able to generate highly reliable tests of broad domains of knowledge.

## Oral examinations

Used for generations of learners in the medical education continuum, "orals" test for breadth and depth of knowledge, and clinical management or judgment.  Further, they are flexible, can assess long-term problems or evolving cases, and can incorporate real practice data such as x-ray or laboratory test results. Their use is ubiquitous.  Their precision is enhanced by inclusion of structured questions, which can improve reliability to acceptable levels.[16]

A variation of the oral examination is the "triple-jump" exercise,  used to determine self-directed learning skills as a component of problem-solving, and developed by the undergraduate medical doctorate program of McMaster University, Hamilton, Canada.[17] It is a three-part oral examination consisting of these components:

- *A vignette or clinical problem to test hypothesis generation, data gathering and interpretation, current knowledge, early problem formulation, and ability to identify learning issues.*

- *An intermediary step comprised of searching the literature, using either a personal or institutional library, or other learning resources.*

- *A final component, permitting the learner to present final conclusions about the case and findings from the literature, thus permitting an assessment of information-retrieval or self-directed learning skills, final problem formulation, management skills, and self-assessment ability.*

## Direct observation

Direct observation is useful when particular skills (such as those manifested in surgery or interviewing) are the object of assessment. Observation has been applied to objective, structured clinical examinations (discussed in chapter 8) as well as other, more practice-based clinical encounters.[16]

It should be noted, however, that direct observation poses some difficulties,[18] and provides only indirect inferences about physician cognitive processes. Nonetheless, observation has been shown to be useful, particularly in the clinical setting, mediated by a one-way mirror, audiotape or videotape, or occasionally, physical presence in the same room with the assessed clinician and his or her patient. In these instances, the observer or the means to observation need to be as unobtrusive as possible. There is evidence that observation is best guided by previously developed checklists, rating scales, or algorithms, which improve the assessor reliability.[13]

## Global rating scales

Rating scales are most frequently used in circumstances or areas in which achieving hard, objective assessments is problematic. Such areas, and therefore uses, include ethical behavior, self-assessment ability, professional responsibility, and interpersonal relationships. Such scales may be simple, consisting of two dimensions (such as "unacceptable" and "acceptable"), or more complex, longer, multipoint scales, representing a range of behaviors. Evidence exists that developing clear descriptions of the behaviors exemplified at the ends of the scale, indicating (if appropriate) other points on the continuum, and ensuring adequate assessor training are necessary ingredients in the successful application of global rating scales.[19]

## Other measures

Those interested in competency assessment have developed, over nearly three decades, a host of other measures. These include essay and modified essay questions, patient management problems, computer, and other technical simulations such as mannequins. They also include the use, in a variety of formats and settings, of standardized or simulated patients, explored in detail in the next chapter. Their utility in practice-based learning depends on these factors: validity, reliability, credibility, comprehensiveness, precision, feasibility, and, ultimately, usefulness in the context of physician learning.

## Measurements in the Practice Site

There are also a host of measures useful in the assessment of physician performance in the practice setting. These include: adaptation of measures developed for competency assessment to the clinical environment, the use of process measures such as chart review (explored in chapter 9) and other data, such as that provided by utilization review, and end-point data (eg, morbidity and mortality statistics) relative to health or patient care outcomes.

Of the first set of measures, the use of direct observation in the clinical setting has been displayed in an early study by Delaney et al,[20] which examined operative technique. Here, faculty surgeons in pairs achieved high interrater reliability with the use of explicit checklists. Standardized patients may also be used in the practice environment, testing performance.

Apart from chart review, there are a number of process variables that form the second set of measurement tools, and which may be used to monitor and observe clinical performance. These measures include utilization data, summarizing the use of resources such as laboratory, radiological, or other clinical services. Of these, bed utilization or length-of-stay figures for patient care (among other measures) have assumed economic importance in North America health care.

The third set of measures are those related to patient outcomes. While not directly or linearly linked to physician performance, such measures as morbidity, mortality, patient compliance, quality of life, and level of pain control (among other clinical outcomes) figure prominently in health services research and quality assurance. These measures have shown potential for shaping educational interventions,[21] and for assessing the impact of CME on physician learners and their patients.

## An Example of a Comprehensive Assessment System: Screening, Diagnosis, and Remediation

While the tools employed by the peer review process of the College of Physicians and Surgeons of Ontario are not unique in themselves, their integrated application provides an example of the use of many of these measurement tools. Their use also serves as the only North American example of a comprehensive, systematic approach to the delineation of competency and learning needs and their linkage to educational strategies.

Almost two decades old, the first step in the province-wide attempt to maintain and assure clinical competency was the institution of a screening, Physician Assessment Program. Here, peer physicians visited the offices of colleagues on a random basis to review practice records and other clinical practices.[22] Pilot work confirmed that the following factors predicted poor physician performance (and high learning need): age over 65 years, solo practice, and lack of certification by or membership in a professional college or specialty society. These findings led to a more targeted, cost-effective approach.[23]

Despite the institution of such a program, difficulties were acknowledged by its authors: an almost-exclusive reliance on physician charts, the potential for automatically equating poor record keeping with poor clinical skills, and the problem inherent in an almost exclusively norm-based assessment. These issues led to the development of a second-stage, more diagnostic activity, termed the Physician Review Program, using a test center based at a university health sciences facility. This program employed many measures described above, and was used to further assess the competency of those physicians (and others) identified in the first, office-based, stage. These measures (chart-stimulated recall, standardized patients, oral examinations, and multiple-choice examinations) were tested for predictive validity and reliability in three groups of physicians: (1) volunteers (self-referrals); (2) randomly selected, community-based physicians; and (3) those referred from the College of Physicians and Surgeons of Ontario. Although some measurers appeared more sensitive than others, all measures successfully distinguished between the members of these three groups.[24,25]

Finally, the project has demonstrated some problems in its "treatment" phase--the reeducation of physicians at very low levels of competence. This third stage, designing remedial education for those physicians deemed to be in need, has been termed "formative"; conclusions regarding what forms of education work best in what particular learning or clinical circumstances have yet to achieve statistical, educational, or clinical significance.[25]

# Conclusions and Implications

This combination of theory and practical applications of clinical competence leads naturally to a discussion regarding two sorts of issues in the assessment of learning needs in practice. The first set has to do with the research issues related to both new understandings in self-directed learning and self-reflection, and more traditional constructs of competency and performance assessment. The second set of issues relates to the imbedding of assessment into the practice of CME providers and their physician clients. A framework for this discussion is shown in the Table.

## Research Implications

To set boundaries for a discussion of competency assessment, and to provide an analysis of its component parts, a matrix or grid may be helpful. Displayed in the accompanying Table, this grid outlines two axes—a horizontal axis sketching the nature of the learning need as perceived by the physician himself or herself, and/or verified by external means, and a vertical axis containing three dimensions of assessment (those related to self-awareness or ability to reflect on one's practice, competence, and performance). Research questions relative to the introduction of the dichotomy of perceived versus verified learning or practice needs are discussed in each of the three dimensions of competence.

## Self-learning and self-reflection

Beyond those tools useful in the practice setting (measuring the performance or behavior of practicing physicians), and those useful in the competency assessment environment (measuring abilities of the physician), there is a need to develop tools to measure or assess the presence of self-reflection or self-learning. The application of such tools, passing methodological criteria hurdles, would ensure that physicians, at some internal level: (1) recognize their learning deficiencies in the context of patient care or professionalism; (2) possess the ability to reflect on their practices; and (3) measure these needs against external and internal standards set by peers, regulatory bodies, patients, policies, the literature, and (perhaps most of all) themselves.

This aspect of competence, relating both to self-reflection and self-directed learning, may also be viewed as a necessary but not sufficient element in the learning physician's armamentarium. While it has been explored extensively (in this book and elsewhere), significant need exists to develop testable models of self-directedness and self-reflection, derived from the model of reflective practice proposed by Schön,[10] or from other models. Schön has highlighted the failure of educational systems to assess the abilities of trainees or graduates to manage complex and non-routine aspects of practice.[11]

Research questions relate to the ability of the physician to perceive his or her learning needs with or without being presented with feedback from objective assessment strategies. For example, when confronted with evidence that the physician "missed" an element of surprise in a clinical encounter, how does he or she perceive the feedback? Are there differences in the form of feedback which would alter his or her response? Are there differences in training, age, or style of practice which would affect his or her learning? What learning is required to make the correction? How is this accomplished?

There are several ways in which reflection on one's clinical practices and subsequent self-directed learning may be measured:

- *Observational studies of physician learning in situ (for example) on the hospital ward or in the clinic. While such observational techniques have been widely used and their difficulties well described,[18] their application to physician learning patterns may be useful. For example, what does the physician do when confronted with a problem for which he or she has no immediate answer, or with a patient whose case is perplexing?*

- *Retrospective studies (for example of charts, identifying gaps in knowledge or skill, articulating and exploring areas in which attitudinal problems may be apparent). The critical incident technique, described initially by Flanagan,[26] may be particularly useful here.*

- *Use of other competence tools to stimulate exploration of reflective and/or self-assessment abilities. Structured interviews may be valuable in this regard. One method has been described by Feightner and colleagues,[27] who employed a variety of stimuli (such as videotapes of the clinical encounter or charts) to prompt discussion of clinical reasoning.*

- *Employing feedback from performance-derived data to test physicians' self-assessment skills, ability to use "surprise" or new information, and other attitudes relative to learning.*

## Other research questions in competency and performance assessment

There are a large number of research questions which pertain to the measurement of competence and performance.

First, do these tools and the constructs from which they are derived provide sufficient and accurate representations of the abilities of the competent clinician? Are there other models of human behavior which need to be applied here, missed by the theories of adult learning and professional competence described in this book and elsewhere?

Second, in the context of currently held relevant models, there are methodological questions which deserve pursuit. To what extent are assessment tools valid? That is, to what extent do they match external references or gold standards such as measures of performance (concurrent validity); are they associated with later outcome measures (predictive validity)? To what extent are these tests precise, ie, display features of reliability, consistency, repeatability, and objectivity? And, to what extent are these tests comprehensive, ie, covering most or all aspects of a particular component of competence or performance?

Third, are questions related to "do-ability," in part research questions, but ultimately questions which direct those interested in physicians as learners to incorporate these measures into everyday educational and clinical practice. To what extent are these test maneuvers credible, ie, possess face validity, clinical relevance, or believability? To what extent are these tests feasible, bearing in mind economic considerations, location, practice variability, and acceptance by professional associations?

Table 7.1

**Parameters in the Assessment of Self-directed Learning, Competence and Performance**

| | Dimension/Domain Assessed | | |
|---|---|---|---|
| | Self-directed Learning and Reflection | Competency (Knowledge, Skills, Attitudes) | Performance (Action or Behavior) |
| Measurement methods | Observation; chart review; clinical debriefing; interviews | Multiple-choice questions; self or other-directed; oral examinations; observations; global rating scales; other measures | Observation; standardized patients; process data claims; utilization review, (laboratory, X-ray, or other), chart review; outcome data (morbidity/mortality figures; patient satisfaction, quality of life) |
| Location | Learner-centered (in practice setting or elsewhere) | Competency assessment sites | Practice |
| Potentially interested parties | Physician professional association; medical and educational facilities; CME providers | | Insurance carriers; governments; quality assurance/peer review organization agencies |

Fourth, perhaps most importantly, are questions linking assessment to educational interventions and learning strategies. Having identified learning needs and deficiencies, what are the best strategies to offer or provide CME? What are the relevant elements of motivation (explored in chapters 3 and 11), perception of the assessment process, and ownership over the remedial educational process?

## Practice Implications:   Imbedding Assessment and Learning into the Clinical Environment

Several interrelated recommendations for both clinical practice and the practice of physician education deserve discussion. They are outlined in the table above.

First, self-analysis, self-reflection, and self-assessment must occur continuously within the physician's own practice site and within his or her own personal practice configuration. Can these skills be developed early and tested frequently, throughout the medical education continuum? While Schön's model has been referenced here, other models may exist, and there is a clear need for the development of tools that are useful in the assessment of this important, self-directed aspect of physician learning. The development and testing of these tools requires support by, in practice, collegial relationships with peers, consultants, and other members of the caregiver team. While owned primarily by the physician himself or herself, they must be fostered by medical faculties, and modified and encouraged by professional and specialty associations.

Second, competency assessment, with its heavy emphasis on tool development, and testing of reliability, validity, and other methodological parameters, requires further development and application in a controlled setting, most likely away from the practice site (eg, in a medical school CME unit), at least in the immediate future. Depending on the owners or proponents of such measures, this may occur increasingly in sites selected by professional associations or licensing bodies, and may, once issues of reliability and validity have been addressed, find homes in practice settings such as HMOs.

However, among the major difficulties inherent in moving from physician self-assessment to a more comprehensive use of objective assessment measures, is the issue of "incompetence" and its implications for relicensure, recertification, and practice. This term, its implication and application, forms a major impediment to the formation and development of regular means by which physicians may undergo or take part in assessments of their clinical abilities. This issue needs to be addressed by parallel and mutually complementary activities—extensive efforts at clarifying methodological issues related to the testing methods, and simultaneous attempts to make their application in learning and practice settings more natural, less punitive, and supportive or encouraging of education. Such activity requires the full cooperation of researchers and practitioners of CME, as well as the close involvement of professional associations, licensing bodies, and others.

Third, performance measures show every indication of increasing application in the practice site as directed by the interrelated forces of health care reform--quality assurance, concurrent quality improvement, and health economics. Though differences exist in the US and Canadian health care systems, both countries experience similar forces (explored in the foreword) driving these systems to be more aware of health economic issues, and to monitor both health care process and outcomes. To these powerful forces are added the growing evidence-based care movement in both countries,[28] calling for strict adherence to rational management strategies based on the best available evidence in clinical care. The development of practice guidelines is one example of this movement. Other examples will follow as an integrated approach develops, linking health care providers, learner assessment programs, practice organizations, professional and regulatory bodies, insurance carriers, health sciences faculties, and CME providers.

### References

1.  Sackett DL, Haynes RB, Tugwell P. *Clinical Epidemiology: A Basic Science for Clinical Medicine.* Boston, Mass: Little, Brown and Co; 1985:247.

2.  Chomsky N. *Aspects of a Theory of Syntax.* Cambridge, Mass: MIT Press; 1965.

3.  Norman GR. Defining competence: a methodological review. In: Neufeld VR, Norman GR, eds. *Assessing Clinical Competence.* New York, NY: Springer Publishing; 1985:15-35.

4.  Miller GE. The assessment of clinical skills/competence/performance. *Acad Med.* 1990;65:563-567.

5.  Senior JR. Toward the measurement of competence in medicine. *Qual Rev Bull.* 1977;3:19-21.

6.  Lloyd JS. *Definitions of Competence in Specialties of Medicine.* Chicago, Ill: American Board of Medical Specialties; 1979.

7.  American Board of Internal Medicine. Clinical competence in internal medicine. *Ann Intern Med.* 1979;90:402-411.

8.  Wakeford R, Bashook P, Jolly B, Rothman A. *Directions in Clinical Assessment: Report of the First Cambridge Conference.* Cambridge, England: Cambridge University School of Clinical Medicine; 1985.

9.  Barrows HS, Colliver JA, Vu NV. *The Clinical Practice Examination: Six-Year Summary.* Springfield, Ill: Southern Illinois University School of Medicine; 1992.

10. Schön DA. *The Reflective Practitioner.* New York, NY: Basic Books; 1983.

11. Schön DA. *Educating the Reflective Practitioner: Toward a New Design for Teaching and Learning in the Profession.* San Francisco, Calif:: Jossey-Bass; 1987.

12. Nungester RJ, Dillon GF, Swanson DB, Orr NA, Powell RD. Standard-setting plans for the NBME comprehensive part I and part II examinations. *Acad Med.* 1991;66:429-433.

13. Neufeld VR, Norman GR. *Assessing Clinical Competence.* New York, NY: Springer Publishing; 1985.

14. Hubbard JP. *Measuring Medical Education: The Tests and Experience of the National Board of Medical Examiners.* Philadelphia, Pa: Lear and Fibger; 1978.

15. Marshall JR. CHECKUP: computerized home evaluation of clinical knowledge understand and problem solving. *Teach Learn Med.* 1989;1:38-41.

16. Grava-Gubbins I, Khan SB, Rainsberry P. *A Study of the Reliability of the 1985 Simulated Office Orals.* Toronto, Canada: The College of Family Physicians of Canada; 1985.

17. Painvin C, Neufeld VR, Norman GR, Walker I. The 'triple jump' exercise: a structured measure of problem-solving, and self-directed learning. *Proc Conf Res Med Ed.* Washington, DC: Am Assoc Med Coll; 1979.

18. Kent RN, Foster SL. Direct observational procedures: methodological issues in naturalistic setting. In: *Handbook of Behavior Assessment.* New York, NY: Wiley; 1977.

19. Streiner DL. Global rating scales. In: Neufeld VR, Norman GR, eds. *Assessing Clinical Competence.* New York, NY: Spring Publishers; 1985:199-141.

20. Delaney PV, Quill RD, Kaliszer M. Assessment of operative surgical skills. *J Inter Med Assoc.* 1978;71:13-17.

21. Davis DA, Thomson MA, Oxman AD, Haynes RB. Evidence for the effectiveness of CME: a review of 50 randomized controlled trials. *JAMA.* 1992;168:1111-1117.

22. McAuley RG. Results of the peer assessment program of the College of Physicians and Surgeons of Ontario. *Can Med Assoc J.* 1984;131:557-560.

23. McAuley RG, Paul WM, Morrison GH, Beckett RF, Goldsmith CH. Five-year results of the peer assessment program of the College of Physicians and Surgeons of Ontario. *Can Med Assoc J.* 1990;143:1193-1199.

24. Davis DA, Norman GR, Painvin A, Lindsay E, Ragbeer MS, Rath D. Letter from Ontario: attempting to ensure physician competence. *JAMA.* 1990;263:2041-2042.

25. Norman GR, Davis DA, Lamb S, Hanna E, Caulford P.  Competency assessment of primary care physicians as a part of a peer review program. *JAMA.*  1993.

26. Flanagan W.  The critical incident technique. *Psychol Bull.*  1954;51:327-358.

27. Feightner JW, Neufeld VR, Norman GR, Barrows HS.  Solving problems: how does the family physician do it? *Can Fam Phys.*  1977;23:67-71.

28. Sackett DL, Haynes RB, Tugwell P. *Clinical Epidemiology: A Basic Science for Clinical Medicine.*  Boston, Mass/Toronto, Canada: Little Brown; 1985.

# Chapter 8

# Competency-based Assessment Using Standardized Patients and Other Measures

*Murray Kopelow*

# Competency-based Assessment Using Standardized Patients and Other Measures

*"The key to competent performance, I believe, is evaluation—not as a coercive stimulus applied periodically by licensing bodies or professional societies but as an indispensable personal tool to assess past performance and determine learning needs."[1]*

Assessments of physicians' abilities may be the most powerful tool for identifying educational needs. Frameworks for clinical assessment have been proposed and are described earlier which equate knowledge with knowing, competence with knowing how, and performance with showing how.[2] Competence and performance have something to do with doing, differentiated by the location of the measurement. In this chapter, performance is defined as that which occurs in the practice site, while competence takes place in the test environment. The latter measurements are thus more indirect and performed outside of actual practice. Performance (practice-based) assessments include peer review by chart audit,[3-5] and direct practice observation by trained standardized patients[6] and are discussed in a subsequent chapter on performance assessment.

The objectives of this chapter are to discuss and review the history and applications of competency assessment in CME with an emphasis on standardized patients. Several additional methods for the assessment of competence, including chart stimulated recall and structured oral examinations, are briefly discussed. Finally, educational measurement issues and ideas for future research directions are presented.

## The Tools of Competency-based Assessment

The study of competence in professional practice is important as a tool to assist in understanding the maintenance of clinical skills and to identify areas of educational need, not only within the scope of an individual practitioner but also in the profession as a whole.

*Chart stimulated recall* utilizes the physician's own record in an interactive session between a physician and an examiner. The record is reviewed and the physician and the examiner discuss the physician's approach to (and management of) the patient. The thinking of the physician at different stages of clinical management, as documented in the record or stimulated by the discussion, is explored. While the assessment is anchored to the physician's practice through the medical record, it can be compared to predetermined or normative criteria at each stage of the process. A description of what the physician actually did in practice is obtained.[7,8]

*Structured oral examinations* move one step further away from actual practice. A clinical vignette initiates the interaction between examiner and physician. The physician is walked through the data collection, problem solving, and management issues relevant to the case in question and actions taken by the physician are compared to criteria anchored to peer performance and expectations. A description of what the physician would do in practice is obtained and compared to that of the examiners or mentors or set by other criteria. Other oral examinations are unstructured versions of the same format; here the physician discusses and manages clinical scenarios but is scored against the examiner's own internal standards.

Other competency-assessment maneuvers employ a variety of *practice or patient simulations.* Written simulations in the form of patient management problems present a clinical scenario and offer the opportunity to move through the patient encounter by exposing with a special marker the chosen action or response (the so-called latent-image response), which discloses a further piece of clinical information, or the consequences of a specific action. Patient management problems have fallen out of favor as a reliable stand-alone evaluation tool but have been shown to be of value as a learning device and measure of change after CME programming.[9] Other simulations of the clinical encounter have been done on paper,[10] computer,[11] with mechanical devices,[12] and with standardized patients both in an examination setting (measuring competence) and in a practice setting (measuring performance).[13-15]

## Standardized Patients

Standardized patients are lay persons trained to portray the role of a patient involved in a clinical encounter with a health care provider in a reproducible and accurate manner. These standardized patients may have fixed physical findings such as a heart murmur or joint restriction or may be taught to simulate abnormalities in the examination such as abdominal tenderness, cough, or gait abnormalities. The encounter is assessed using a list of actions, usually presented as a checklist, which are deemed important for success in that encounter. The simulator and/or the assessor complete the checklist at the end of the encounter, recording actions which might be categorized into history, physical examination, information sharing, diagnosis, test selection and management, or other categories. If one makes the measurements in a test environment, competence is measured. If the same patient enters a physician's practice in an undetected manner, then performance is measured. Assessments by standardized patients can thus bridge the gap between competence and performance.

Standardized patients were first described by Barrows and Abrahamson in 1964.[16] As a neurologist, Barrows saw the potential in having a person reproducibly and accurately portray a patient with a specific medical problem to clinicians who could then participate in a standardized learning experience. Subsequently others,[17-19] described the use of standardized patients in teaching and evaluation, based on the original description by Barrows and Abrahamson. Since then, the use of standardized patients has spread. It has been reported that about 85% of North American medical schools use standardized patients in some form in their undergraduate medical programs.[20] While this activity has usually been termed "teaching and learning" it could be considered competency-based self assessment, or assessment by observation, set in a directed learning environment. The learner practices a specific skill and then assesses how successfully that skill has been learned.

Competency-based assessment using standardized patients has been popularized recently within the so-called multi-station examination standardized patient (MSESP) format. The MSESP format, although first described in 1984,[18] was based on earlier work on the objective structured clinical examination (OSCE).[21] Subsequently, two forms of the examination developed, the so-called "long case"[22] and "short-case" formats.[18]

In the long-case format, the assessment is built from the juxtaposition of patient scenarios that are of a length that approximates the time spent with a patient in real practice (for example 15 to 25 minutes). The short-case examination was designed to fit standardized patients into the OSCE format, which usually means 5 to 10 minutes per station, or problem or patient. The two formats developed as the result of the needs and past experiences of the educators who first took advantage of them. The short cases were first used to evaluate clinical clerks during training to look at basic clinical skills such as examination of a joint or taking a focused history. The long cases developed to assist more senior (end-of-clerkship) students to evaluate their clinical skills at the level of a full encounter with a patient.

In the long-case format, an acute arthritis problem might be presented as follows: *"You are about to see a 14-year-old girl with a sore knee. Please perform a focused history and physical examination and communicate your findings and plan to the patient. You have 20 minutes to complete the encounter."* In the short-case format, the challenge to the physician might be as follows: *"Please take an appropriate focused history relevant to the patient's chief complaint of sore knee. You have 5 minutes."* Although both encounters produce real information about the learner's competence and potential performance in practice, the information gained may differ in each case.

## Measurement Issues

The formulation of these two cases and their use in medical education raises several questions about measurement. Tests need to be accurate (valid) and reproducible (reliable). A good test has a credible appearance (face validity), is built from clinical issues that relate to actual practice (content validity), and produces scores that correlate with other measurements made on the same individuals (concurrent validity) and/or with future scores or success in practice (predictive validity). The MSESP format has faired well in this area of validity testing. MSESPs that are built from well-trained standardized patients, portraying valid cases, give results that trainees and practicing physicians indicate are true reflections of their ability: they are being tested while doing what they do every day in practice. Data exist from studies which show that scores achieved on MSESP, relate directly to scores on other forms of evaluation, as well as to future success in specialty training programs.[22-24]

The reliability (reproducibility) of the measurements made on these assessments has also been the subject of study. The precision of the measurement and the confidence in the decisions made at the pass mark, or cutting score, are very important. Reliable measurements are based on the examiner being increasingly sure of the reproducibility of the measurements as the learner is measured and remeasured (or tested and retested). If the physician scores 50% on a one-station examination, the examiner cannot indicate what the mark on the next station might be, nor what the candidate's ability actually is. If the candidate achieves an average 50% on a 6-hour, 20-station examination, with scores that range from 45% to 55%, one could be reasonably sure that the score is a true reflection of ability. Thus, both the number of cases and the total examining time are important factors in determining the reliability of the MSESP format.[25]

What is being measured in the examination is also an issue. Data exist to show that, when history, physical examination, and interpersonal skills are measured, acceptable reliabilities are easier to reach than when diagnosis, test selection, and management are included.[25] Deleting the latter three skills from the assessment for fourth-year medical students does not necessarily compromise the validity of the evaluation. However, if diagnosis and management are absent from the assessment of a practicing physician, the first comment might be: "What good was assessment? Is not the objective to arrive at the correct diagnosis and appropriate treatment plan?" It is difficult to argue with this challenge. Therefore, using the MSESP format as a pass/fail examination to determine the maintenance of practice eligibility for practicing physicians becomes complicated. As one moves to maximize reliability, compromises in face and content validity are made that might ultimately detract from the examination, perhaps negating all the inherent advantages of the method.

# Current Applications

## Certification and Qualification

In most jurisdictions, physicians are certified competent by a medical school, specialty board, or professional college. The qualification, or license to practice, is provided by the local licensing authority. Ongoing certification and maintenance of certification requirements vary widely across these jurisdictions, and within these variable administrative structures standardized patients have found many applications. In some, the local medical school assists physicians in identifying needs and in designing educational programs.[26] In other settings, interested parties have cooperated to fill the same need.[27,28]

We know that standardized patient assessments measure something different than other forms of examinations. They do this in a valid and reliable manner. MSESP formats involving a large number of sites and candidates tested simultaneously are possible to stage.[28,29] Some medical schools in Canada and the United States have used this form of assessment for graduating medical students.[22,30] Both countries are developing the same type of examination at the entry-to-practice level, and some jurisdictions apply this examination to graduates of foreign medical schools applying for entry-to-practice programs.[31]

## Educational Needs Assessment in CME

In response to licensing authorities' requirement for personalized CME programs, some university CME departments have been able to design programs of assessment and evaluation that operate as individualized educational needs assessments. Usually the physician is offered many different forms of assessment, each trying to deal with a component of the physician's ability. Standardized patients have been used in this way, both to evaluate the physicians' interpersonal and data collection skills as well as their diagnostic, test selection, and management talents.[27,28] These studies suggest that physicians cover fewer history items and perform a more limited physical examination in the office than in the examination situation,[13-15] generating more abbreviated histories and physical examinations than deemed acceptable by a matched set of peers.[15] However, carefully crafted standards are difficult to establish. Other researchers have used standardized patient assessments to measure physician ability with locally established guidelines for clinical practice by introducing undetected standardized patients into the physicians' practices.[32]

## Implications for the Future

### Research Questions

Questions need to be answered with respect to the administration, development, psychometrics, and application of standardized patients in the assessment of competence for physicians.

First, how should MSESP formats be presented to physicians? The literature describes a difference in the measurements made on the same physician in the office and test center using this technology. What is the cause of that difference? What are the specific differences between what is done in the office and what is done in the examination setting?

Second, how should standards be set for the measurement of competence using standardized patients? The application of practice guidelines as performance standards has produced very low scores for practicing physicians in MSESP formats, on the other hand, using peers to set standards on a case-by-case basis is complicated and may not allow for local peculiarities in practice. There is a need to analyze the components of acceptable standards of practice and apply them to this assessment format.  Of importance to those involved in standard setting and in making pass/fail decisions for physicians are these questions:  "What constitutes a pass?"; "What is 'good enough'?";  and "What pattern of action, questions, or interventions represents acceptable clinical behavior?"

The third set of question arises from issues of standardized patient training.  How much training is required to make the patient accurate in his/her portrayal?  How similar do different simulations have to be in order to ensure that the same challenge is being presented to all the physicians?  Standardized patient training time varies between centers.  The desired level of accuracy achieved by training is unknown and also variable. It is important to establish the essential components of the challenge of a case and the appearances of one case that would distinguish it from another similar one, and to relate these components to the training and development of standardized patients.

Fourth, and finally, scores on standardized patient cases are usually broken down into subscores, such as history, physical examination, test selection, management, and interpersonal skills. In spite of the overall measured reliability of these assessments being in the acceptable range (less than 0.6), the subscore reliabilities may fall short of this mark.[13-15]  In order to give learners useful information about their competence and educational needs, reproducible subscores are necessary.  Work needs to be done in this area.  For example, can interpersonal skill measurements be broken down into subscores?  A global report of good or bad interpersonal skills does little to assist the physician in identifying special needs.  We need to establish a way to give feedback on components of interpersonal skills (such as sensitivity and the ability to include the patient in the decision-making process).  Reliable measurements of the patient's perceptions of the interpersonal skills of a physician involved in an encounter can be captured using a checklist with a Lickert-type rating scale.[33]

## Standardized Patient-based Competency: Assessment for Practicing Physicians

It may be that the quality of the CME will improve as practice-based needs assessment and  monitoring for changes in practice become more a routine component of the development of CME programming.  Self-directed CME curricula based on an individual's perceived and real educational needs will, without question, be a major part of the foundation for CME in the future.  As the ability to measure competency and performance in a safe, reliable, and valid manner becomes widely accepted, such competency assessment practices may become the norm rather than the exception.  Physicians might, in the future, integrate regular assessment into their learning strategies so that they can maximize the efficiency of their CME activities.  These movements will be driven by several environmental forces including:  pressures placed on physicians to maintain skills in high-risk areas such as critical care, neonatology, and obstetrics  by their  liability insurance carriers and hospital privileges panels; certification bodies which are increasingly articulating the position that physicians may not be maintaining their competence; and last, government and consumer discussion of mandatory recertification through reexamination, or health care reform priorities.

There are other ways to relieve these anxieties other than by mandatory recertification. Voluntary participation in effective self-directed CME programming that includes periodic self-assessment of competence (and perhaps performance) would be an important solution. Specialty societies could include competency assessment modules at scientific meetings and assemblies, and hospital boards could ask that medical rounds include competency assessment on a regular basis. Of equal importance is the inclusion of such programming into medical school and residency training programs in a nonpunitive manner. The model exists for this in those CME departments that provide physician enhancement programs. In these departments, the feedback of the competency assessment is formative in nature, providing the individual with real needs on which to build an individualized educational program.

If there is so much pressure to institute such a worthwhile form of educational needs assessment, what forces impede its implementation? Physicians and their advocacy organizations are remarkably cautious about anything that documents or records a physician's competence or performance primarily because the information may not be secure, physician restrictions may ensue, and the information may not be accurate. We have not been able to demonstrate to physicians in practice that we can accurately measure their clinical "goodness." We can achieve a reliable or precise measure, and can be 95% sure that we will get the same number tomorrow, but are not yet sure what the number means. It is a truism that "precision with no accuracy is a dangerous misuse of statistics." Nowhere is this truer then in the assessment of physician competence and performance. Until further work has been done on establishing practice standards and transferring these to the standardized patient testing environment, caution in the application and interpretation of results is warranted.

Perhaps, in the future, competency assessment will be looked at as an indispensable personal tool to be incorporated into the lives of practicing physicians. This will only occur after physicians see that the measurements are valid and reliable and that the information is safe in the hands of the assessors. At that time, physicians will not view competency assessment as a coercive stimulus, and the profession will have incorporated it into the fabric of a lifelong learning program that all professionals will be expected to construct in order to maintain competence and practice.

## References

1.  Squires BP. Competence, evaluation and learning, *Can Med Assoc J.* 1989;144:257.
2.  Miller GE. The assessment of clinical skills/competence/performance. *Acad Med.* 1990;65:S63-S67.
3.  Borgiel AEM, Williams JI, Anderson GM, et al. Assessing the quality of care in family physicians' practices. *Can Fam Phys.* 1985;31:853-862.

4.  Cruft GE, Humphreys JW, Hermann RE, Meskauskas JA. Recertification in surgery: 1980. *Arch Surg.* 1981;116:1093-1096.

5.  McAuley RG, Henderson HW. Results of the peer assessment program of the College of Physicians and Surgeons of Ontario. *Can Med Assoc J.* 1984;131:557-561.

6.  Russell NK, Boekeloo BO, Rafi IZ, Rabin DL. Using unannounced simulated patients to evaluate sexual risk assessment and risk reduction skills of practicing physicians. *Acad Med.* 1991;66:S37-S39.

7.  Parboosingh J, Ararad D, Lockyer J, Watson M. The use of clinical recall interviews as a method of determining needs in continuing medical education. *Proc Annu Conf Res Med Educ.* Washington, DC. 1987;26:103-108

8.  Maatsch JL, Huang R, Downing SM, Munger BS. Studies of the reliability and validity of examiner assessments of clinical performance: what do they tell us about clinical competence? In: Hart I, Harden R, Walton H. *Newer Developments in Assessing Clinical Competence.* Montreal, Canada: Heal Publications; 1986:352-360.

9.  Marquis Y, Chaoulli J, Bordage G, Chabot JM, Leclere H. Patient management problems as a learning tool for the continuing medical education of general practitioners. *Med Educ.* 1984;18:117-124.

10. Sriram TG, Chandrashekar CR, Isaac MK, et al. Development of case vignettes to assess the mental health training of primary care medical officers. *Acta Psychiatr Scand.* 1990;82:174-177.

11. Norcini JJ, Meskauskas JA, Langdon LO, Webster GD. An evaluation of a computer simulation in the assessment of physician competence. *Eval Health Prof.* 1986;9:286-304.

12. Sullivan MJ, Guyatt GH. Simulated cardiac arrests for monitoring quality of in-hospital resuscitation. *Lancet.* 1988;2:618-620.

13. Norman GR, Neufeld VR, Walsh A, Woodward CA, McConvey GA. Measuring physician's performances using simulated patients. *J Med Educ.* 1985;60:925-934.

14. Rethans JJ, Van Leeuwen Y, Drop R, Van der Vleuten C, Sturmans F. Competence and performance: two different concepts in the assessment of quality of medical care. *Fam Pract.* 1990;7:1-7.

15. Kopelow ML, Schnabl GK, Hassard TH, et al. Assessing practicing physicians in two settings using standardized patients. *Acad Med.* 1992;67:S19-S21.

16. Barrows HS, Abrahamson S. The programmed patient: a technique for appraising student performance in clinical neurology. *J Med Educ.* 1964;39:802-805.

17. Stillman PL, Swanson DB. Ensuring the clinical competence of medical school graduates through standardized patients. *Arch Intern Med.* 1987;147:1049-1052.

18. Petrusa ER, Blackwell TA, Rogers LP, Saydjari C, Parcel S, Guckian JC. An objective measure of clinical performance. *JAMA.* 1987;83:34-42.

19. Kretzschmar RM. Evolution of the gynecology teaching associate: an education specialist. *Am J Obstet Gynecol.* 1978;131:367-373.

20. Stillman PL, Regan MB, Philbin HL. Results of a survey on the use of standardized patients to teach and evaluate clinical skills. *Acad Med.* 1990;65(5):288-292.

21. Harden RM, Gleeson FA. Assessment of clinical competence using an objective structured clinical examination (OSCE). *Med Educ.* 1979;13:41-54.

22. Barrows HS, Williams RG, Moy RH. A comprehensive performance-based assessment of fourth-year students' clinical skills. *J Med Educ.* 1987;62:805-809.

23. Rutala PJ, Fulginiti JV, McGeagh AM, Leko EO, Koff NA, Witzke DB. Predictive validity of a required multidisciplinary standardized-patient examination. *Acad Med.* 1992;67:S60-S62.

24. Distlehorst LH, Verhulst SJ, Vu NV, Barrows HS. The use of performance-based assessment scores and traditional measures in prediciting first-year residency performance. *Proc Ann Conf Res Med Ed.* Washington, DC. 1988:176-181.

25. Van der Vleuten COM, Swanson DB. Assessment of clinical skills with standardized patients: state of the art. *Teach Learn Med.* 1990;2(2):58-76.

26. Kopelow ML. A multistation examination using standardized patients as a needs assessment in CME. Presented at the Third Congress on CME; April 20, 1990; San Antonio, Tex.

27. Bunnell KP, Kahn KA, Kasunic LB, Radcliff S. CPEPP: development of a model for personalized continuing medical education. *J Contin Educ Health Prof.* 1991;11:19-27.

28. Norman GR, Davis DA, Painvin A, Lindsay E, Rath D. Comprehensive assessment of clinical competence of family/general physicians using multiple measures. In: Bender W, Heimstra R, Scharpbier A, Zwierstra RP, eds. *Teaching and Assessing Clinical Competence.* Groningen, Holland: Boekwerk; 1990:357-363.

29. Grand Maison P, Lescop J, Rainsberry P, Brailovsky C. Large-scale use of an objective structured clinical examination for licensing family physicians. *Can Med Assoc J.* 1992;146:1735-1740.

30. Klass D, Hassard T, Kopelow M, Tamblyn R, Barrows H, Williams R. Portability of a multiple-station performance-based assessment of clinical competence. In: Hart IR, Harden RM, eds. *Further Developments in Assessing Clinical Competence.* Montreal, Canada: Canadian Health Publications; 1987:434-442.

31. Cohen R, Rothman A, Ross J, Domovitch E, Jamieson C, Jewett M. A comprehensive assessment of graduates of foreign medical schools. *Ann Roy Coll Coll Phys Surg Canada.* 1988;21:505-509.

32. Gonzalez-Willis A, Rafi I, Boekeloo B, et al. Using simulated patients to train physicians in sexual risk assessment and risk reduction. *Acad Med.* 1990;65(9):S7-S8.

33. Schnabl GK, Hassard TH, Kopelow ML. The assessment of interpersonal skills using standardized patients. *Acad Med.* 1991;6:S34-S36.

Chapter 9

# Performance Assessment:

## The Role of
## Chart Review
## Analysis
## and CME

*Jocelyn Lockyer*
*Van Harrison*

# Performance Assessment:

## The Role of Chart Review, Analysis, and Continuing Medical Education

*In what may be called the natural method of teaching, the student begins with the patient, continues with the patient, and ends his studies with the patient, using books and lectures as tools, as means to an end.*[1]

History teaches us that experience is the best teacher. In the context of practice, it is the medical record that facilitates the analysis of that experience. The review of medical record data is probably the most frequently used, formal method for identifying potential problems in patient care. Medical records, particularly the hospital record of inpatient care, contain more information about a care episode than is routinely accessible from any other source. Such opportunities to make observations from practice have resulted in important practice research and in new ways of practicing medicine and surgery, and have facilitated important administrative changes.

## Conducting a Chart Review

Derry et al[2] describe chart review as a multistage process involving six steps: (1) selecting a topic; (2) establishing target standards or criteria against which a level of performance can be measured; (3) observing practice by collecting, analyzing, and presenting data; (4) comparing performance with targets; (5) implementing required changes through discussions, written policies, or other mechanisms; and (6) repeating the review to ensure that changes have been implemented and that quality of care has been enhanced.

In the first phase, topics (eg, diseases, procedures, or medication use) are selected for review. In considering a topic for an audit, reviewers generally choose a disease or procedure for which an audit has the potential to facilitate changes in patient management that will benefit the community, hospital, or physician (eg, reducing length of stay, reducing the cost of drugs, or reducing mortality or morbidity). In some cases, the topic is selected to determine compliance with "appropriate" care. Although many chart reviews occur in smaller practice settings, large databases involving multiple sites may be reviewed to identify geographic variations in care. In either case, the chart review itself is a necessary first step in developing strategies to identify the reasons for variations and from appropriate care levels and to develop corrective strategies.

Most review teams consider the *purpose* of the audit. If the review is primarily to educate health care professionals, the criteria selected often reflect the optimum steps in providing appropriate care. In this instance, the criteria (and associated review process) are likely to be more complex, frequently requiring algorithms that are useful both as an overall instructional guide and for problem identification.

Greenfield[3] suggests that the *timing* of the review is also important. When algorithms are applied prospectively, the criteria may direct care. Thus they must be logical, complete, and able to include information not routinely recorded in medical records. When the criteria and review are applied retrospectively, they focus on selected aspects of care that can be more readily assessed from data already present in the medical record. When the review is concurrent (eg, while the patient is still in the hospital), the review of care may produce immediate feedback to the physician that has the potential to alter the care of a particular patient. When the review is truly "retrospective," the feedback will only change care for patients in treatment at a later date.

In the second stage of the audit process, target *standards* or *criteria* for care are established, against which the level of performance may be measured. Both explicit and implicit criteria are used.[4,5] *Explicit* criteria are written descriptions of conditions and actions that constitute appropriate care for the condition under consideration. These criteria, frequently presented as checklists or logic trees, are then used to determine whether care was appropriate. *Implicit* criteria are never formally stated; it is assumed that proficient clinicians know and recognize steps in appropriate care. While the application of explicit criteria produces more uniform results across reviewers and the criteria provide a specific guide for teaching correct actions, no one set of criteria is likely to cover all possible clinical contingencies. In contrast, although applying implicit criteria may result in unreliable, unguided judgments about care provided, the reviewer can take into account those factors that are unique to a specific case. It is increasingly common to employ explicit criteria to identify cases in which problems are likely, then to confirm whether or not a problem has actually occurred through a peer review of the identified case, using implicit criteria.

Explicit criteria assume importance in the education of physicians; they are more amenable to CME targeted to large groups, using organized presentations of substantial amounts of information. These criteria may be based on algorithms for care originally developed for instructional purposes. When applied to relevant medical data they clearly identify what appropriate care should be performed or what inappropriate care should be stopped. In contrast, implicit criteria are more helpful for one-on-one education, or when assessing needs for unique individual problems.

In establishing criteria, Lohr[4] suggests that consideration be given to employing criteria that are both substantive and amenable to implementation. Substantive attributes include scientific grounding, latitude of variations included, clarity, acceptability, sensitivity, and specificity. Implementation attributes include feasibility, ease of use, flexibility, and the ability to be evaluated and modified. In general, the greater the extent to which a criteria set and its implementation in the review process possess these attributes, the more useful the criteria and results will be in directing CME and other change activities.

The third stage requires the collection, analysis, and presentation of results. In the fourth stage, performance is compared to that of the target (ie, the previously agreed upon standard of performance). Generally, at the fifth stage, this analysis and ensuing discussion on the part of the peer review team or committee will result in recommendations for future action. Finally, the sixth and final stage requires audits to be repeated to ensure that progress is being made. For studies involving large databases to assess geographic variation in clinical management, all of the steps involved in an audit may not be carried out, although most studies make recommendations for further analysis and investigation.[6-8]

# Limitations of Practice Review

Practice review has a number of limitations. Tugwell and Dok[9] have noted medical records are primarily used by physicians to aid memory. As such, they often do not document all of the management steps taken by the practitioner. The failure to record actions in charts consistently leaves the auditor with uncertainty as to whether an action was done but not recorded, or not done at all.[10-12] Furthermore, when information about clinical decision making (eg, the rationale behind the selection of one drug over another or the choice of one procedure instead of another) is required, record reviews are most often inadequate. It has been suggested that such reviews should be supplemented by other methods (such as clinical recall interviews,[13] questionnaires,[14] or observational techniques[15]) to obtain a more complete picture of the management decision making.

Tugwell and Dok[9] have also noted difficulties in reviews of charts used by several members of a health care team; it is often difficult in these cases to determine who made various decisions or initiated investigations or treatment. However, in cases in which performance about an institutional unit is being examined and compared to national data, chart reviews of this nature may be satisfactory.

Within the ambulatory setting, chart audits can pose special problems. Often there are logistical difficulties in identifying homogeneous samples as there may not be incentives to implement methods for retrieving charts with similar problems and diagnoses.[9] As outpatients make repeated visits, often over several years, accommodation has to be made for multiple providers, concurrent illness, patient compliance, and temporal issues.[12,16] Even when physicians are committed to audit, many work in settings without age, sex, and diagnostic registers.[17] Opportunity for discussion of results in such settings, an integral part of the audit process, is frequently compromised by patient care commitments.[17]

Other impediments to chart review include cost and location of the review activity. Chart audits can be expensive.[10,14] Professionals must design the study; data must be collected, collated, analyzed, and compared; and there must be a forum for discussing the findings and using them to facilitate needed change.[17] Despite other practice pressures, it is clear that, for effective change to accrue from a review, doing the work at a local level helps ensure enthusiasm for conducting the audit and acting upon the results.[2,18]  Greer[19] has observed that adoption of innovation most frequently occurs following validation by trusted local experts because the innovation must be seen as appropriate for their circumstances.  Similarly, Mugford et al[20] noted that feedback from an audit was most likely to influence clinical practice if it was part of a strategy to target decision makers who had already agreed to review their practice, and if it was presented close to the time of decision making.

Computer systems, thought to be the answer to problems with audit logistics, are often inadequate for the task unless funding is available for programming and data analysis.[14]  Even when simple solutions, such as binding a chart in a different format, are proposed to facilitate review, there can be a lengthy delay in implementation.[10]  Finally, physician distrust of medical audit is well known.  Physicians fear that review may lead to criticism, ridicule, and legal action[10] and, as a result, avoid the chart review process.

## Factors Encouraging the Review of Data From Medical Records

Despite the limitations of medical record audits, there are factors which have encouraged the development of care improvement through the review of data from medical records.  First, there exists an increasing need to assess and improve care and, second, there is the inherent convenience of using an existing, enduring data source.

The societal and political interest in assessing and improving the quality of care has increased in parallel with the proportion of economic resources devoted to health care. Significant energy has been devoted to research on assessing and improving care, and in developing and enforcing regulations relative to patient care.  The extensive review of data from medical records has been fostered largely by governmental agencies and by agencies accrediting health care facilities. In the United States, governmental efforts have sought to assure that, under Medicare and Medicaid, appropriate services are provided *(quality assurance)* and that unnecessary resources are not used *(utilization review)*.  From 1970 to 1975, the Experimental Medical Care Review Organizations (EMCROs) were funded and administered through the National Center for Health Services Research and Development.  These organizations comprised voluntary associations of physicians who developed and evaluated methods for assessing and assuring quality of care for both inpatient and ambulatory services. In 1975, EMCROs were replaced by Professional Standards Review Organizations (PSROs) administered by the Health Care Funding Agency (HCFA).  These local physician organizations performed studies to assure that physicians and institutions achieved quality-of-care objectives, including medical care evaluation studies, quality review studies, and hospital utilization review. Finally, PSROs were felt to be ineffective in producing change and, in 1984, gave way to utilization and quality control Peer Review Organizations (PROs) empowered not only to review representative samples of all hospital cases for selected conditions but also to generate educational recommendations.[4]

Hospital accrediting bodies have also influenced the use of medical record review to target care improvement. The two most prominent agencies in the United States and Canada are the Joint Commission on the Accreditation of Hospitals and the Canadian Council on Hospital Accreditation, respectively. For many years, with increasing emphasis during the last decade, they have required hospitals to set up processes to monitor patient care, identify and resolve problems, and to evaluate the impact of quality assurance acuities. These processes include the review of medical records both retrospectively and concurrently.

These efforts have resulted in a substantial literature concerning the assessment and improvement of care. This literature deals with conceptual and research issues, methods of chart audit, and utilization review. It also contains many studies that have used data from medical records (or derived databases) to assess care and employed educational strategies to improved care.[4,5,9,20-23]

# Uses of Chart Audit

## 1) For Self-assessment

Chart audit has been used by many physicians for self assessment. Early in the century, Osler[24] suggested that physicians:

> *"Begin early to make a three-fold category--clear cases, doubtful cases, mistakes. And learn to play the game fair, no deception, no shrinking from the truth, mercy and consideration for the other man, but none for yourself, upon whom you have to keep an incessant watch ... it is only by getting your cases grouped in this way that you can make any real progress in your post collegiate education; only in this way can you gain wisdom with experience. It is a common error to think the more a physician sees, the greater his experience and the more he knows."*

Generally, physicians conducting audits of their own practices keep notes in a file indexed by condition so they can compare their experiences and lessons with colleagues and the medical literature. The experience of Holdsworth[25] in auditing records is typical of this process. He examined the records of vascular patients under his care for a 5-year period to determine postsurgical complication and mortality rates. He noted that, while audit for the individual surgeon was important, he required national statistics against which he could compare his work. Similarly, physicians in a group practice may exchange charts on a regular basis with colleagues to audit patient records. Furthermore, Williams (cited by Manning and DeBakey[26]) has described the review of charts diagnostic and therapeutic plans by an invited expert.

## 2) For Assessing Physician Competence

Chart audit has also been helpful in assessing physician competence by others interested in quality assurance. Licensing authorities have used audit to perform overall assessments of competence. In two studies,[27,28] chart audit was used as part of a peer assessment of family physicians and specialists in Ontario, Canada. These studies showed serious deficiencies in the medical records and care provided by a small number of practitioners and enabled the researchers to identify subgroups of physicians who were at a higher risk of delivering suboptimal care.

Audit may be coupled with other tools in the assessment of physician competence. McGuire[29] indicates that interpretation of chart data can be variable and a large number of cases (and/or judges) are necessary to obtain a reliable estimate of competence. Consequently, there is hesitation about using chart audit for the purposes of assessing overall individual competence and predicting future performance. Thus, audit may be more useful in identifying extreme individual deficiencies and widespread deviations.

Gerbert and Hargreaves[15] examined physician interview, patient interview, chart audit, and videotaped observation to examine physician performance. While they found that all methods were of reasonable cost and that all were acceptable to physicians, chart audit and videotaped observation had poor content validity. They concluded that no one method provided an accurate picture of physician behavior and that a combination of methods was desirable. In a later study, Gerbert et al[30] compared physician interview, patient interview, chart audit, and videotaped observation for their ability to analyze medication regimens in patients with chronic obstructive pulmonary disease. Interviews with physicians and videotaped observation were the best data sources, followed by chart audit and patient self reports. Similarly, Norman et al[31] used multiple measures to assess the clinical competence of family/general practitioners. Their measures included discussions about specific charts selected at random (ie, chart-stimulated recall), standardized patients, an objective structured clinical examination, multiple-choice examination, and structured oral examination. They concluded that oral examinations, standardized patients, and chart-stimulated recall were able to discriminate between groups of physicians and were valid methods of assessing physician competence.

## 3) Community-based Chart Audit

Chart audit can also provide baseline data on how physicians and surgeons manage conditions within a specified community. Information about coexisting morbidity and complication rates and mortality has been central to improving patient outcomes. There are a number of studies in which audit has played an important role in determining physician baseline performance and in which educational and other interventions have improved patient management practices. Wylie-Rosett et al[32] used chart audit in conjunction with staff interviews and observations to evaluate and improve the standards of care for diabetes. Similarly, Brien et al[33] determined that the neurologic morbidity and mortality associated with carotid endarterectomy in their public teaching institution was 20%, similar to results from other hospitals. They developed a standardized protocol in an attempt to improve surgical outcome following carotid endarerectomy. Over a 10-year period, adherence to the protocol reduced major neurologic morbidity and mortality rate to 3%. In a multicenter study involving carotid endarterectomy and establishing baseline data, Fode et al[34] determined that the use of electroencephalographic monitoring during surgery was the largest single determinant of better outcome following surgery.

Chart reviews have been important in providing data to examine changes in the way physicians manage specific diseases over time. Stross[35] used chart audit to assess changes in the way that chronic airway obstruction was managed over a 6-year period and then surveyed physicians to determine the sources of information they had used as they changed their practices. Chart audit has also been helpful in developing predictive models for care. Maher et al[36] studied the survival from acute renal failure requiring renal replacement therapy in critically ill patients admitted to an intensive care unit. They developed diagnostic criteria that predicted the likelihood of survival. They concluded that the use of these criteria, calculated as a score, could be helpful in patient assessment and would enable comparisons of studies at different sites.

Still others, concerned about the appropriate selection and cost of therapeutic agents for specific diseases, have used audit to determine medication use. An examination by Parrino[37] of the use of antibiotics in his institution determined of the subgroup of physicians responsible for the majority of antibiotic costs—those who used less expensive antibiotics and those who prescribed multiple antibiotic therapy. Mishriki et al[38] were able to determine the incidence of postoperative infections for individual surgeons. Their study was useful in identifying the need for extra supervision and training of junior staff and peer review for senior clinicians. Similarly, Ambrose et al[39] carried out a prospective audit of sepsis in operations for inflammatory bowel disease to determine the best combination of antibiotics to prevent postoperative infection.

Comparisons with experience in other hospitals can be helpful in determining acceptable patient care practices and outcomes. Extensive studies have been undertaken in Manitoba, Canada, to compare surgical rates both from community to community and from community to international standards, in an effort to ensure that unnecessary surgery was not being performed, that complication rates were not inordinate, and that surgical procedures were cost effective.[40,41] The analyses were helpful in revealing large differences in surgical and complication rates between communities.[40,42]

Last, chart audit can be helpful in alerting physicians and other staff to problems that they might not otherwise detect. The prevalence of alcoholism in hospitalized patients is one example. Baird et al[43] conducted a retrospective chart audit and found that physicians identified a prevalence rate of 4.3%. However, chart review using specific criteria for the diagnosis of alcoholism was able to raise the estimated prevalence to 15.9%.

## 4) To Assess the Adoption of Guidelines

A further use of chart review has been the examination of physician adoption of practice protocols and guidelines developed by government, specialty society, and local bodies. One of the most extensive studies to examine guideline adoption was conducted by the US National Institutes of Health. In this study, Kosecoff et al[44] reviewed medical records throughout the state of Washington with respect to 12 recommendations made by their Consensus Development Program. The authors concluded that consensus conferences failed to stimulate change in physician practice, despite moderate success in reaching the appropriate target audience. Such studies have been helpful in determining that dissemination alone rarely leads to change in physician practice behavior, a concept explored in more detail in chapter 12.

Other studies have attempted to use audit as part of a motivational tool for effecting change in physician behavior. Lomas et al[18] compared two interventions that attempted to stimulate adoption of contemporary guidelines promoting a trial of labor following cesarean section. One group experienced chart review with feedback, while the other was exposed to the influence of trained opinion leaders. There was no change in performance among the chart audit group.

McMillan et al[13] used chart audit as a "barometer" of progress in assessing the adoption of guidelines for the use of phototherapy in infants jaundice (hyperbilirubinemia). In this study, a number of educational techniques were employed as a preliminary intervention. When subsequent chart audits showed that adoption levels were less than optimal, a follow-up intervention incorporating chart-stimulated recall interviews with physicians about cases in progress facilitated behavior change.

For large databases, chart review with concomitant statistical analysis has been helpful in determining those factors that appear to act as barriers to the adoption of guidelines. For example, Goldman et al[45] compared Quebec women who underwent vaginal birth after cesarean section to women with repeated cesarean sections by using chart audit techniques to identify the factors that favored vaginal delivery. Their analysis identified physician characteristics (related to type of practice and degree of hospital specialization) that predicted obstetrical or surgical patterns relative to the question of cesarean section. Such information can be useful in developing targeting strategies with the most likelihood of success.

# Assessing Small- and Wide-Area Variations in Care

The most promising new area to emerge in analysis of care has become possible with the advent of large databases and sophisticated computer processing systems. Large-scale databases that draw on and computerize the information found in charts have been useful in examining variations in clinical practice, often described as small- and wide-area variations in care. Such studies draw on Medicare data, private insurance data, and aggregate hospital statistical data.

A number of studies have demonstrated that variations occur from procedure to procedure, hospital to hospital, and city to city. Chassin et al,[6] using data from Medicare beneficiaries, measured geographic differences in the use of more than 100 medical and surgical procedures in 13 large areas of the United States. They found large and significant differences in the use of services. For over half of the procedures there were at least threefold differences between sites with the highest and lowest rates of use. Similarly, Leape et al[46] studied Medicare data related to the appropriateness of the use of coronary angiography, carotid endarterectomy, and upper gastrointestinal tract endoscopy in 23 adjacent counties in one state by comparing this data to criteria derived by an expert panel. They found wide variability from hospital to hospital. In coronary angiography, for example, rates varied from 13 to 158 per 10 000 Medicare patients and inappropriate use of the procedure varied from 8% to 75% between counties. In a study of orthopedic procedures, Keller et al[7] found that rates of use in an area tended to vary depending on the lack of agreement about optimum treatment. In that study, feedback to the physicians reduced the variation. Similarly, an international study demonstrated a large variation in cesarean sections rates in 21 countries.[47]

In addition to determining variations in the use of a surgical procedure, audit has been helpful in looking at adverse events that occur in hospitals. For example, Brennan et al[48] conducted a large study involving medical records from a random selection of hospitals in New York and determined that certain types of hospitals have significantly higher rates of adverse events due to substandard care. O'Connor and colleagues[8] conducted a prospective regional study to examine the observed differences in in-hospital mortality associated with coronary artery bypass grafting. Significant variability was observed in both medical centers and surgeons.

While much of the literature to date in this area has simply identified that variation occurs, the next generation of research will no doubt focus on methods of reducing variation through educational and administrative strategies. As O'Connor et al[8] note, observed differences do not appear to be solely the result of differences in case mix and may reflect differences in currently unknown aspects of patient care.

# Chart Review and Continuing Medical Education

CME is one of the methods used to correct deficiencies identified through chart review. The results of chart review can be used in conjunction with CME in at least three ways[24]:

1) *results of deficiencies from the review of physicians' charts can be used by those physicians to plan a group-oriented CME activity such as a lecture or workshop;*

2) *results of screening or peer review of charts can be used to provide individualized feedback and consultation to a physician; or*

3) *results of a variety of different types of chart review (particularly in hospitals) can be communicated to physicians responsible for designing CME activities. These CME planners integrate this diverse information into the selection of CME topics and the planning of CME activities.*

No information has been systematically collected concerning the extent to which CME offices and planners have drawn on chart review to develop interventions that facilitate physician learning or practice change. The first suggested method, using the results of chart audit to design formal CME activities, is probably the least frequently used of the three. Comparatively few systematic studies regarding specific care activities are undertaken with the expected outcome the planning of a CME activity. Sandlow et al[49] confirm this phenomenon. Despite having done more than 185 medical audits in more than 120 health problem areas, virtually none of the studies identified deficiencies in physician performance for which a formal CME program would be the preferred remediation.[49] The second method occurs fairly frequently. Case finding using simple screening criteria are often used to identify outlier cases whose physicians then undergo peer review. Physicians are contacted with increasing frequency by peers in hospitals and from third-party payers with information on the improvement of clinical or administrative aspects of patient care. The last method has grown in favor among CME planners and occurs with increasing regularity. Effective CME providers use several methods to assess the needs of the target audience. The planners may use results from several methods of chart review (eg, screening studies, studies of specific aspects of care, or tumor conferences) in determining which needs are most important and most appropriately addressed through CME activities.

The linkage between chart review and CME involves an individual who interprets the chart review results and then develops an appropriate individual or group CME activity. However, criteria for chart review are often not sufficiently complex to reflect the total care process, and the information relevant to decision making may not be part of the chart. Consequently, it may be difficult to use solely the data from a review study to develop a program with enough specificity and examples to convince participants they need to change their care practices, particularly in instances where physicians are unaware of their own compliance with guidelines.[50]

Just as chart review is only one method to assess need for a CME activity, CME activities are only one method to bring about change suggested from the results of chart review. Other methods for change include instituting incentives and disincentives for physicians and implementing other types of administrative and organizational changes. It is increasingly important to consider all of the options that can be used to disseminate information to improve care. Such dissemination is more likely to be successful if used in conjunction with computer-based feedback or reminders, opinion leaders, chart review, or practice rehearsal activities.[51]

# Future Trends for Chart Review and CME

## Implications for Practice

The review of data from medical records is likely to increase rapidly in the face of health reform imperatives. Concerns about reducing the costs and assuring the quality of health care continue to fuel the development of clinical guidelines and policies, databases to review care, and the dissemination of strategies or interventions.

These trends are apt to affect CME in noticeable ways. More criteria for the management of many conditions and the utilization of services are likely to be developed and their introduction and updating will be an important part of CME activities. Physicians' care patterns are likely to be increasingly reviewed and monitored with systematic, individualized feedback assuming a more important component in the individual physician's ongoing education. Performance data are more likely to be available and aggregated on local, regional, and national levels to provide guidance for CME activities at each of those levels.

In both the United States and Canada, federal, state, and provincial governments have initiated programs to develop and disseminate clinical practice guidelines and standards of care. These initiatives are shared by third-party payers, medical societies, and health care organizations.[52] Particular emphasis has been placed on developing criteria for high-risk, high-cost, high-volume, and problem-prone services. These efforts will produce criteria and algorithms that can be used directly as the content for CME activities. To the extent the criteria are applied in routine chart reviews, the results will provide the basis for ongoing feedback in local CME activities.

Perhaps an even greater expansion is likely to occur in the databases developed from medical records. Several partial ways have been developed to assemble data in more retrievable formats. For example, US federal agencies are currently determining the feasibility of developing a Uniform Clinical Data Set, comprising approximately 1600 items to be abstracted from a representative sample of all hospital medical records.[4,23] A similar process is occurring within an equivalent Canadian organization, the Hospital Medical Records Institute. Uniform data sets afford the opportunity to develop a central database for several types of review activities. Other initiatives include the linkage of several years of Medicare claims files to monitor aspects of care over several episodes of ambulatory and hospital care. For example, a diabetic's condition could be monitored to see if the person's physician is obtaining regular, relevant blood tests. Finally, computerized medical records show promise in structuring and recording medical care information not only to improve care directly but also to facilitate the review of care. These innovations are likely to increase the recording and review of relevant care data over the episodes of care and may expand the results available for incorporation into CME activities.

## Implications for Research

Chart review has been a helpful tool in assessing physician competence and practice on an individual, group, national, and international basis. Additional research will be required to use the work of chart review to improve continuing medical education and physician practices. There are at least three ways that research can be helpful.

First, research is needed to clarify characteristics of criteria for care (ie, practice parameters) that make CME a more effective method for change. Detailed criteria about patient evaluation and management are more likely to provide the basis for CME activities than are simple case-finding screens. A number of characteristics of criteria and their use can be examined to identify which characteristics or combinations of characteristics are particularly relevant to change through CME.

Second, research is needed to incorporate new databases into CME development. As audits are done and databases are created, this information should be available for planning CME purposes.

Third, research is necessary to relate CME to other methods for changing physician performance. It is essential that researchers better understand the circumstances under which CME is likely to be effective by itself. Similarly, it is important to learn when CME is likely to be more cost-effective than other methods of changing behavior (such as computerized reminder systems and opinion leaders) and when CME should be combined with other methods of behavior change.

In addition to considering research required by the evolution of chart review, the evolution of CME itself should be considered. Research is needed to understand how to combine results of chart review with other forms of needs assessment in developing CME activities. Gerbert and Hargreaves[15] found that chart review was more helpful in needs assessment when combined with other techniques. Work should continue to examine the potential of the clinical recall interview (also known as chart-stimulated recall[53]), to improve the data available to assess physicians both individually and in groups. This method involves interviewing physicians about specific cases[54] in an effort to uncover information not normally found in charts. So far, studies have shown the technique to be fairly unobtrusive, sensitive to the dynamics of performance, reliable, and valid.[31,55]

# Conclusion

Chart review has proven itself helpful as a method of assessing physician competence. Charts are an integral component of patient care and are readily available for use as an assessment tool by the individual physician wishing to measure his/her own performance or by others trying to assess an individual or a group of clinicians. Limitations to chart review include the lack of recording of some types of data and the potential difficulty in locating and extracting relevant data that are recorded.

Increasing emphasis has been placed on assuring quality of care with the subsequent development of more explicit criteria for care (ie, practice parameters), the development of databases containing information relevant to assessing care, and the development of methods to disseminate and implement clinical guidelines. The results of chart audit provide both direct and indirect means to plan CME activities.

Future research is needed in a number of areas, including linking CME and other methods in order to make changes suggested by chart review results, and combining chart review and other assessment methods to develop more appropriate CME activities. The ultimate goal, of course, in using chart review to initiate changes through CME, is the improvement of patient care. As Osler[1] stated, an ongoing assessment of the patient is the key to improving the health of the patient; books, lectures, and guidelines are only tools to improving care.

## References

1. Osler W. The hospital as a college. In: *Aequanimitas, With Other Addresses to Medical Students, Nurses and Practitioners of Medicine.* 3rd ed. Philadelphia, Pa; Blackiston Co; 1945:315.

2. Derry J, Lawrence M, Griew K, Anderson J, Humphreys J, Pandher KS. Auditing audits: the method of Oxfordshire Medical Audit Advisory Group. *B Med J.* 1991;303:1247-1249.

3. Greenfield S. Measuring the quality of office practice. In: *Providing Quality Care: The Challenge to Clinicians.* Goldfield N, Nash DB, eds. Philadelphia, Pa: American College of Physicians; 1989:183-198.

4. Lohr KN, ed. *Medicare: A Strategy for Quality Assurance.* Washington, DC: National Academy Press; 1990:1.

5. Donabedian A. *Explorations in Quality Assessment and Monitoring: The Criteria and Standards of Care.* Ann Arbor, Mich: Health Administration Press, 1982:2.

6. Chassin MR, Brook RH, Park RE, et al. Variations in the use of medical and surgical services by the Medicare population. *N Engl J Med.* 1986;314:285-290.

7. Keller RB, Soule DN, Wennberg JE, Hanley DF. Dealing with geographic variations in the use of hospitals: the experience of the Maine Medical Assessment Foundation Orthopedic Study Group. *J Bone Joint Surg Am.* 1990;72:1286-1293.

8. O'Connor GT, Plume SK, Olmstead EM, et al. A regional prospective study of in-hospital mortality associated with coronary artery bypass grafting. *JAMA.* 1991;266:803-809.

9. Tugwell P, Dok C. Medical record review. In: Neufeld VR, Norman GR, eds. *Assessing Clinical Competence.* New York: Springer Publishing Co; 1985:142-182.

10. Gabbay J, McNicol MC, Spiby J, Davies SS, Layton AJ. What did audit achieve? Lessons from preliminary evaluation of a year's medical audit. *B Med J.* 1990;301:526-529.

11. Charny MC, Roberts GM, Beck P, Webster DJ, Roberts CJ. How good are case notes in the audit of radiological investigations? *Clin Radiol.* 1990;4292:118-121.

12. Payne BC. The medical record as a basis for assessing physician competence. *Ann Intern Med.* 1979;91:623-629.

13. McMillan DD, Lockyer JM, Magnan L, Akierman A, Parboosingh JT. Effect of educational program and interview on adoption of guidelines for the management of neonatal hyperbilirubinemia. *Can Med Assoc J.* 1991;144(6):707-712.

14. Yudkin PL, Redman CW. Obstetric audit using routinely collected computerized data. *Br Med J.* 1990;301:1371-1373.

15. Gerbert B, Hargreaves WA. Measuring physician behavior. *Med Care.* 1986;24:838-847.

16. Crombie IK, Davies HT. Audit of outpatients: entering the loop. *Br Med J.* 1991;302:1437-1439.

17. Webb SJ, Dowell AC, Heywood P. Survey of general practice audit in Leeds. *Br Med J.* 1991;302:390-392.

18. Lomas J, Enkin M, Anderson GM, Hannah WJ, Vayda E, Singer J. Opinion leaders vs audit and feedback to implement practice guidelines: delivery after previous cesarean section. *JAMA.* 1991;265:2202-2207.

19. Greer AL. The state of the art versus the state of the science: the diffusion of new medical technologies into practice. *Int J Tech Assess Health Care.* 1988;4:5-26.

20. Mugford M, Banfield P, O'Hanlon M. Effects of feedback of information on clinical practice: a review. *Br Med J.* 1991;303:398-402.

21. Donabedian A. *Explorations in Quality Assessment and Monitoring: The Definition of Quality and Approaches to its Assessment.* Ann Arbor, Mich: Health Administration Press; 1980.

22. Donabedian A. *Explorations in Quality Assessment and Monitoring: The Methods and Findings of Quality Assessment and Monitoring. An Illustrated Analysis.* Ann Arbor, Mich: Health Administration Press; 1985.

23. Lohr KN, ed. *Medicare: A Strategy for Quality Assurance: Sources and Methods.* Washington, DC: National Academy Press; 1990:2.

24. Osler W. The student life: a farewell address to Canadian and American medical students. *Med News.* 1905;87:629-630.

25. Holdsworth JD. Five-year vascular audit from a district hospital. *Br J Surg.* 1991;78(5):601-606.

26. Manning PR, DeBakey L. *Medicine: Preserving the Passion.* New York, NY: Springer-Verlag NY Inc; 1987.

27. McAuley RG, Henderson HW. Results of the peer assessment program of the College of Physicians and Surgeons of Ontario. *Can Med Assoc J.* 1984;131:557-561.

28. McAuley RG, Paul WM, Morrison GH, Beckett RF, Goldsmith CH. Five-year results of the peer assessment program of the College of Physicians and Surgeons of Ontario. *Can Med Assoc J.* 1990;143:1193-1199.

29. McGuire C. Perspectives in assessment. *Acad Med.* February 1993;68:3S-8S.

30. Gerbert B, Stone G, Stulbarg M, Gullion DS, Greenfield S. Agreement among physician assessment methods: searching for the truth among fallible methods. *Med Care.* 1988;26(6):519-535.

31. Norman GR, Davis DA, Painvin A, Lindsay E, Rath D, Ragbeer M. Comprehensive assessment of clinical competence of family/general physicians using multiple measures. In: *Pro Conf Res Med Educ.* Washington, DC. 1989;75.

32. Wylie-Rosett J, Villeneuve M, Mazze R. Professional education in a long-term-care facility: program development in diabetes. *Diabetes Care.* 1985;8:481-485.

33. Brien HW, Yellin AE, Weaver FA, Carroll BF. A review of carotid endarterectomy at a large teaching hospital. *Am J Surg.* 1991;57(12):756-762.

34. Fode NC, Sundt TM Jr, Robertson JT, Peerless SJ, Shields CB. Multicenter retrospective review of results and complications of carotid endarterectomy in 1981. *Stroke.* 1986;17(3):370-376.

35. Stross JK. Information sources and clinical decisions. *J Gen Intern Med.* 1987;2:155-159.

36. Maher ER, Robinson KN, Scoble JE, et al. Prognosis of critically ill patients with acute renal failure: APACHE II score and other predictive factors. *Q J Med.* 1989;72:857-866.

37. Parrino TA. The nonvalue of retrospective peer comparison feedback in containing hospital antibiotic costs. *Am J Med.* 1989;86:442-448.

38. Mishriki SF, Law DJ, Johnson MG. Surgical audit: variations in wound infection rates of individual surgeons. *J R Coll Surg Edinb.* 1991;36:251-253.

39. Ambrose NS, Alexander-Williams J, Keighley MR. Audit of sepsis in operations for inflammatory bowel disease. *Dis Colon Rectum.* 1984;27:602-604.

40. Roos LL Jr, Cageorge SM, Roos NP, Danzinger R. Centralization, certification and monitoring: readmissions and complications after surgery. *Med Care.* 1986;24:1044-1066.

41. Roos LL, Fisher ES, Sharp SM, Newhouse JP, Anderson G, Bubolz TA. Postsurgical mortality in Manitoba and New England. *JAMA.* 1990;263:2453-2458.

42. Roos NP, Roos LL. High and low surgical rates: risk factors for area residents. *Am J Public Health.* 1981;71(6):591-600.

43. Baird MA, Burge SK, Grant WD. A scheme for determining the prevalence of alcoholism in hospitalized patients. *Alcohol Clin Exp Res.* 1989;13:782-785.

44. Kosecoff J, Kanouse DE, Rogers WH, McCloskey L, Winslow CM, Brook RH. Effects of the National Institutes of Health Consensus Development Program on physician practice. *JAMA.* 1987;258:2708-2713.

45. Goldman G, Pineault R, Bilodeau H, Blais R. Effects of patient, physician and hospital characteristics on the likelihood of vaginal birth after previous cesarean section in Quebec. *Can Med Assoc J.* 1990;143:101-124.

46. Leape LL, Park RE, Solomon DH, Chassin MR, Kosecoff J, Brook RH. Does inappropriate use explain small-area variations in the use of health care services? *JAMA.* 1990:263:669-672.

47. Notzon FC. International differences in the use of obstetric interventions. *JAMA.* 1990;263:3286-3291.

48. Brennan TA, Hebert LE, Laird NM, et al. Hospital characteristics associated with adverse events and substandard care. *JAMA.* 1991;265:3265 -3269.

49. Sandlow LJ, Bashook PG, Maxwell JA. Medical care evaluation: an experience in continuing medical education. *J Med Educ.* 1981;56:580-586.

50. Rosser WW, Palmer WH. Dissemination of guidelines on cholesterol: effects on patterns of practice of general and family physicians in Ontario. *Can Fam Physician.* 1993;39:280-284.

51. Davis DA, Thomson MA, Oxman AD, Haynes RB. Evidence for the effectiveness of CME: a review of 50 randomized controlled trials. *JAMA.* 1992;268:1111-1117.

52. Kelly JT, Toepp MC. Practice parameters: development, evaluation, dissemination and implementation. *Quality Rev Bull.* 1992;18:405-409.

53. Munger BS, Reinhart MA. Field trial of multiple recertification methods. In: Lloyd JS, Langsley DG, eds. *Recertification for Medical Specialists.* Evanston, Ill: American Board of Medical Specialties; 1987:71-88.

54. Parboosingh J, Avard D, Lockyer J, Watson M, Pim C, Yee J. The use of clinical recall interviews as a method of determining needs in continuing medical education. In: Proceedings of AAMC Research in Medical Education Conference; November 6-12, 1987; Washington, DC; 103-108.

55. Maatsch JL, Huang R, Downing SM, et al. *Predictive Validity of Medical Specialty Examinations.* Executive Summary for National Center of Health Services Research, Grant No HS02038-04; 1983.

# Section II

# Annotated Bibliography

**Barrows HS.** An overview of the uses of standardized patients for teaching and evaluation of clinical skills. *Acad Med.* 1993;68:443-451.

> This review of standardized patients focuses on their development, uses, and roles, and finds increasing acceptance in medical education as a means of prompting self (and other) assessments and learning.

**Colliver JA, Williams RG.** Technical issues: test application [of standardized patients]. *Acad Med.* 1993;68:454-460.

> The evidence from a literature review of standardized patient studies confirms their reliability, reproducibility, and validity, and outlines other technical issues, such as their influence on learning.

**Derry J, Lawrence M, Griew K, Anderson J, Humphreys J, Pandher KS.** Auditing audits: the method of the Oxfordshire medical audit advisory group. *Br Med J.* 1991;303:1247-1249.

> The authors develop a coding system for the audit cycle used prospectively in assessing audits reported to medical audit advisory group coordinators.

**Donabedian A.** *Explorations in Quality Assessment and Monitoring. Volume I: The Definition of Quality and Approaches to its Assessment, Volume II: The Criteria and Standards of Care, and Volume III: The Methods and Findings of Quality Assessment and Monitoring. An Illustrated Analysis.* Ann Arbor, Mich: Health Administration Press, 1985.

> These three volumes are a major review of the field of assessing the quality of health care. The review includes conceptual definitions and methods used to assess and improve health care. It also reviews the results of studies using the various approaches.

**Gerbert B, Hargreaves WA.** Measuring physician behavior. *Med Care.* 1986; 24:838-847.

> Four methods of obtaining information on physician behavior in the ambulatory care of chronic obstructive pulmonary disease are reviewed: physician interview, patient interview, chart audit, and videotaped observation. While the content validity of the two interview methods is reasonably good, chart audit and videotaped observation appear to have poor content validity and require other methods to improve their usefulness.

**Harden RM.** What is an OSCE? *Med Teacher.* 1988;10:19-22.

The objective structured clinical examination (OSCE) is described in detail. It is an approach to the assessment of clinical competence, using brief, structured, clinical scenarios adopted from clinical encounters.

**Kosecoff J, Kanouse DE, Rogers WH, McCloskey L, Winslow CM, Brook RH.** Effects of the National Institutes of Health Consensus Development Program on Physician Practice. *JAMA.* 1987;258:2708-2713.

The effects of the National Institutes of Health Consensus Development Program on Physician Practice are investigated by reviewing the medical records of patients treated in hospitals throughout the state of Washington with respect to 12 recommendations. The authors note that the program failed to stimulate change in physician practice, despite moderate success in reaching the appropriate target audience.

**Leape LL, Park RE, Solomon DH, Chassin MR, Kosecoff J, Brook RH.** Does inappropriate use explain small-area variations in the use of health care services? *JAMA.* 1990;263:669-672.

The authors compared the appropriateness of coronary angiography, carotid endarterectomy, and upper gastrointestinal tract endoscopy to their rates of use in 23 adjacent counties in one state. Appropriateness was assessed by means of a detailed review of the medical records of Medicare beneficiaries using preset criteria developed by an expert panel.

**Lohr KN, ed.** *Medicare: A Strategy for Quality Assurance, Volume II: Sources and Methods.* Washington, DC: National Academy Press; 1990.

This is one of two volumes which report a major federal review of quality assurance for health care. It reports on relevant methodologies, as well as the history, current forces, policy issues, future considerations, and recommendations regarding quality assurance activities.

**Marshall J.** Assessment during postgraduate training. *Acad Med.* 1993;68:S23-S26.

The author reviews the process of assessing both undergraduates in medical school and physicians in postgraduate training, contending that this traditional and still dominant process is inadequate because of its limitations. It focuses narrowly on end-point evaluation, using predominantly multiple-choice questions, rather than on identifying deficiencies during the training period so that trainees are able to correct these deficiencies before their end-point evaluations. An example of a more valid process of assessment is the set of tests employed by the Royal Australian College of General Practitioners to assess the skills of family practice physicians by using behavioral ratings.

**McAuley RG, Paul WM, Morrison GH, Beckett RF, Goldsmith CH.** Five-year results of the Peer Assessment Program of the College of Physicians and Surgeons of Ontario. *Can Med Assoc J.* 1990;143:1193-1199.

The office practices of physicians selected through stratified random sampling by the College of Physicians and Surgeons of Ontario registry were assessed by peers. General and family physicians presented more serious deficiencies on chart review in one or both areas than specialists. Predictors of physician performance were: age, membership (in a specialty society), and type of practice (solo vs group).

**McGuire C.** Perspectives in assessment. *Acad Med.* 1993;68:S3-S8.

Success in predicting the course of any phenomenon under study is valued precisely because it furnishes the basis for influencing the phenomenon or, where that is not possible, for mitigating its consequences. This is especially urgent with respect to the psychosocial complexities of medical education related to clinical practice and measured by reliably predictive assessment measures.

**McMaster University, Program for Educational Development.** *Evaluation Methods: A Resource Manual.* Hamilton, Canada: McMaster University Faculty of Health Sciences; 1987.

A comprehensive and useful reference to issues related to the use of assessment measures such as rating scales, essays, multiple-choice questions, oral examinations, objective structured clinical examination, and direct observations. The "triple-jump" exercise is explored in some detail as it pertains to self-directed learning skills.

**McMillan DD, Magnan L, Lockyer JM, Akierman A, Parboosingh J.** Effect of educational program and interview on adoption of guidelines for the management of neonatal hyperbilirubinemia. *Can Med Assoc J.* 1991;144:707-712.

The authors report on physicians interviews regarding; (1) whether physicians adhere to the guidelines for the management of neonatal hyperbilirubinemia, (2) influences on their decisions to investigate and treat the condition, and (3) the effect of an educational program and clinical recall interview on compliance with the guidelines.

**Mugford M, Banfield P, O'Hanlon M.** Effects of feedback of information on clinical practice: a review. *Br Med J.* 1991;303:398-402.

This review article makes the claim that feedback audit is most likely to influence clinical practice if it is (a) part of a strategy to target decision makers already agreed to review their practices, and (b) presented close to the time of decision making.

**Nash DB, Markson LE, Howell S, Hildreth EA.** Evaluating the competence of physicians in practice: from peer review to performance assessment. *Acad Med.* 1993;68:S19-S22.

This article describes three programs for such physician evaluation: (1) the program of US Healthcare, a national managed health care company; (2) the DEMPAQ (Developing and Evaluating Methods to Promote Ambulatory Care Quality) project; and (3) a project initiated by the American College of Physicians in Philadelphia, Pennsylvania, to assess both medical competence and technical performance in the hospital setting.

**Neufeld VR, Norman GR.** *Assessing Clinical Competence.* New York, NY: Springer Publishing; 1985.

This book defines competence, outlines methods for its determination, explores methodological considerations, and concludes by offering suggestions for the application of these methods across the continuum of medical education.

**O'Connor GT, Plume SK, Olmstead EM, et al.** A regional prospective study of in-hospital mortality associated with coronary artery bypass grafting. *JAMA.* 1991;266:803-809.

A prospective regional study was conducted using observed differences in in-hospital "mortality" as evaluation end-points, relative to coronary artery bypass grafting. Significant variability was observed among medical centers and among surgeons.

**Oddi LF.** Development and validation of an instrument to identify self-directed, continuing learners. *Adult Ed Q.* 1986;36:97-107.

This study describes the personality characteristics of self-directed, continuing learners; the development of an assessment instrument; its refinement; and its testing on graduate students. Its test-retest reliability, internal consistency, and descriptions of construct validity suggest its use as a valid tool for identifying self-directed continuing learners.

**Parboosingh J, Avard D, Lockyer J, Watson M, Pim C, Yee J.** The use of clinical recall interviews as a method of determining needs in continuing medical education. 1987;26:103-108.

The study examines the feasibility of using information collected by chart audit and clinical recall interviews to identify the learning needs of physicians relevant to a selected care practice—in this case, physician recognition of intrauterine growth retardation during routine antenatal care.

**Payne BC.** The medical record as a basis for assessing physician competence. *Ann Intern Med.* 1979;91:623-629.

This is a review of medical audit used for assessment of physician performance. The authors note that the confounding of outcome measures (by compliance issues, natural history of disease, severity of illness, status of defense mechanisms, and performance of ancillary services) does not make audit an attractive, single measure of physician performance.

**Sanazaro JP.** Measurement of physicians' performance using existing techniques. *The Western J Medicine.* 1980;133:81-88.

Professional auspices are needed for the development and application of methods that can provide continuing assurance that the clinical activity of physicians corresponds to contemporary standards. The author proposes a system of incentives provided to physicians to promote their participation in voluntary programs of self-assessment, in the form of performance assessment credits, comparable in definition to CME.

**Slater CH.** An analysis of ambulatory care quality assessment research. *Eval Health Prof.* 1989;12:347-378.

This article offers a framework that distinguishes quality as an attribute of the processes of medical care from effectiveness as the results of that care. The review of process-outcome studies in the light of this framework reveals not only a confusion of concepts but a variety of methodological and measurement problems. This article proposes a minimum set of elements to be considered in developing a valid quality assessment method.

# Section III

# The
# CME
# Enterprise

"Apart from the ill-fated war on [drugs], nothing approaching such major interdisciplinary exercises as the Manhattan Project, NASA's space program, or the short-lived boosts in educational efforts following Sputnik's launch, has ever been contemplated as medicine's response to the intellectual, scientific and economic revolution engulfing our entry into the information age."

White K, ed.
*The Task of Medicine Dialogue at Wickenberg.*
Menlo Park, Calif:
HJ Kaiser Fnd Pub;
1988.

# Introduction to Section III

The subject matter of this section is the traditional domain of CME—the provision of activities, programs, and interventions which form the product of the CME enterprise. We use the term "enterprise" both here and in the title of the final chapter of this section to demonstrate the size and scope of the CME delivery system in North America. Like all enterprises, we believe that this one is successful only insofar as it meets the demands of its consumers—in this case, the needs or wants of the practicing physician and his or her patient population. Its size, complexity, and mechanisms certainly attest to its energy and abilities.

The provision of CME may appear relatively straightforward to most of us. After all, very few of us haven't attended continuing education courses or programs of one stripe or another, and most of us have experienced undergraduate teaching programs in a wide variety of disciplines or fields. So we know (or think we know) what constitutes effective teaching and learning. This short vignette illustrates why our understanding may not necessarily stand up to scrutiny:

*A recent PhD graduate (in Adult Education) has joined the faculty of medicine at Midway Medical College. Assigned one-half time to the CME office, he determines, along with the CME committee, that a useful exercise would be to analyze the impact of the relatively extensive conference program mounted by the college. Employing a structured interview technique in several post-conference focus groups, he asks the question, "What changes will you make as a result of attending this course?" While many physicians indicate changes in drug therapy or new investigations, he is surprised to hear such comments as:*

- *"No changes. I don't really see the need to make any as a result of this course."*

- *"I won't make any changes. I've incorporated many of these new drugs into what I prescribe already. I suppose I could talk to one of the faculty members I met today if I had a question."*

- *"No, I don't think I'll change my practices. My patients are somewhat different from the ones talked about here."*

- *"I already am practicing what the faculty talked about today. I usually just attend these courses to check if I'm out-of-date."*

- *"I've learned about the drugs, but I don't think I'll start prescribing them until more of my colleagues have. The side effects are pretty scary."*

This example raises two sets of issues and questions. First are the questions related to the individual needs and agendas of physicians attending CME courses. These patterns of self-directed learning or self-determined curricula in individualized CME are explored by John Premi in chapter 10. Similarly, reasons for participation in CME activities are examined by Donald Moore and colleagues in chapter 11. Second, this vignette (containing answers pretty close to what other researchers have found in similar focus groups) also reflects considerations of the adoption of innovation, the effect of peers on learning and change, and other considerations described in section I.

A not-so-futuristic example, provoking thoughts about the effectiveness of CME or other educational strategies is this one:

> *The Ethica Health Corporation has appointed its vice president of quality assurance as its new President and CEO. She and her executive committee have approved a new strategic plan, one which is tightly linked to the funding of hospital departments and programs. Specifically, the plan indicates that "funding of programs will flow in direct proportion to their proven effect on patient care and health care outcomes." While all departments are affected by the recommendation of the strategic plan, two are particularly touched by it—the quality assurance and the CME offices.*

"Affected by" may be a mild term here; certainly these departments (and any of us who are involved in the physician-as-learner process) need to consider the effect of CME activities on physician performance, and the effect these changes have, if any, on patient or health care outcomes. The two offices, CME and quality assurance, may even begin to contemplate merging. The CME office will certainly begin to look critically at its product, which to date has incorporated rounds and occasional conferences. This perspective on the CME enterprise is considered in chapter 12, which explores the issue of effectiveness and attempts to broaden the definition of CME and to describe the new face of CME.

As much as we need to look at the effects of specific CME interventions, we need to examine the providers of physician continuing education and their interrelation-ships. The type, range of activity, and scope of these providers is best demonstrated by a final vignette:

> *The Chautaqua County Medical Association has undertaken a survey of its members, all 300 of them, to determine practices and problems in CME. It has also surveyed relevant hospitals, medical schools, specialty societies, and professional associations or groups within the state. Regarding the physicians, 20% are family or general (FPs/GPs), and almost 80% are specialists.*
>
> *Of the FP/GP group, half attend sessions mounted at the local medical school, and a third attend local hospital rounds. A handful participate in*

*outside conferences such as those mounted by the American Academy of Family Physicians or other primary care groups.*

*Of the specialists, only a few attend the local medical schools' conferences, though some have taken clinical traineeships or miniresidencies. Most go to larger centers for conferences organized in their specialty or in a related one. Several individuals have gone to large, week-long refresher courses at the medical school or elsewhere. Most attend their own local rounds, where the topic is relevant. Both groups indicate a heavy dependence on reading and consulting with local or medical school colleagues as major sources of learning. Noticeably absent from these results are: recognizable patterns of attendance relative to local needs; responses to health care reform; and any indication of organization at the county or state level of the providers' activities.*

There are several things apparent from this imaginary, but not necessarily imaginative, survey. First, there are a wide variety of "providers" from local hospitals to big medical schools to even bigger professional associations. Second, there appears to be a heavy reliance on local activities, including reading, talking with colleagues, and hospital rounds, especially among FPs/GPs, who rely on local activities to a greater extent than their specialist colleagues. Third, none of this quite extensive activity appears to be interrelated or organized, either in the sense of a basis-in-practice need, health care policy changes, or as a result of learning opportunities collaboratively planned and organized. These issues, along with the question of accreditation, are the driving forces behind chapter 13, by Paul Mazmanian and Willard Duff. This chapter also produces the concept of regional learning centers, produced by the effective collaboration of several groups, including medical faculty.

There are a number of ways we can study the subject matter raised by these three scenarios. They are represented by methods adopted by the chapter authors. The use of previously developed models is seen frequently in this, and earlier sections. Tyler's model of curriculum development forms the root of the accreditation process described in chapter 13; a model of individualized learning is modified from that developed by Kolb, in chapter 10; and chapter 11, on factors affecting participation in CME, develops a modification of Cross's construct regarding participation in adult education.

Finally, in an attempt to overcome the deficiencies inherent in the sequential discussion of individual studies, CME researchers have adapted the biomedical "literature review" model to the study of CME. These form the basis of the chapter on effective CME interventions (chapter 12). We believe that, where such reviews establish strict searching and screening criteria to locate and analyze the relevant literature, their findings can be useful. While these models, studies, and reviews are not exhaustive, they do point to the depth and breadth of the so-called CME literature, and indicate new directions—in research and practice—useful for those with an interest in physician learning and its outcomes.

# Chapter 10

# Individualized Continuing Medical Education

*John Premi*

# Individualized Continuing Medical Education

*CME, like any educational process, involves the complementary activities of teaching and learning. Traditionally, CME has emphasized those aspects of the process that relate to teaching, but is now beginning, along with continuing education in other professions, to focus more of its attention on aspects of learning. Because learning is the* sine qua non *of any educational process, this shift in emphasis represents a rational, evolutionary development. It also represents a marked change from the way CME has been conceptualized and practiced in the past.*

The objective of this chapter is to identify and describe the substance and implications of that change in thinking about CME. To this end, a brief historical review of the role of the individual in medical education will be presented, incorporating a selective review of the educational literature critiquing this role. This will be followed by the presentation of a conceptual model of individualized learning, and a discussion of the research and practice implications of this model. In the chapter, the practice of CME dedicated to a learner-centered model is referred to as *individualized CME*. It is defined as the educational practice that assists and enhances the learning process by which a physician conceives, plans, implements, completes, and evaluates CME activities designed to maintain and enhance his or her medical practice competency.

A fundamental presupposition of individualized CME is that all physicians have the actual or potential capacity for self-directed lifelong learning and, therefore, the ability to maintain an acceptable, qualitative level of practice throughout their professional careers. However, there is a wide spectrum in the capacity of practicing physicians to actualize their self-directed learning potential. Some possess very sophisticated and effective learning strategies and have the capacity to articulate and meet their entire personal learning needs. However, others do not, and require ongoing educational help and/or supervision. Regardless of the extent of the differences between physicians in their ability to plan and direct their individual CME activities, they are all considered to be part of the study and practice of individualized CME.

The notion that all physicians have the potential to maintain their competency throughout their practice careers may seem idealized and somewhat unrealistic, but it is, in fact, current hard reality. Once qualified, physicians are held personally responsible for the maintenance of their professional knowledge and skills; further they are expected to accomplish this goal without readily available or formal educational assistance. This expectation is based on the assumption that physicians have the ability, either innately or by acquisition, to continue to learn effectively throughout their practice careers.

Most professional medical organizations and individual physicians implicitly accept this assumption, believing that few physicians fall below the acceptable standard of practice, and that those who do are the authors of their own fate, due to neglect of their own learning strategies or practices.  The possibility that a physician may not be able to take advantage of the learning opportunities that are available or, in some other way may be educationally handicapped, does not seem to have been considered as a possible alternative explanation.  Given the realities of medical education in North America, this position is difficult to understand.  Learning how to learn has not been (and for the most part, is still not) part of the undergraduate or postgraduate medical curriculum in North American medical schools.

# The Individual in Undergraduate and Graduate Education

In general, undergraduate medical education in North America is driven by a standard curriculum with both the content and method of instruction largely determined by tradition and faculty.  Evaluations with feedback are designed to determine the degree to which a student has learned a finite, relatively well-circumscribed knowledge base, and to provide guidance for remediation if necessary.  In residency, programs are grounded in a defined series of clinical experiences from which learners are expected to determine their own learning needs.  However, considerable assistance is usually provided to them in the identification and fulfillment of these learning needs by their supervisory clinical faculty, and by means of periodic in-training evaluations designed to provide both summative and formative feedback.

Thus, in both undergraduate and graduate education, learners are given considerable direction regarding what needs to be learned, periodic review of how the learning is progressing, and, when necessary, assistance and support in the clinical application of what is learned.  At the conclusion of these educational experiences, learners are given qualifying examinations, based on reasonably well-defined bodies of knowledge and skills.  These assure (or attempt to assure) that newly qualified physicians are able to compare their knowledge base with a recognized and accepted external standard, and usually with that of their peers.  What they are not given are instruction or courses on how to become independent lifelong learners.

Learning how to identify one's own learning needs, how to satisfy those needs independently, how to evaluate the efficiency or effectiveness of the learning process, and  how to critically appraise the quality of the information learned have not traditionally been an explicit part of medical education.  In addition, faculty at all levels of medical education are generally chosen for their clinical or research expertise rather than their knowledge of educational process, with the result that learning skills, if they are learned at all, are done so primarily through precept and example, and not with the same academic rigor with which clinical material is learned.  When one considers all of these factors—the students' lack of experience in unsupervised personal curriculum planning, an undergraduate and residency system that provides opportunities for individual feedback and support (but does not extend these opportunities into practice), the lack of formal training for students in learning how to learn, and a faculty not primarily trained in education—it seems presumptuous to expect that all physicians would possess the requisite knowledge and skills for effective, self-directed, lifelong learning.

# The Individual in Traditional CME

And yet, this seems to be the presumption on which much of the current CME enterprise is founded. In general, CME programs concentrate on the dissemination of information about new scientific discoveries to practicing physicians, usually in large group sessions. Programs are developed with the full expectation that the members of these audiences have the capacity to selectively identify the information related to their own individual needs and to subsequently translate that information into clinical practice.

In CME, audiences are often viewed as homogeneous entities rather than what they really are—groups of disparate individual physicians, perhaps sharing a common interest in the particular topic being presented, but, in other ways, almost certainly very different. Individual physicians in any audience represent a wide variety of backgrounds, needs, attitudes, experiences, and, perhaps most important of all, different learning aptitudes and styles. It is generally not seen as part of the CME mandate to take these differences into consideration during traditional formal course planning. The emphasis remains on information transfer, with rarely (or no) provision made to help individual learners identify or meet their own learning needs or to help them integrate new knowledge into their individual practices. The unproven expectation, in spite of their lack of formal training in self-directed learning, is that all practicing physicians are able to accomplish this independently.

Were there evidence to support the effectiveness of formal, didactic CME in maintaining the competence of practicing physicians, there would be no need to address these apparent dificiencies. Such evidence, however, is lacking. In a study of Canadian family physicains, Dunn and colleagues[1] were unable to demonstrate any correlation between the quality of care in a physician's practice and his or her participation in traditional CME. Further, a recently published review of 50 randomized controlled studies in CME concluded that the widespread concerns about the effectiveness of traditional CME methods are justified—there was little evidence to support their efficacy in either changing physician behavior or health care outcomes.[2]

Other concerns about CME effectiveness arise from two additional studies which examined the knowledge and performance of practicing physicians. The first described a randomized study of peer review among Canadian physicians in which significant deficiencies in physician performance and knowledge were much more widespread than previously believed, particularly in those in practice the longest.[3] The second study, in which a group of practicing US internists wrote the same board examinations as a group of residency candidates just completing their training, confirmed the Canadian findings.[4] This latter study demonstrated that the knowledge deficits of the physicians characteristically reflected a failure to acquire information discovered since their entry into practice, rather than an erosion of knowledge acquired during the undergraduate or postgraduate training period.

What emerges from these studies is the concept that a significant number of practicing physicians are either unable or unwilling to use current CME resources to maintain or enhance their professional competency. Is this the result of the presumed deficiencies in the current approach to CME or a manifestation of careless or negligent educational planning and/or performance on the part of the physicains involved? There is no obvious answer, but a selective review of the educational literature does provide some insights into the question. It also provides insights into what constitutes effective educational practice, which components of this practice are missing or inadequately represented in current CME programming, and how this information can be used to develop a new and more effective paradigm for CME.

## Evidence From the Literature

There is considerable evidence that simply making information available to physicians does not guarantee change in their clinical behavior. Whether the information is the product of a consensus conference in which it has been sanctioned by the leaders in its field,[5,6] or specifically designed for the target audience to whom it is delivered,[7,8] appears to make no difference to its impact on physician performance. One might argue that simple exposure to information might not have provided sufficient opportunity for learning to occur, but even the demonstration that physicians have acquired the knowledge in question is not necessarily followed by behavior change.[7-9] If the primary goal of CME is to change physician behavior, a model based mainly on the conveyance of new scientific information is clearly not an effective one.

However, there is considerable evidence to support an alternative model that uses learner experience as the foundation for continuing learning. The first step in the process of using experience as a stimulus to learning is the development of learning needs, explored in some detail in section II. To identify learning needs that accurately reflect deficiencies in performance, the learner must be able to both reflect on, and accurately interpret, his or her experience. These are difficult tasks and there is evidence to suggest that, while this may easily be achieved with some of the simpler issues that occur in practice,[10] there may be significant problems where the issues are complex or poorly defined.

Several studies have revealed important differences between what practitioners know, what they do, and what they think they do. This has been demonstrated in the provision of preventative care,[11] in the performance of repeat cesarean sections,[5] and in the prescribing of benzodiazepines.[12] In each case, physicians' basic knowledge in the clinical area in question was adequate, but their estimates of how they actually performed when they applied that knowledge to clinical practice exceeded that which occurred in reality. It is clear that physicians' basic knowledge and their clinical performance do not necessarily bear a one-to-one relationship. Further, and perhaps more importantly, physicians may not be aware of a perception/reality gap. From an educational perspective, however, the provision of feedback, identifying the perception/reality gap in a constructive way, can result in a more accurate reframing of the experience.[12,13] In one study, such feedback led to positive behavioral changes in clinical performance.[12]

In contrast, simply providing feedback without providing assistance in engaging with (or constructively reframing) the information seems to produce no change in behavior, or one that does not endure over time,[14-17] even in the face of a financial incentive.[16] When feedback has been provided with appropriate additional educational input (such as information that is relevant to the problem[15] or an opportunity to discuss relevant issues with a mentor by means of a chart review), behavior changes have been demonstrated.[15-17] Some of these changes have been shown to endure.[16] These studies provide evidence for the importance of defining learning needs from practice experience, and the potential effectiveness of providing appropriate educational assistance to help learners accomplish this task. There are other studies, however, that have displayed more mixed results. These studies highlight the importance of another component of the educational process important in facilitating behavior change, that of practice integration.

In the first of these trials, Ray and his colleagues[18] used physician educators to provide feedback on practice performance to a group of practicing physicians known to be prescribing diazepam inappropriately. While some reduction in prescribing was seen in all physicians in the study, those who employed a schedule detailing steps in the withdrawal of diazepam (ie, information on practice integration) showed a much greater change than those who did not. In another study by the same author, however, an attempt to reduce the prescribing of antipsychotic medication in nursing homes by using similar educational methods did not change physician behavior. The authors concluded that the unique practice environment of a nursing home and their failure to consider it in their educational intervention probably underlay the negative results.[19]

It is clear that factors other than strictly medical issues strongly influence how drugs are prescribed in nursing homes (eg, the views of the nursing staff), and failure to deal with these factors presumably creates an insurmountable barrier to the hoped-for changes. This conclusion is supported by a second, similar study by Avorn et al[20] that took these factors into consideration in the development of an educational intervention which subsequently demonstrated positive results. In this study, the education program included needs assessment and academic detailing and was directed at all relevant health care providers, not just physicians. These examples provide evidence for the effectiveness of supplying educational interventions which help learners overcome the barriers of translating knowledge into practice, regardless of whether the barrier existed in the learner or in the practice environment.

When intervention studies considered the learning and information needs of practitioners, as well as potential problems in practice integration, they were able to realize desired behavior changes in study subjects. The nursing home study by Avorn et al,[20] another by Inui et al[21] (which improved patient hypertensive outcomes by training in and demonstrating patient compliance issues), and a further study by Klein et al[22] (which changed prescribing behavior for the treatment of urinary tract infection) all paid careful attention to physician experience, needs assessment, the provision of appropriate information, and practice integration. If the objective of CME is to change physician behavior, then a comprehensive and integrated educational approach seems to be the recipe for success.

One study that appeared to follow this recipe, and yet failed to show the expected results in improving health care outcomes, is worthy of special consideration.[9] The objective of this study was a reduction in the blood pressure of patients with uncontrolled hypertension who were receiving treatment. Physicians in the study were given computer-generated information about the blood pressure of hypertensive patients in their rosters or an educational program on patient compliance, or both. Results included an increase in the number of patient visits in all groups and improved knowledge about patient compliance in the cohorts who received the educational package, but no statistical differences in changes in the blood pressures of the patients being treated by any of the study groups. Noticeably absent from the educational intervention used in this study, however, was an opportunity for the physicians in the educational groups to observe how to apply the newly acquired information on compliance in clinical settings, or to receive any feedback on their attempts to do so. Comparing this study to a similar trial where such opportunities were provided and in which significant reductions in patients' blood pressures did occur, the importance of providing opportunities for procedural knowledge, when necessary, is strongly supported.[21] Research in other areas of medical education has also demonstrated that effective techniques in the teaching and learning of professional interpersonal skills are those which provide opportunities to practice the new skills and receive feedback on those attempts.[23-25]

One other intervention of demonstrated effectiveness is not as easily described as an educational approach. Educational influentials or opinion leaders appear to be effective educational tools for changing physician behavior.[26,27] How they accomplish educational tasks is not clear, although several possibilities exist, best described within the context of the physician experience, learning needs, and practice integration. First, opinion leaders by definition have the respect of their colleagues and provide both sanctioning and role modeling for new behavior. Second, because opinion leaders are peers of those they seek to influence, it is likely that they have reasonable insights into the learning needs and practice idiosyncrasies of their prospective learners and thus are able to format and highlight information in a constructive and useful way. Finally, opinion leaders most likely understand issues of practice integration and are able to develop appropriate strategies to deal with them.

# Toward a Model of Individualized Learning

Thus, the current CME model has inherent deficiencies, primarily because it fails to deal with some crucial aspects of the educational process required to enhance change in physician behavior.  A selective review of the literature focusing on studies that demonstrated changes in physician behavior as a result of an educational intervention has revealed a number of educational strategies that seem to be the key to overcoming these deficiencies and, thus, facilitate change.  The remainder of the chapter will describe a conceptual model to illustrate the relationship between these various educational maneuvers and the more traditional view of CME, followed by a discussion of the service and research implications of such a construct.

Because one of the first objectives of a new educational model would be to compensate for the deficiencies in existing CME methods, emphasis is on individual learners rather than audiences, and on the process of education rather than its content.  In such a model, the role of CME faculty consequently shifts from being solely providers of information to becoming learning facilitators; and learners, instead of being passive participants in what to them is an obscure educational process, become actively engaged in the identification and fulfillment of their own learning needs.

These needs will be described in terms of practice rather than knowledge.  To do otherwise would be to misconstrue the central role of professional practice, which is to set what is wrong, right (not simply know about, or describe it).[28]  Although the practice of medicine, like all professional practice, is anchored in the basic sciences, it is itself an applied science and is, therefore, first and foremost, a normative activity.  It is what the physician does to (and for) patients and not what he or she knows that is of primary importance to society at large.

What physicians do in practice also has other important educational implications because practice activities give rise to experience, and experience, as shown by the studies described previously, is a powerful determinant of human behavior.  Since it may be argued that changing physician behavior is the ultimate goal of CME, the role of experience must be taken into consideration in the development of a new model.  This position is consistent with, and supported by, one of the major tenets of adult learning which, for several decades, has emphasized the role of experience of the individual in the learning process.[29]  It is also consistent with the conclusions of a recent review of the problem-solving literature by Schmidt et al,[30] which suggests that what physicians actually do in practice is more related to their previous clinical experience than to their fund of medical knowledge.

How can all of these disparate elements be brought together to form a new CME model that would facilitate the achievement of the objectives implied in our definition of individualized CME?  One way to accomplish this objective is to adapt the experiential learning model as described by Kolb.[31]  This model makes it possible to consider all of the important parts of the individualized learning process as well as the relationship between them.  It also makes possible a comparison between a new orientation of CME and the traditional approach.

The figure is a schematic representation of the adaptation of Kolb's experiential learning model. The process represented in this model can start at either the experiential level or the new knowledge level. The former is typical of learning initiated by the practice situation while the latter is typical of learning occurring as a result of exposure to new knowledge, eg, in reading a journal article or attending a traditional CME event.

## Figure 10.1

## The experiential learning model

### (adapted from Kolb)

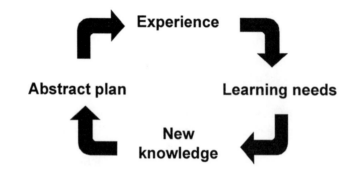

For a practice experience to initiate the process, it must be followed by a critical reflection of the event in order to identify the relevant issues, or questions, that arise from the experience in a manner described by Schön[32] as "reflection-on-action." These issues, or questions, must then be converted into true learning needs, either by refining them into researchable questions, or translating them into specific objectives for acquiring new skills or attitudes. When the physician is able to identify these learning needs, without formal outside help, they are described as *perceived* learning needs. When the physician is not primarily able to identify these needs on his or her own and does so only with the help of outside resources (eg, chart audit, chart-stimulated recall, or personal feedback), they are described as *unperceived or misperceived* learning needs. The term "unperceived" is used when the physician remains totally unaware of the identified issue, whereas the term "misperceived" is used when there is a discrepancy between what the physician believed the situation was, and what it was in reality. Because learning can only occur when the learner acknowledges a learning deficit, unperceived and misperceived needs must be converted into perceived needs before learning will proceed.

In the new model, the clarification of learning needs through critical reflection is followed by a search for knowledge that will satisfy these needs. Knowledge in this context includes both factual and procedural knowledge, that is the "what" and the "how to" of medical practice, as well as knowledge about one's own personal attitudes, the culture of the practice venue, the formal or informal standards of the local medical community, and other influences on the application of new learning to practice.

The next phase of experiential learning is molding the new information into an abstract plan. This maneuver requires an intimate knowledge of the practice situation, since any proposed changes in diagnostic or management plans must take into consideration what has gone before, as well as patient needs and wishes. In preparation for this step, careful consideration of these factors will often identify potential obstacles, or pitfalls, to the planned changes, making it possible to prepare tactics or strategies to deal with them before they actually occur. In attempting to implement practice changes, having a well-thought-out strategy, with opportunities to plan (and, where necessary, to practice) complex tactical maneuvers, greatly enhances the potential for success. A good abstract plan includes both what is to be done and how it is to be done, with consideration given to potential barriers to its implementation.

The final phase is the process of the actual application of the abstract plan to the specific problem that gave rise to the process. This represents practice integration and gives rise to a new experience and the potential for new learning. When learning continues to occur as a result of this process, it is useful to conceptualize this ongoing process as a spiral rather than a circle demonstrating the concept of learning as a continuous process.

When the process is initiated through the introduction of new knowledge, it is influenced by a very different set of circumstances. Where there are no predetermined, practice-generated learning needs, the learner must be able to visualize the clinical application of that knowledge without the benefit of the stimulus that those needs usually provide. Alternatively, the learner must store the information in his or her random memory with the hope that a fortuitous event will allow its use before it is lost to recall. This represents a much more abstract process, one which would appear to render the learning process more difficult and less efficient.

# Implications for CME

## 1) Practice

The foregoing promotes the hypothesis that the educational approach most effective in changing physician behavior and/or health care outcomes concerns itself in a major way with the specific educational needs of individual physicians, preferably within the context of their own practices. The most obvious, simplest, and yet most profound implication of this for the practice of CME is that it must reorient itself to thinking in terms of how it can best help physicians learn how to do new things (or how to do old things better) rather than in terms of telling them what is new, or what we think they may have forgotten. This change of orientation, which means changing the focus of CME from audiences to individuals, and from teaching to learning, does not necessarily connote a system of one-on-one teaching. The concept of individualized CME is quite compatible with having learning activities conducted in groups (either large or small), as long as the learning objectives of the individuals in those groups may be achieved in that format.

Described within the framework of the experiential learning model, the essential task of CME educators is to help physicians fuse new knowledge and previous experience into more effective clinical behavior in managing health care problems. Since the processes through which this will occur are the critical reflection of previous experience to develop authentic learning needs, and the integration of new learning into practice, it is by helping physicians do these things more effectively that CME providers can be of most help to practitioners in the field.

While, undoubtedly, creative research in the area of learning needs assessment will uncover new methods to help physicians more accurately identify their educational needs, there are already examples of how the currently used approaches could be improved. Learning needs assessments are generally conducted by means of surveys of prospective or current course attendees by requesting them to describe their current and future needs. A second method in common use is to have one or more representatives of the target audience become members of the planning group so that they can provide the planning group with their perspective of the learning needs of the target audience. Neither method addresses unperceived or misperceived needs in a systematic way, clearly an important omission.

One simple way of facilitating the inclusion of such needs in a program is to provide more opportunities for audience participation and discussion. Questions by members of the audience, particularly if they are case based, are more likely to reflect true learning needs than unfocused surveys. Further, they also provide an opportunity for speakers to diplomatically identify and address unperceived or misperceived needs that may be implicit in question. A recent report by De Buda and Woolf[33] outlines how the use of questions can be effectively incorporated into the traditional approach to CME by mandating that the time allocated for questions be equal to that allocated for prepared presentations.

Using individual learner's practice experience as the basis for an educational program is another way of increasing the fidelity of learning needs. This has been done by case discussion from which a group was able to develop a customized learning agenda[34] and also by asking participants to bring their own charts to a CME event and auditing them themselves, using a standardized schema provided at the program.[35] Both of these examples demonstrate how CME programs can provide opportunities to address unperceived and/or misperceived needs.

Finally, it should be possible to increase the quality of information that comes from current survey approaches by posing better-directed and more relevant questions. For example, a few years ago an unpublished survey, in which the author was involved, was carried out in Ontario in preparation for the development of a comprehensive program in geriatrics for family physicians. A trained interviewer phoned a randomly selected group of family physicians and asked them to identify their learning needs in geriatrics. Responses to those questions could easily be cataloged by traditional medical systems, such as cardiology or gastroenterology. However, each physician was asked a final practice-based question, ie, to describe the specific health care problems he or she experienced with the last elderly patient seen. Without fail, the answers related to process issues such as problems of patient compliance with medication, concerns about polypharmacy and the potential for drug interactions, and worries about how to support the frail elderly who live alone, along with other problems not easily categorized within a traditional medical framework. The anecdote, in addition to illustrating how the implied direction of a question may influence the answers it elicits, also suggests that practicing physicians are prepared to share more personal practice information with CME providers if the latter are prepared to signal their willingness to receive it.

The description of the application of needs assessment to practice can also be applied to the issue of practice integration. Specific examples about what facilitates the translation of knowledge to practice behavior have been given, and what has been said about the use of questions in better defining learning needs can be equally applied to the subject of practice integration. What is most important at this point, however, is not the development of a laundry list of specific interventions (the objective of chapter 13) but the incorporation of the concept that authentic learning needs and practice integration must be considered in the development of every CME intervention. Once program planners have made that conceptual shift, methods for dealing with the issues will follow.

## 2) Research in CME

If CME providers are to redirect their educational strategies to help individual physicians learn more effectively, then a research agenda for individualized CME must include, if not emphasize, studies that will yield information to clarify and support this activity. This new direction places much more emphasis on the study of physicians, their learning activities, and the environment and context in which they practice and learn. This research agenda also expands the breadth and depth of studies done on physicians and their practices and must include, as Watts[36] has suggested, studies on the doctor-patient relationship, the practice venue, the "art" of medicine, and other factors that exist in practice that influence the provision of medical care.

Research in CME has been moving into studies of individualized CME for some time. The studies by Fox et al[37] that explore the factors influencing changes in practicing physicians perhaps provide the best single example of this kind of research, although studies relating to the adoption of innovation (the subject of chapter 2) provide several more.  The major contribution of this research is insight into the factors influencing that learning and change which occurs in the physician's practice of clinical medicine.

The model presented in this chapter offers an opportunity to conceptualize the steps in the individual learning process and the relationship between them.  For example, in ascertaining learning needs, how and why does experience give rise to the identification of learning needs?  What starts and stops the process?  What are the barriers and facilitators to this process?  Are the skills required inherent, or learned?  These questions, and others, can be applied to each of the processes represented by arrows in the schematic drawing of the model (see figure 10.1).

While research into these fundamental questions is important to provide insight into basic issues of physician learning, the most urgent need for research in individualized CME is at the applied level.  Several examples of effective educational interventions were cited in this chapter; few, if any, of these have been converted into ongoing CME programs.  By their description, there is no doubt that these educational interventions were labor intensive and financially expensive to develop, and thus not "practical" in a CME world where cost recovery at the outset is the *sine qua non* of remaining operational.  But without developing and testing such interventions, how is progress to be made?

There is substantial evidence that much of CME currently available is ineffective, but because of its availability, familiarity, and its ability to produce revenue, it remains popular.  Effective CME, examples of which have been provided in this chapter, that engages the individual learner and enhances the potential for behavior change is unfamiliar, not readily available, and will almost certainly be expensive, at least in its developmental phase.  The CME enterprise in its broadest sense must come to grips with this paradox and find the motivation and resources to develop new educational initiatives incorporating the philosophy and spirit of individualized learning.  It is only in this way that more effective programming can be developed, evaluated, and refined.  It is only in this way we can make the quantum leap from a dissemination-oriented system of CME to one that directs its energies to helping individual learners realize the goal of maintaining competency through a program of self-directed, lifelong learning.

### References

1.   Dunn EV, Bass MJ, Williams JI, et al.  Study of relation of continuing medical education to quality of family physician's care. *J Med Educ.* 1988;63:775-784.

2.   Davis DA, Thomson MA, Oxman AD, Haynes RB.  Evidence for the effectiveness of CME: a review of 50 randomized controlled trials. *JAMA.* 1992;268:1111-1117.

3.   McAuley RG, Paul WM, Morrison GH, et al.  Five-year results of the peer assessment program of the College of Physicians and Surgeons of Ontario. *Can Med Assoc J.* 1990;143:1193-1199.

4.  Ramsey PG, Carline JD, Inui TS, et al.  Changes over time in the knowledge base of practicing internists. *JAMA*. 1991;266:1103-1107.

5.  Kosecoff J, Kanouse DE, Rogers WH, et al.  Effects of the national institutes of health consensus development program on physician practice. *JAMA*. 1987;258:2708-2713.

6.  Lomas J, Anderson GM, Domnick-Pierre K, et al.  Do practice guidelines guide practice? the effect of a consensus statement on the practice of physicians. *N Engl J Med*. 1989;321:1306-1311.

7.  Sibley JC, Sackett DL, Neufeld V, et al.  A randomized trial of continuing medical education. *N Engl J Med*. 1982;306:511-515.

8.  Pinkerton RE, Tinanoff N, Willms JL, Tapp JT.  Resident physician performance in a continuing education format:  does newly acquired knowledge improve patient care? *JAMA*. 1980;244:2183-2185.

9.  Dickinson JC, Warshaw GA, Gehlbach SH.  Improving hypertension control:  impact of computer feedback and physician education. *Med Care*. 1981;19:843-854.

10. Covell DG, Uman GC, Manning PR.  Information needs in office practice:  are they being met? *Ann Intern Med*. 1985;103:596-599.

11. Premi JN.  Health maintenance procedures in family medicine:  do family doctors do what they think they do? *Can Fam Phys*. 1978;24:663-671.

12. Rosser WW.  Using the perception-reality gap to alter prescribing patterns. *J Med Educ*. 1983;58:728-732.

13. Premi J.  An assessment of 15 years' experience in using videotape review in a family practice residency. *Acad Med*. 1991;66:56-57.

14. Tierney WM, Miller ME, McDonald CJ.  The effect on test ordering of informing physicians of the charges for outpatient diagnostic tests. *N Engl J Med*. 1990;322:1499-1504.

15. Manning PR, Lee PV, Clintworth WA, et al.  Changing prescribing practices through individual continuing education. *JAMA*. 1986;256:230-232.

16. Martin AR, Wolf MA, Thibodeau LA, et al.  A trial of two strategies to modify the test-ordering behavior of medical residents. *N Engl J Med*. 1980;303:1330-1336.

17. Everett GD, deBlois CS, Chang PF, Holets T.  Effect of cost education, cost audits, and faculty chart review on the use of laboratory services. *Arch Intern Med*. 1983;143:942-944.

18. Ray WA, Blazer DG, Schaffner W, et al.  Reducing long-term diazepam prescribing in office practice. *JAMA*. 1986;256:2536-2539.

19. Ray WA, Blazer DG, Schaffner W, Federspiel CF.  Reducing antipsychotic drug prescribing for nursing home patients: a controlled trial of the effect of an educational visit. *Am J Public Health*. 1987;77:1448-1450.

20. Avorn J, Soumerai SB, Everitt DE, et al.  A randomized trial of a program to reduce the use of psychoactive drugs in nursing homes. *N Engl J Med*. 1992;327:168-173.

21. Inui TS, Yourtee EL, Williamson JW.  Improved outcomes in hypertension after physician tutorials. *Ann Intern Med*. 1976;84:646-651.

22. Klein LE, Charache P, Johannes RS.  Effect of physician tutorials on prescribing patterns of graduate physicians. *J Med Educ*. 1981;56:504-511.

23. Wolf FM, Woolliscroft JO, Calhoun JG, Boxer GJ.  A controlled experiment in teaching students to respond to patients' emotional concerns. *J Med Educ*. 1987;62:25-34.

24. Verby JE, Holden P, Davis RH.  Peer review of consultations in primary care:  the use of audiovisual recordings. *Br Med J*. 1979;1:1686-1688.

25. Maguire P, Roe P, Goldberg D, et al.  The value of feedback in teaching interviewing skills to medical students. *Psychol Med*. 1978;8:695-704.

26. Strass JK, Hiss RG, Watts CM, et al. Continuing education in pulmonary disease for primary care physicians. *Am Rev Respir Dis.* 1983;127:739-746.

27. Lomas J, Enkin M, Anderson GM, et al. Opinion leaders vs audit and feedback to implement practice guidelines. *JAMA.* 1991;265:2202-2207.

28. Cervero RM. The importance of practical knowledge and implications for continuing education. *J Contin Ed Health Prof.* 1990;10:85-94.

29. Knowles M. *The Adult Learner: A Neglected Species.* Houston, Tex: Gulf Publishing Company; 1984.

30. Schmidt HG, Norman GR, Boshuizen HPA. A cognitive perspective on medical expertise: theory and implications. *Acad Med.* 1990;65:611-621.

31. Kolb DA. *Experiential Learning.* Englewood Cliffs, NJ: Prentice-Hall, Inc; 1984.

32. Schön DA. *Educating the Reflective Practitioner.* San Francisco, Calif: Jossey-Bass Publishers; 1987.

33. De Buda Y, Woolf CR. Saturday at the university: a format for success. *J Contin Ed Health Prof.* 1990;10:279-284.

34. Premi JN. Problem-based, self-directed continuing medical education in a group of practicing family physicians. *J Med Educ.* 1988;63:484-486.

35. Craig JL. The OSCME (Opportunity for self-assessment CME). *J Contin Ed Health Prof.* 1991;11:87-94.

36. Watts MSM. CME or PME? *J Contin Ed Health Prof.* 1990;10:129-136.

37. Fox RD, Mazmanian PE, Putman RW. *Changing and Learning in the Lives of Physicians.* New York, NY: Praeger Publishers; 1989.

# Chapter 11

# Participation in Formal CME:

## Factors Affecting Decision-making

*Donald Moore, Jr*
*Nancy Bennett*
*Alan Knox*
*Robert Kristofco*

# Participation in Formal CME:

## Factors Affecting Decision Making

*Physicians typically manage patients on the basis of their own knowledge and experience. Occasionally, physicians encounter patients with challenging problems and seek to supplement their knowledge and experience base with information from others.[1]*

## Forces Impacting on Attendance at Formal CME Activities

This is the heart of the physician learning experience. Physicians seek information from a variety of sources and obtain it in a variety of formats. These sources include medical schools, hospitals, professional organizations, the pharmaceutical and medical equipment industries, and colleagues. While physicians seem to use multiple sources, their preferences appear to differ according to individual characteristics, such as age, specialty and stage of career, practice setting, and content of the problem.[1-4] Formats selected by physicians include conventions, symposia, and conferences, as well as rounds, journals, textbooks, informal conversations, patient referrals, audiotapes, videotapes, and computer software.

Formal CME activities such as conferences and symposia remain an important part of physician information-seeking strategies.[5-9] Participation in these activities represents a significant expenditure of physician time as well as public and personal resources. However, there is a less-than-complete understanding of the decision-making process that physicians use to select formal CME activities they wish to attend. Many of the studies about physician participation in CME reported in the literature focus on marketing-related concerns, such as time, place, price, and content. This is useful at one level for CME planners, but perhaps a more important concern remains obscured—how does physician decision-making about participation in formal CME relate to problems or challenges encountered in practice? In addition, how does physician decision-making about participation in formal CME relate to the ongoing process of information seeking that is a part of the professional life of most physicians?

Further, the most commonly asked question in the reported research has been: "What are the factors that affect physician attendance at formal CME activities?" Researchers have asked these questions primarily about "traditional" formal CME activities. Richards and Cohen[10] described a formal CME activity as one that is a continuous series of formal activities, lasts for 1 to 5 days, and frequently requires out-of-town travel.

There are four broad clusters of findings related to attendance at formal CME activities described in these studies. These findings relate to reasons, purposes, obstacles, and facilitators of attendance.

## Reasons for Participation

Reasons for participation include more general motivations that result in decisions to participate in CME activities. The most commonly reported of these reasons can be described as "professionalism,"[11-13] which may be regarded as a collection of forces that initiate and propel physicians to participate in CME.[14] These forces include concern about providing the best possible care for patients and the values of education as an approach to maintaining professional competency.[15]

Schein[16] articulates two distinguishing characteristics of professionals—a specialized body of knowledge and skills and their commitment to ongoing improvement of those competencies through participating in continuing education activities. In recent years, it has become common to attribute increased participation in short courses, conferences, and workshops to a general concern about the effects of the biomedical information explosion on professional competency. In addition, increased concern has been expressed about the deterioration of the knowledge base of practicing physicians.[17] Physicians have reported that they attend continuing education activities to maintain and improve professional knowledge and skills in order that they can provide the best possible care to their patients.[18] This motivation emerges from the inner standards of excellence that drive professionals to perform at optimal levels.

## Purpose of Participation

In contrast, purposes stated by physicians for their participation in CME activities are more specific than reasons, and relate directly to anticipated outcomes. Some of the literature confuses reasons for participation which relate more to psychological motivation, and purposes for participation which incorporated the notion of benefits derived from anticipated outcomes.[14,19] Purposes of participation can be categorized by means of their desired outcomes. Three are described here: educational outcomes, regulatory outcomes, and social outcomes.

Educational outcomes have been described in several ways. In studies, physicians have reported that they wished to gain "information in general,"[20] an "expansion of general knowledge,"[5] and (closely related to the first two) "general knowledge of program material."[20] A more commonly reported purpose of CME participation was to gain information related to a specific technique or treatment.[20-22] Some physicians also reported wanting to acquire clinical and technical skills within a specialty.[5]

The most frequently cited purpose was to "keep up with advances in medicine."[15,21,23-26] Other educational purposes reported include: to validate previous learning,[10] to review or refresh previous learning,[20] and to prepare for board examinations.[5,20] Some physicians saw participation as part of a remedial program to correct deficiencies in their performance.[5]

Regulatory outcomes related primarily to obtaining CME credit and certifying attendance in response to requirements of medical license, hospital privileges, or professional society membership.[15,20,21] According to Wolf and colleagues[15] some physicians reported that their attendance at CME activities was a means to reduce the possibility of malpractice. Stross and Harlan[27] reported that no major changes occurred in CME participation patterns as a result of mandatory CME requirements.

Social outcomes related primarily to the physician's desire for a change of pace from busy office practice.[15,21,26] Recreational benefits, such as combining a vacation with CME, socializing with other physicians, or returning to academic medicine have also been reported.[15,23,24,26] Physicians indicated financial gain as the least important reason for attending CME.[15]

## Obstacles to Participation

The decision to participate is predetermined to a large degree by the number of commitments related to work, family, and the community.[28] In general, occupational responsibilities are the greatest obstacle to participation in continuing education; family and community responsibilities appear to be less important.[29]

The most common obstacle to participation reported in the literature is related to constraints of practice. Many physicians report that a heavy patient load prevents more widespread participation in continuing education activities.[5,21,25,30-36] Because most CME activities are scheduled during the week, there are conflicts with patient care responsibilities. Many physicians reported difficulties in arranging coverage. If a physician feels that time can be taken off from seeing patients, enrolling in a CME activity is possible. Practice arrangements may contribute significantly to the ability of an individual physician to participate. Other obstacles reported by physicians have included conflicts with family and community responsibilities,[25,30,31,36] cost (including travel and tuition cost), as well as loss of patient income.[5,30,36] Kotre and colleagues,[33] however, found that cost was not a major hindrance in attending a formal CME activity.

## Facilitators of Attendance

Two major factors facilitate physician attendance in CME activities—opportunities and positive attitudes toward CME. While a majority of physicians surveyed indicated that there were formal CME activities within a reasonable traveling distance,[10] problems of access to a regular comprehensive CME program is a problem, particularly in rural areas. Physicians in one state suggested that attendance would increase if relevant CME programs occurred within a 50-mile radius.[23]

Although formal continuing education activities may be available, an individual decision to participate is affected by the perception of the effectiveness of education generally and of a specific continuing education activity in particular.[37] Kristofco and colleagues[23] reported that physicians relied on the information contained in program brochures to help them judge the worth of a formal CME activity.

Physicians have reported that they considered CME a valuable experience and have developed a positive attitude toward participation.[26,38] In a well-designed study, Rothenberg and colleagues[5] concluded that physicians regarded attending formal CME activities as very useful and that all physicians spent several days and often as much as 2 weeks each year attending such events.  Mann and colleagues[12] reported that the physicians in their study regarded formal continuing education opportunities available to them as good, but that medical school programming was, in most cases, better than hospital-based programming.  Several studies[9,39] have shown that physicians consider professional society meetings to be the best formal CME experience. In another survey,[8] physicians reported that they preferred hospital-based CME programming for information about routine care, but medical school and specialty society CME programming for knowledge about the management of exceptional patients.

# A Model Describing Decision-making to Attend Formal CME Activities

There is a common-sense notion here, supported by the literature—the decision to attend formal CME activities is a complex process in which many variables interact. Figure 11.1 depicts this process by combining a synthesis of the research on physician participation in formal CME and adapting Cross's model[40] describing participation in general adult education.

The process depicted follows an algorithm conceptualizing the decision-making process physicians use when considering participating in formal CME activities. The decision of an individual to attend continuing education activities is the result of an awareness of need that emerges from discrepancies in the practice setting.[41] Professionalism appears to be the driving force behind the recognition of such discrepancies.  Allington and Kouzekanani[42] reported that the physicians in their study used a variety of approaches to identify discrepancies in their practice, or educational needs.  Fox and Harvill[43] reported that, if physicians decide this need is great enough, they will consider attending continuing education activities as a way to meet that need.  If a positive attitude toward formal continuing education exists, it is likely that participation in a formal continuing education activity would be considered.  Finally, individual decisions to participate in an educational activity relate to expectations about achieving specific educational goals as well as to opportunities and obstacles.  Decisions to participate appear to be influenced by perceptions of beneficial educational, regulatory, and social outcomes.  Factors related to opportunity such as timing, applicable topics, reputation of faculty, size of community, practice arrangements, and location as well as attitude toward CME, appear to be important.  Obstacles to participation include costs to participation and the constraints of practice.

## Figure 11.1

## Attendance at formal CME activities
### Outline of physician decision making

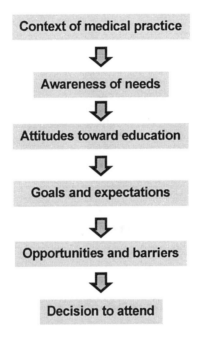

Nakamoto and Verner[30] reported that, once the decision is made to participate in a formal CME activity, the most powerful consideration in determining which formal continuing education activity to attend was subject matter, followed by well-known speakers and conference location.  Other important considerations included length of the course (most physicians preferred short courses of 1 to 3 days), varied formats (lectures, group discussions, and "hands-on" experiences), and sponsor (the most popular sponsor in this study was the state medical society; medical school CME was considered too academic). Registration fees do not appear to be a major barrier.  Allington and Kouzekanani[42] reported that physicians ranked considerations for selecting a formal CME activity in the following descending order—topics, location, dates, objectives, faculty, recreational opportunity, sponsoring organization, and fee.

The model has some shortcomings.  It has not been tested.  And, because it is derived from a synthesis of the literature, it reflects the weaknesses of the methodologies employed by researchers. Specifically, findings from these studies suffer from a number of design problems that make comparison among them, and generalization to all physicians, difficult.  For example, samples in these studies were restricted to single CME activities.  In addition, sampling was most often not randomized and, in many cases, response rates were low.  Further, the issues examined varied from study to study, and there was little attempt to replicate, synthesize, or test the results of previous studies.

There is another factor that complicates the development of a model for participation in formal CME. Findings from research on participation in general adult education (such as the model developed by Cross[40]) may not be directly transferable to CME.[19] Some considerations in studying participation of professionals differ from adult education studies in general. For example, level of education appears to act as a constant for professionals, but it is the strongest predictor in adult education studies. In addition, occupational status shows little variability in studying the participation of professionals. It may be that because participation in CME is so much a part of the professional way of life of physicians, the decision is not so much *whether* to participate, but *where* and *how* to participate. In a Canadian context, Lockyer and associates,[44] however, reported that certification status with a specialty society has predicted attendance by family physicians at local CME courses.

Finally, and probably most important, many of the studies reported in the CME literature focused only on participation in traditional, formal CME activities. Recent research suggests, however, that CME is a much broader enterprise than formal conferences and symposia, and that participation is more complex than simply enrolling in a course.

# Formal CME and Physician Information Seeking

Because attendance at formal CME activities forms part of a broader search for information related directly to problems or opportunities for improvement in clinical practice, this searching process includes not only participation in formal conferences, but reading, consulting with peers and experts, and other forms of self-directed learning.[42,45-49]

## Physician Information Seeking

Information-seeking strategies are initiated by physicians to deal with uncertainty in the clinical encounter. Patients present to physicians with a variety of health care problems which, combined with patient characteristics, may create uncertainty. On the other hand, physicians bring to clinical encounters their own experiences and characteristics which shape their reactions to the uncertainties and variables that emerge during the encounter.[50]

In a study of six professional groups, Schön[51] reported his observations of reactions of these professionals to situations of uncertainty and ambiguity. He described the characteristic mode of professional practice, which he called "knowing-in-action" or "tacit knowing," as actions, recognitions, and judgments which professionals know intuitively how to carry out. This tacit knowing is stored in frames. When intuitive performance yields the results expected (ie, the professional encounter fits the frame), professionals tend not to be conscious of the process.  However, when intuitive performance leads to surprises (where the frames do not fit as expected), professionals may respond by "reflecting-in-practice," and developing a response to the uncertainty caused by the lack of fit.  When the situation is outside the range of ordinary expectations, and when the professional is unable to use another similar frame, a new frame may be constructed and a "frame experiment" may be conducted.  In many cases, the new frame can be constructed and the experiment conducted on the basis of experience and previous understandings.  In other cases, however, the professional seeks information to help design and/or implement a new frame.  This model is explored in some detail in chapter 6.

In a recent study, Gerrity et al[52] suggested that an important component of physician reaction to uncertainty appeared to be stress.  While the authors caution that the relationship between stress and performance of a task is complex, they suggest that stress related to uncertainty may influence physicians to pursue behavior that will reduce the stress.  Havelock[53] described a similar phenomenon called "need reduction" behavior.  In this case, individuals who felt "uncomfortable" about lack of information sought that information from a variety of sources.

Means[54] applied a variant of the need reduction model to the information-seeking behavior of family physicians in Michigan.  He found that the strongest factor initiating information seeking was cognitive dissonance (ie, anxiety felt by the physician due to a current deficiency in understanding).  To reduce that anxiety, these family physicians used a combination of sources that included print material (such as journals and texts), interaction with colleagues, non-print materials (such as audiotapes and telephone access services), and formal CME activities.  These sources appeared to be used in sequence, starting with texts, and then journals and conversations with colleagues.  Formal CME activities usually came last in the sequence.  The findings of recent studies have challenged elements of this sequence, suggesting that physicians currently place less emphasis on reading materials[55] and more emphasis on collegial communications within a medical community.[56]  Covell and associates[57] also concluded that physicians were more likely to seek information from colleagues than from journals or other written materials.  Gruppen[2] has suggested that physicians seek out other physicians because they provide timely advice targeted to the particular problem they were confronting without having to search out and synthesize a mass of information for themselves.

In a report describing how physicians change their practice behavior, Geertsma and his colleagues[58] also identified an initial stage of discomfort that they called *priming.*  In this stage, physicians experienced dissatisfaction with some aspect of practice behavior, which appeared to operate as a catalyst for a search for information to improve that behavior.  While a wide variety of information sources were identified by physicians who participated in the study, in most cases, journals and interactions with colleagues were the most common sources of information to effect a change in practice behavior.  Formal CME activities were used more *after* a change was made, perhaps for reinforcement.  Lockyer and colleagues[59] also reported that physicians used multiple sources of information when making a change in practice behavior.

Fox and colleagues[45] demonstrated support for the notion that learning is driven more by some form of internal comparison of present and projected states than by any other motivations. Fox and Harvill[43] reported, however, that if physicians conclude this need is great enough, they will consider participation in continuing education activities as a way to reduce that need. These studies suggest that a discrepancy between actual and expected outcomes in the clinical setting serves as the catalyst for physician information seeking. Some of these studies also suggest that physicians seek information in a wide variety of formats from a number of sources. Finally, while it is not clear how large a discrepancy is necessary before a search for information is started, nor how large that discrepancy is before formal rather than informal sources are used,[41] it does appear that a positive attitude toward formal continuing education will likely lead to a consideration of participation in such activities.[29]

## The Place of Formal CME in the Information-seeking Process

Putnam and Campbell[60] reported that physicians they studied sought information from a number of sources—journals, formal CME courses, and colleagues. They also reported that the information-seeking strategies of these physicians were driven by a desire to change, caused by the presence of an innovation and/or a growing dissatisfaction with the results of currently used methods of providing care. The physicians in the study went through three phases of information seeking to make these changes—preparing to change, making the change, and solidifying the change. Stages described by Geertsma et al[58] parallel the first two phases.

Further, Putnam and Campbell[60] reported that the physicians in their study selected different sources for information in each of the three phases of change. Participation in a formally organized CME activity was the most frequent way these physicians prepared to change, although reading journals and discussing issues with colleagues were almost as important in the first phase. A considerable number of those who sought information from other physicians did so from recognized experts in the field. In the "making-the-change" phase, the most popular source of information was colleagues. Although used less extensively than in the preparation phase, formal CME programs were also an important resource. Unlike the other two phases, a greater proportion of physicians relied on their peers or colleagues as information sources when solidifying the change. Formally organized CME activities continued to be an important information source, but local CME activities played a larger role in this phase. After declining in importance as an information source in the second phase, journals were used more frequently for solidifying new clinical practices. In a study of physicians attending a formal CME course, Gruppen and colleagues[1,61] found that, in the early stages of information seeking for a challenging problem, textbooks or journals were used first, followed by consultation with colleagues and specialists. Northrup and colleagues[62] reported similar findings.

The work reported by Putnam and Campbell[60] is an elaboration of research done by Greer.[56] Greer found that change occurs in a medical community only after consensus is reached within it. This consensus is usually achieved after considerable exchange of information occurs among physicians, their peers, and local experts in such settings as corridor conversations and the doctors' lounge. Physicians in the Putnam and Campbell study reported that their colleagues were important sources of information, particularly in the latter two phases of change in which refinement and reinforcement (consensus) took place. In addition, Putnam and Campbell demonstrated the applicability of the adopter or diffusion categories identified by Rogers[63] in the literature related to the adoption of innovation, more fully discussed in chapter 2. Some of the physicians in the Putnam and Campbell study initially sought information from experts, perhaps "innovators" or early adopters in the community. In later phases of change, discussion may have taken place among "early adopters." Other studies have also suggested the applicability of the diffusion model to physician learning and changing.[64] Extensive work at the University of Michigan, for example, has identified the "educational influential" or opinion leader as a key actor in the dissemination of information to the medical community.[65,66]

# New Directions in Research on Participation in CME

There are three important conceptual areas that shape the future formulation, discussion, and examination of issues related to physician participation in formal CME. The three areas include an expanded definition of participation, a broadened definition of CME, and the recognition that participation is a complex, transactional phenomenon.

## Expanded Definition of Participation

There are two parts of an expanded definition of participation. First, the concept of participation should include the notions of initial enrollment, persistence, and application as defined by Knox.[37] Initial enrollment includes learning about potential educational opportunities and decisions about becoming involved. Persistence occurs when a learner continues his or her involvement until the reasons for enrolling are accomplished. Application is the integration of new information and capabilities into the learner's knowledge base and behavior. This conceptual framework expands research concerns about participation beyond concentration on issues related to initial enrollment, to issues related more to educational and patient care outcomes.

Second, recent research suggests that the important question to examine has not been "attendance at formal CME programs" but "physician participation in CME." The study reported by Fox et al[45] indicated that physician participation in CME was a multidimensional phenomenon affected by a wide variety of external influences and by internal motivation.  Attendance at formal CME activities is part of a broader search for information; this broader search for information is related directly to the clinical reasoning process (ie, the practice of clinical medicine).  The search includes not only participation in formal conferences, but reading, consulting with peers and experts, and other forms of self-directed learning.  More meaningful research on physician participation in CME will result from a broader definition of CME.

## Broadly Defined CME

CME is broader than formal CME conferences or large group sessions. Goldfinger's letter[67] in the *New England Journal of Medicine* described learning by "contamination" as a response to the study published by Sibley and colleagues,[68] which criticized the impact of episodic, formal CME.  This letter underscored the fact that the CME of any physician is a dynamic interaction of multiple information-gathering strategies, both formal and informal, structured and unstructured.  The evidence for the multiplicity of these strategies is considerable.  Means[54] reported that family physicians in Michigan used a combination of print sources, colleagues, formal CME activities, and nonprint media to obtain information to address practice-related concerns.  The study by Rothenberg and colleagues[5] provided important evidence that physicians use a wide variety of CME activities to obtain the information they need to improve performance.  Manning and DeBakey[46] interviewed selected physicians and also confirmed that physicians employed a wide range of information-seeking strategies to answer questions in practice.  In addition to the fundamental strategies of reading and consulting, they reported examples of  discussions with peers and mentors, practice audits, teaching, writing, and computers as ways by which physicians obtained information.  Fox et al[45] suggested that there were important interactions among all these activities.  Therefore, any meaningful examination of participation must consider activities included in a broader definition of CME.

The relationships among the components of a broader definition of CME have become more complicated. Recent studies have provided evidence that physicians have expressed disenchantment with reading journals,[55] once considered the mainstay of physician self-directed learning.[5,69,70] A study by Greer[56] suggested that interaction among peers in local medical communities may be a more important mode of CME than previously thought.  Laxdal and colleagues[71] obtained similar results.  Owen and colleagues[72] reported that British general practitioners found collegial interaction to be the most valuable source of CME.

There are differences in information-seeking strategies among physicians.  Gruppen and colleagues[1,61] suggested that the strategies physicians used varied with both the setting and the content of the problem.  Curry[73] reported that different specialties preferred different information-seeking strategies. In her study, family physicians preferred refresher courses and hospital-based conferences while specialists chose reading journals and attending national conventions.  There is also increasing evidence that the selection of one CME format rather than another might also be related to the learning styles of individual physicians.[74] Some physicians may prefer formal CME activities while others prefer reading journals or consultation with colleagues.

## Participation as a Complex-Transactional Phenomenon

Findings from previous research on participation suggest that the decision to participate in formal CME was the result of a complex interaction of internal and external forces. Knox[37] suggested that these forces emerge from three sources—the participant (internal), the CME provider (external), and the societal context within which both exist. Internal influences emerge from professionalism and other factors, and often include a desire to improve or a concern about performance in a specific area of practice. External influences derive from the environment of medical practice and may include technological change or a shift in patient mix. Any examination of physician participation must consider issues related to these three sources of influence.

## A Modified Participation Model

Figure 11.2 depicts a proposed model describing physician decision-making regarding participation in CME. The revised model extends the model in Figure 11.1 by reflecting the complexities of multiple influences, considering an expanded definition of participation beyond attendance, and including decisions about different forms of CME arising from a consideration of a broader definition of CME.

The process that is depicted in Figure 11.2 shows that the decision of an individual physician to participate in continuing education activities is the result of the interaction of a complex array of internal and external influences.[14,28,37,45,60] Internal influences emerge from professionalism and could include a desire to improve or a concern about performance in a specific area of practice. Some external influences emerge from the environment of medical practice and could include technological change or a change in patient mix. Other external influences emerge from CME providers whose promotional materials describe CME opportunities. These influences create an awareness of need. Fox and Harvill[43] reported that if physicians conclude that this need is great enough, they will consider participation in continuing education activities as a way to reduce that need.

Awareness of a need is the first step in defining a change in practice behavior. Several studies have demonstrated that change in practice behavior occurs in three phases and that a different format of CME is used predominantly in each phase. The revised model reflects these findings by including "phase of change" and "CME formats" in the algorithm.

As in the initial model, positive attitudes toward a particular CME format will likely lead to participation in that format. Individual decisions to participate in an educational activity relate to expectations about achieving specific educational goals (eg, improved patient care) as well as to opportunities and obstacles. Decisions to participate appear to be influenced by perceptions of beneficial educational, regulatory, and social outcomes. Factors related to opportunity such as timing, applicable topics, reputable faculty, size of community, and practice arrangements and location as well as attitude toward CME appear to be positively related. Obstacles to participation appear to be related to constraints of practice and cost.

The findings reported by Nakamoto and Verner[30] in their study of attendance at formal CME activities require reexamination in light of changes to the algorithm reflected in Figure 11.2. While subject matter may continue to be the most power-

## Figure 11.2

## Participation in CME activities
### Outline of physician decision making

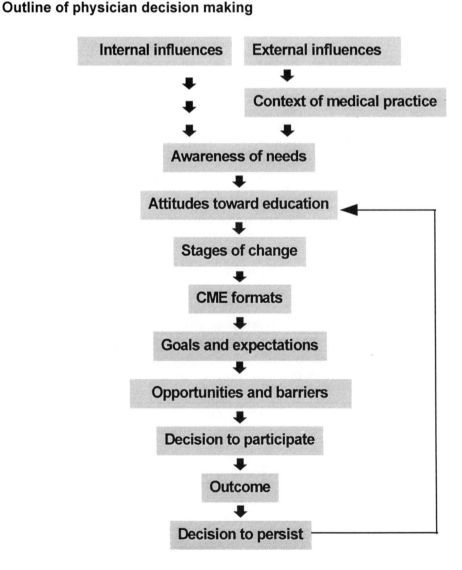

ful consideration, other considerations (such as well-known speakers, location, and length of the activity) may not be as relevant to other CME formats.

Finally, consideration of an expanded definition of participation is incorporated into Figure 11.2. This broadened definition assumes importance if the suggestion that initial enrollment is the beginning of a multi-phase practice change process is true. According to Knox,[37] physicians will continue participating in CME activities throughout the change process if their expectations of educational and patient care outcomes (application) are accomplished.

# Research Questions and Directions

Early research in the area of CME participation focused on marketing issues related to attendance at formal CME activities. More recent research focuses on participation in formal CME as part of a continuum of information-seeking strategies related to specific problems in practice. While the need remains to continue basic market research, new broader, and more powerful, research questions can be formulated on the basis of this proposed model, leading to increased understanding of physician participation.

It is important to formulate these questions in the terms of issues important to potential users of the findings of research studies. There are three audiences for the results of research on CME participation—physician participants, CME providers, and the organizations and individuals in the societal context of CME and health care. Physicians might find information about how all the parts of CME fit together useful in their decision-making regarding what kind of CME format or activity will best meet their specific, practice-related educational needs. CME providers might find research information about physician participation in various CME formats useful in their efforts to attract and retain physician participants as well as to develop and offer other program and learning support functions. Information about how all the parts of CME fit together may inform health policy makers about the positive relationship between CME and physician performance and health outcomes. Questions related to each of these areas are explored in the following section.

## Issues Related to Physician Participants

(1) How do exemplary physicians move from recognition of educational need to participation in CME activities?

(2) How do exemplary physicians sequence and select various types of CME activities?

(3) What is the relationship between participation in informal and formal CME activities?

(4)  It is increasingly recognized that physicians make changes in their practice behaviors to make the transition from "novice" to "expert" physician. How does a physician make decisions about participating in CME to support this transition?

(5)  What expectations do physicians have regarding outcomes or benefits of participation in various CME activities?

(6)  How does the diffusion-adoption model apply to physician decision-making participation in CME events or engaging in other learning activities?

(7)  How does an educational influential effect change in practice sites? How does a practicing physician "use" such an individual, if at all? What is the role of such individuals in promoting participation in formal and other activities?

(8)  Is there a model for decision-making related to purchasing a commercial product that would shed light on physician decision-making about participating in CME?

(9)  How consciously does a physician perform personal needs assessment? Are educational needs carefully identified? Is the process implicit or explicit? How aware are physicians of their "real" educational needs? Is the decision-making process to participate in CME more intuitive than systematic?

(10) What is the relationship between the learning style of an individual physician and his or her decision to participate in a particular form of CME?

(11) What is the relationship between specialty and participation in CME?

(12) How is the decision to participate in CME activities linked to questions of location and method?

(13) Does participation in "local CME" facilitate or inhibit participation in formal conferences elsewhere?

(14) Does physician participation in CME satisfy the purpose for participation, ie, does participation meet physician needs and expectations? What are the expectations for participation?

(15) Is there evidence that supports the belief that physicians prefer CME programs that are "practical" and relevant to their practice over those of a more academic nature?

(16) How do the experiences of physicians in medical school influence how they learn in practice? Does a certain kind of medical school

experience facilitate or hinder accepting new ways of learning?

(17) Do physicians use different information-seeking strategies for routine and difficult patient problems? Does the content of the information to be obtained influence the selection of an information-seeking strategy?

(18) How do educational, regulatory, and social purposes for participation interact?

## Issues Related to the CME Provider

(1)  It is increasingly recognized that most, if not all, physicians make the transition from "novice" to "expert." How does a CME provider design CME to help physicians make this transition? How will this redesign influence physician participation?

(2)  Is the relationship between formal and informal CME changing? What are the implications for providers of formal CME?

(3)  Using a marketing segmentation approach, what variables or groups of variables are most useful in predicting participation patterns? What is the interaction among these variables?

- *needs/interests*
- *specialty*
- *practice setting*
- *year of graduation*
- *program characteristics*
- *how information about the activity is obtained*

- *available opportunities*
- *stage of practice*
- *medical school attended*
- *frequency of local attendance*
- *faculty/speakers*
- *sponsors*
- *attitude toward education*

(4)  How does educational quality and program design influence decision-making to participate? How do physicians define educational quality? What are important features of educational quality? Some features include: educational process, methods, and technology; program "white space" (opportunity for interaction with colleagues); prerequisites/preparation for application; and perceived transferability. Are there others? What are their interactions?

(5)  Does CME provider decision-making take into account the interaction of an organized body of knowledge with participant experience and action? Do the learners know what they don't know? Do providers take this deficiency into account?

(6)  Does actual and/or potential collaboration among CME providers influence physician decision-making about participation?

## Issues Related to the Societal Context of Health Care

(1)  How does the practice setting impact on participation?  There are three subsets of this question:

- *What impact will the current trends toward blending work and learning, as evidenced by the adoption of continuous quality improvement approaches in health care, have on physician participation in CME?*

- *What is the relationship between physician participation in CME and organizational and system learning in hospital and practice settings?*

- *What are the implications for the CME enterprise of the increase in the corporate nature of medicine?  Will CME be prescribed to match a corporate-determined physician role?*

(2)  What impact do health care reform and evolving practice arrangements have on CME participation patterns?

## General Issues

(1)  How will the potential conflict of expectations for CME participation among potential physician participants, CME providers, and policy makers affect participation?  A relevant and researchable question relates to mandatory continuing education.  While this policy has resulted in increased enrollments in CME courses in which it has been implemented, its impact on persistence and application issues are not clear.

(2)  How do the underlying organizational and funding arrangements for CME prevent CME providers from changing to meet the needs and expectations of participation? What is the role for CME providers when participation is considered more broadly?

(3)  Do cultural values such as individualism and equity have an impact on participation?

In summary, physician participation in CME is a more complicated phenomenon than previous efforts in marketing style research on attendance have suggested. Recent studies have shown that the decisions of individual physicians to participate in formal CME activities are part of an ongoing search for information that includes a variety of other CME formats.  This search for information is typically undertaken to accomplish change in practice behaviors, and to improve patient outcomes. Practice change occurs in three phases, and it appears that different CME formats are selected in each.  Formal CME activities appear to be more popular when physicians initiate change and as sources of reinforcement after the practice change has been accomplished.

The research questions posed here reflect some of the multidimensionality of physician participation in CME and other learning opportunities. Findings from research projects that investigate these questions will enhance understanding of physician decision-making about participation. This improved understanding should help individuals who plan and organize formal CME programs improve their offerings, effectiveness, and ability to attract and hold participants and information-getting behaviors. And, as physicians perceive increased benefits from participation in these improved CME activities, it is anticipated that physician participation will increase.

## References

1. Gruppen LD, Wolf FM, VanVoorhees C, Stross JK. Information seeking strategies and differences among primary care physicians. *Mobius.* 1987;7:18-26.

2. Gruppen LD. Physician information seeking: improving relevance through research. *Bull Med Libr Assoc.* 1990;78:165-172.

3. Bennett NL, Hotvedt MO. Stage of career. In: Fox RD, Mazmanian PE, Putnam RW, eds. *Changing and Learning in the Lives of Physicians.* New York, NY: Praeger Publishers; 1989:65-78.

4. Savatsky PD, Haitz MC, Stearns NS. Patterns of continuing medical education: a generation unit analysis of physicians in three community hospitals. *Soc Sci Med.* 1981;15A:665-672.

5. Rothenberg E, Wolk M, Scheidt S, Schwartz M, Aarons B, Pierson RN Jr. Continuing medical education activities in New York County: physician attitudes and practices. *J Med Educ.* 1982;57:541-549.

6. Richards RK, Cohen RM. *The Value and Limitations of Physician Participation in Traditional Forms of Continuing Medical Education.* Part 1. Kalamazoo, Mich: The Upjohn Company; 1981.

7. Richards RK, Cohen RM. *The Value and Limitations of Physician Participation in Traditional Forms of Continuing Medical Education:* Part 2. Kalamazoo, Mich: The Upjohn Company; 1983.

8. Mason JL, Kappelman MM, Hornung CA, Massagli MP. *Continuing Medical Education: Utilization and Preferences of Primary Care Physicians.* Baltimore, Md: University of Maryland School of Medicine; 1979.

9. Kotre JN, Mann FC, Vanselow NA. The Michigan physician: his use and evaluation of the professional meeting and postgraduate course. *Mich Med.* 1971;70:111-117.

10. Richards RK, Cohen RM. Why physicians attend traditional continuing medical education programs. *J Med Educ.* 1980;55:479-485.

11. Cervero RM. A factor analytic study of physicians' reasons for participating in continuing education. *J Med Educ.* 1981;56:29-34.

12. Mann FC, Kotre J, Reilly A, Vanselow NA. The Michigan physician and his continuing education. *Mich Med.* 1970;69:981-990.

13. Kotre JN, Mann FC, Vanselow, NA. The Michigan physician and his continuing education: summary and conclusion. *Mich Med.* 1971;70:525-529.

14. Cordes DL. Relationship of motivation to learning. In: Green JS, Suter E, Grosswald SJ, Walthall DB, eds. *Continuing Education for the Health Professions.* San Francisco, Calif: Jossey-Bass Publishers; 1984:52-71.

15. Wolf FM, Gruppen LD, VanVoorhees C, Stross JK.  Dimensions of motivation for continuing medical education of primary care physicians. *Eval Health Prof.* 1986;9:305-316.

16. Schein E. *Professional Education.* New York, NY: McGraw Hill; 1973.

17. Ramsey PG, Carline JD, Inui TS, et al.  Change over time in the knowledge base of practicing internists. *JAMA.* 1991;266:1103-1107.

18. Mann FC, Kotre J, Reilly A, Vanselow NA.  The Michigan physician: his work needs and opportunities. *Mich Med.* 1970;69:1063-1070.

19. Grotelueschen A, Kenny WR, Harnisch DL. *Research on Reasons for Participation in Continuing Professional Education: A Statement of Position and Rationale.* Champaign, Ill: University of Illinois, College of Education; 1980.

20. Duff WM, Cheung MC.  Long-term evaluation of CME. *Contin Med Ed News.* 1979;22:6.

21. DeNio JN, Neth RL, Rising JD.  Continuing medical education: survey of physicians' opinions. *J Kans Med Soc.* 1976;77:109-113.

22. Naftulin DH, Ware JE Jr, Myers VH. Results of a Southwestern study. *Arch Gen Psychiatry.* 1967;24:260-264.

23. Kristofco RE, Hall SA, Chick E.  CME preferences, practices of West Virginia physicians. *West Virg Med J.* 1987;83:223-225.

24. Rising JD, Neth RL. An evaluation of the Kansas Circuit Course for physicians.  *J Kans Med Soc.* 1977;78:129-130.

25. Dohner CW, Hamberg RL.  The CME short course. *Northwest Med.* 1970;69:327-330.

26. Fahs IJ, Miller WR. *Patterns of Continuing Education: Minnesota Physicians.*  St Paul, Minn: Northlands Regional Medical Program; 1968.

27. Stross JK, Harlan WR.  The impact of mandatory continuing medical education. *JAMA.* 1978;239:2663-2666.

28. Knox AB. *Adult Development and Learning.* San Francisco, Calif: Jossey-Bass Publishers; 1977.

29. Miller HF. *Participation of Adults in Education: A Force Field Analysis.* Syracuse, NY: Center for the Study of Liberal Education for Adults; 1967.

30. Nakamoto J, Verner C. *Continuing Education in Medicine.* Vancouver, Canada: University of British Columbia; 1972.

31. Caplan RM, Yarcheski T. Survey of continuing medical education in Iowa. *J Iowa Med Soc.* 1973;64:159-164.

32. Lemon FR.  Continuing education: practices and attitudes of Kentucky physicians:1972. *J Ky Med Assoc.* 1973;71:221-227.

33. Kotre JN, Mann FC, Vanselow N. The Michigan physician and continuing education: looking to the future. *Mich Med.* 1971;70:397-401.

34. Castle CH, Storey PB. Physicians' needs and interests in continuing medical education. *JAMA.* 1966;206:611-614.

35. Peterson O, Andrews LP, Spain RS, Greenberg BG. Analytical study of North Carolina general practice, 1953-1954. *J Med Educ.* 1956;31:1-165.

36. Vollan DD. *Postgraduate Medical Education in the United States.* Chicago, Ill: American Medical Association; 1955.

37. Knox AB. Influences on participation in continuing education. *J Cont Educ Health Prof.* 1990;10:261-274.

38. Bloom B, Hauck WW Jr, Peterson OL, Nickerson RJ, Colton  T. Surgeons in the United States: opinions on current issues related to surgical practice. *Surgery.* 1977;82:635-642.

39. Ferguson KJ, Caplan RM. Physicians' preferred learning methods and sources of information. *Mobius.* 1987;1:1-9.

40. Cross KP. *Adults as Leaners: Increasing Participation and Facilitating Learning.* San Francisco, Calif: Jossey-Bass Publishing; 1981.

41. Fox RD. Discrepancy analysis in continuing medical education: a conceptual model. *Mobius.* 1983;3:37-44.

42. Allington GH, Kouzekanani K. Factors contributing to physicians' selection and participation at continuing medical education activities. *J Cont Educ Health Prof.* 1988;8:7-12.

43. Fox RD, Harvill RM. Self-assessments of need, relevance, and motivation to learn as indicators of participation in continuing medical education. *Med Educ.* 1984;18:275-281.

44. Lockyer J, Jennett P, Parboosingh J, McDougall G, Bryan G. Family physician registration at locally produced courses. *Can Med Assoc J.* 1988;139:1153-1155.

45. Fox RD, Mazmanian PE, Putnam RW. *Changing and Learning in the Lives of Physicians.* New York, NY: Praeger Publishers; 1989.

46. Manning PR, DeBakey L. *Medicine: Preserving the Passion.* New York, NY: Springer-Verlag; 1988.

47. Manning PR, Denson TA. How physicians learned about cimetidine. *Ann Intern Med.* 1980;92:690-692.

48. Manning PR, Denson TA. How cardiologists learn about echocardiography. *Ann Intern Med.* 1979;91:469-471.

49. Stross JK. Information sources and clinical decisions. *J Gen Intern Med.* 1987;2:155-159.

50. Eisenberg JM. Sociological influences on decision-making by clinicians. *Ann Intern Med.* 1979;90:957-964.

51. Schön DA. *The Reflective Practitioner.* New York, NY: Basic Books; 1983.

52. Gerrity MS, DeVellis RF, Earp JA. Physicians' reactions to uncertainty in patient care: a new measure and new insights. *Med Care.* 1990;28:724-736.

53. Havelock RG. *Planning for Innovation through the Dissemination and Utilization of Information.* Ann Arbor, Mich: University of Michigan Institute for Social Research; 1969.

54. Means RF. How family physicians use information sources: implications for new approaches. In: Green JS, Suter E, Grosswald SJ, Walthall DB, eds. *Continuing Education in the Health Professions.* San Francisco, Calif: Jossey-Bass Publishers; 1984:72-86.

55. Williamson JW, German PS, Weiss R, Skinner EA, Bowes F. Health science information management and continuing education of physicians. *Ann Intern Med.* 1989;110:151-160.

56. Greer AL. The state of the art versus the state of the science: the diffusion of new medical technologies into practice. *Intl J Tech Assess Health Care.* 1988;4:5-26.

57. Covell DG, Uman GC, Manning PR. Information needs in office practice: are they being met? *Ann Intern Med.* 1985;103:596-599.

58. Geertsma RH, Parker RC Jr, Whitbourne SK. How physicians view the process of change in their practice behavior. *J Med Educ.* 1982;57:752-761.

59. Lockyer JM, Parboosingh JT, McDougall GM, Chugh U. How physicians integrate advances into clinical practices. *Mobius.* 1985;5:5-12.

60. Putnam RW, Campbell MD. Competence. In: Fox RD, Mazmanian PE, Putnam RW, eds. *Changing and Learning in the Lives of Physicians.* New York, NY: Praeger Publishers; 1989:79-97.

61. Gruppen LD, Wolf FM, VanVoorhees C, Stross JK. Information seeking strategies and treatment decision making. *Proc Conf Res Med Educ.* Washington, DC: Assoc Am Med Coll. 1987;26:203-208.

62. Northrup DE, Moore-West M, Skipper B, Teaf SR. Characteristics of clinical information searching: investigation using critical incident technique. *J Med Educ.* 1983;58:873-881.

63. Rogers EM. *Diffusion of Innovations.* New York, NY: The Free Press; 1983.

64. Coleman JS, Katz E, Menzel H. *Medical Innovation: A Diffusion Study.* New York, NY: Bobbs Merrill; 1966.

65. Hiss RG, MacDonald R, Davis WK. Identification of physician educational influentials (EIs) in small community hospitals. *Proc Ann Conf Res Med Educ.* Washington, DC: Assoc Am Med Coll. 1978;17:283-288.

66. Stross JK, Bole GG. Evaluation of a continuing education program on rheumatoid arthritis. *Arthritis Rheum.* 1980;23:846-849.

67. Goldfinger SE. Continuing medical education: the case for contamination. *N Engl J Med.* 1982;306:540-541.

68. Sibley JC, Sackett DL, Neufeld V, Gerrard B, Rudnick KV, Fraser W. A randomized trial of continuing medical education. *N Eng J Med.* 1982;306:511-515.

69. Curry L, Putnam RW. Continuing medical education in maritime Canada: the methods physicians use, would prefer, and find most effective. *Can Med Assoc J.* 1981;124:563-566.

70. Kotre JN, Mann FC, Morris WC, Vanselow NA. The Michigan physician's use and evaluation of his medical journal. *Mich Med.* 1971;70:11-16.

71. Laxdal OE, Jennett PA, Wilson TW, Salisbury GM. Improving physician performance by continuing medical education. *Can Med Assoc J.* 1978;118:1051-1058.

72. Owen PA, Allery LA, Harding KG, Hayes TM. General practitioners' continuing medical education within and outside their practice. *Br Med J.* 1989;299:238-240.

73. Curry L. Do family physicians differ from specialists? a particular case in continuing medical education patterns. *Can Fam Phys.* 1984;30:2405-2410.

74. VanVoorhees C, Wolf FM, Gruppen LD, Stross JK. Learning styles and continuing medical education. *J Cont Health Prof.* 1988;8:257-265.

**Chapter 12**

# The Effectiveness of CME Interventions

*David Davis*
*Elizabeth Lindsay*
*Paul Mazmanian*

# The Effectiveness of CME Interventions

*"In what is typically an intensive 2- or 3-day short course, [instructors lecture and lecture and lecture] fairly large groups of ...professional people who sit for long hours in an audiovisual twilight, making never-to-be-read notes at rows of narrow tables covered with green baize and appointed with fat binders and sweating pitchers of ice water."*[1]

Philip Nowlen, 1988

## Defining, Characterizing, and Evaluating CME

### The Nature of CME:  Formal or Informal Activities?

When asked for a definition of "CME," most physicians will describe a set of didactic learning activities designed for large groups of physicians, much as those reflected in the quote above.  Such "formal" CME activities are generally planned by principles established by the Accreditation Council for CME (ACCME),[2] follow from physician needs assessment, have stated objectives and evaluation measures, range from several hours to days in length, and are planned for large audiences of physicians using mostly didactic or lecture-centered presentations. Examples of such interventions are everywhere: rounds, conferences, symposia, refresher programs, courses, and other activities familiar to the practicing physician are all considered subsets of formal CME. They are so commonplace in fact, that "CME" has become synonymous with their presence.

This mind set about CME should not surprise the reader, given the presence of several coexisting factors. First, it may be the undergraduate experiences of most traditionally taught physicians that create the belief that such learning experiences are the nature of continuing education as well.  Second, medical schools, the first purveyors of CME, adapted this mode of information transfer to the field of CME, both in early outreach programs and, later, in conferences and courses.[3]  Third, the establishment of guidelines to monitor course quality by the ACCME has also contributed to the phenomenon of equating CME with formal activities: of 11 principles used to accredit providers of CME, the majority assess the production of short courses.[2] Fourth, current potent forces in mandatory CME, relicensure, and recertification encourage attendance at formal events and courses.

Despite this emphasis on traditional CME activity, CME, the way by which physicians learn, is most certainly broader than the CME refresher course, update, or conference.  A survey of Ontario physicians, although a decade old, remains typical of the pattern of physician participation in CME activities.[4]  The Ontario survey divided activities into: (a) those in which physicians were able to participate locally, within the community or practice setting; and (b) those of a more formal nature, often requiring travel. See Table 12.1.  Here, in order, reading journals, consulting with specialists, and other colleagues, using texts, attending rounds and receiving pharmaceutical or audiovisual materials were considered important local resources. Formal activities consisted primarily of formal, traditional CME programs, ranging from scientific sessions of professional associations, through hospital-organized CME events, to clinical traineeships.

Since the Ontario survey, several other CME methods have entered the literature of physician performance change. Documented in a recent review of the trials testing the effectiveness of CME[5] these include: opinion leaders or educational influentials; academic detail visits; chart review or recall with a peer or supervising mentor; computer-generated information; multiphasic, role-reinforcing maneuvers in workshops; and other, more complex methods detailed below. It is the objective of this chapter to pursue the questions of the nature of these interventions, their effectiveness, and implications for research in, and the practice of, CME.

**Table 12.1**

**Ontario Physicians' Participation in CME[4]**
**Percentage of Physicians Reporting:**

**(A) Informal, Local, Community-based CME Activity**

| Activity | % Reporting | Hrs/ Week |
|---|---|---|
| Reading journals | 98.8 | 3.2 |
| Informal consultings | 83.5 | 1.7 |
| Reading texts | 76.0 | 2.3 |
| Attending rounds | 72.9 | 1.7 |
| Using drug company materials | 42.5 | 0.6 |
| Using AV materials | 39.4 | 1.5 |

**(B) Attendance at Formal or Distant CME Programs**

| Activity | % Reporting | Hrs/yr |
|---|---|---|
| Scientific sessions of professional associations, societies, speciality groups | 71.0 | 44.9 |
| Local formal hospital events (rounds, clinic days, inservice) | 52.1 | 28.2 |
| Meetings of local medical societies | 44.6 | 16.8 |
| Medical school CME activities | 43.4 | 36.4 |
| Speakers programs organized by drug companies, other agencies | 41.3 | 16.4 |
| Clinical traineeships | 6.0 | 272.4 |

## Characterizing and Categorizing CME Interventions

Because these CME interventions or strategies are so varied, this chapter proposes to categorize CME and related maneuvers by their educational purpose. Since that purpose is to help physicians change what they know in a subject area and to ultimately change practices, Green's[6] classification of determinants of behavior change in health promotion assists the process of organizing the CME intervention literature. These determinants, derived from the PRECEDE framework, and modified for the purposes of this book, include: predisposing (focused on what physicians know, think, and can do); enabling (techniques which facilitate the desired change in the practice site); and reinforcing factors (reminders or feedback).

The majority of CME interventions fall within the "predisposing" category and are directed at knowledge, skills, or attitudinal changes within the physician learner. For the purposes of this chapter these are referred to as "primary" methods (see Table 12.2). These strategies most often include didactic, formal sessions, as well as printed materials and related information-searching techniques, audiovisual methods, and computer-assisted instruction. Primary interventions also include education directed at how to do something differently (ie, skills). While frequently skills are addressed only at an information-sharing level, educational interventions directed towards skill enhancement may include demonstration and practice of competencies. Finally, attitudes may be addressed by information-sharing methods which include simulations, role play, or other strategies.

The second cluster of methods are termed "secondary." They include CME interventions which provide dissemination methods, such as printed materials, linked to: enabling mechanisms such as algorithms or flow charts, patient educational materials, or methods; reinforcing strategies, which include computer-generated reminders, and feedback to physicians at the conclusion of learning activities; or combinations of the two approaches. It should be noted that this is a working definition only: while used extensively in the health promotion literature, the PRECEDE model has only recently been adapted for use in the categorization of CME interventions,[5] and requires further testing and refinement.

## Measuring Effectiveness

Over a period of several decades, the recognition of the importance of CME has been challenged by the question of its effects on physician competence and performance, and on their intended product, improved health care outcomes: in other words, does CME work? These effects, or inter-relationships, assume greater importance as the body of biomedical literature and as the CME "enterprise" grow, and as regulatory bodies consider more seriously the nature of competence and its relationship to CME. Thus there is considerable need for a careful, critical appraisal of the evidence for the impact of CME interventions. If health care practices based on the best available information are an ideal of clinicians, then, equally, delivery of CME, based on the best evidence about its efficacy, should also become an integral ingredient in CME provision. This chapter, based on the most recent evidence available on the nature and impact of CME, attempts to direct CME practitioners, researchers, and physicians toward that goal.

---

**Table 12.2**

**Primary and Secondary Interventions in Continuing Medical Education**

| Intervention | Synonyms, Examples |
|---|---|
| **Primary** | |
| • Formal CME | Didactic sessions<br>Courses<br>Conferences<br>Rounds |
| • Print materials | Newsletters<br>Bulletins<br>Texts, journals<br>Practice guidelines/clinical<br>   policies |
| • Audiovisual methods | Audiotapes<br>Videotapes<br>Videodiscs |
| • Academic detailing | Physician educator visits |
| • Computer-aided instruction | |
| **Secondary** | |
| • Enabling | Flow charts, algorithms<br>Patient education materials<br>Patient-specific information<br>Question in practice programs<br>Consultation |
| • Reinforcing | Reminders<br>Feedback |
| • Mixed or multipotential<br>methods | Opinion leaders/educational<br>   influentials<br>Chart review |

A basic step in answering questions regarding effectiveness is to identify an appropriate level of impact, given a particular educational intervention. CME literature
reviews assessing this impact are not a new phenomenon. Earlier reviews by
Bertram and Brooks-Bertram,[7] Lloyd and Abrahamson[8] and Stein,[9] focusing on
traditional or didactic aspects of CME, have been complemented by later, more
comprehensive reviews by Haynes and associates,[10] Beaudry,[11] McLaughlin and
Donaldson,[12] and Davis et al.[5] These latter analyses are more catholic in their
interpretation of the definition of CME, and reflect a growing understanding of its
nature and of the expanding body of literature relative to its effectiveness. Most of
these authors conclude that, while there is good evidence that formal CME activities
alter physicians' competence, there is less solid evidence for the translation of these
skills or knowledge into performance changes in the workplace, the office, or
hospital ward. Further, these reviews provide generally weak evidence for the
penetration of changes initiated by formal CME into health care or patient outcomes.

In discussing this literature, verification of the extent or nature of changes made by
physicians as a result of their participation in CME programming forms a significant
question. Dixon's[13] discussion of levels of impact assists this analysis. The most
basic level and most immediate impact is on attendance and perceptions about the
value of a program on the part of participants. The next level of impact includes
changes in physician competence, that is, knowledge skills and attitudes, measured
in the test environment. The third level includes measures related to physician
performance or behavior change in the practice setting. The final level or outcome
measure includes assessments of health care or patient outcomes.

Another significant question in assessing the impact of CME relates to the quality of
evidence about CME interventions. This chapter draws extensively on the literature
relevant to CME interventions, using the Research and Development Resource Base
in CME,[14] described in the Preface. These more general CME studies are of a variety
of designs, study outcomes, methods of descriptions of populations and interventions, and of variable quality, but are helpful in describing interventions and their
effects on the learner. Because the question of effectiveness of specific interventions is so important to this chapter, a subset of that literature is given special
attention. This subset comprises randomized, controlled trials (RCTs) which meet
criteria established by Haynes and colleagues[10] to analyze the effects of specific
interventions at either or both of Dixon's higher two levels of impact—physician
performance/behavior or health care outcomes. (See Table 12.3). A summary of
these trials is referenced throughout this chapter,[5] and is included in this section's
annotated bibliography. Together, the randomized controlled trial and more general
literature comprise the evidence to date about the impact of CME interventions,
methods, and strategies.

Table 12.3

Quantitative Criteria for Selection of Trials for Comparative Purposes (adapted from Haynes et al[10])

### 1) Study Design

Random allocation of individual physicians of functional units of health professionals (eg, wards or clinics) to experimental and control groups

### 2) Intervention

Replicable, complete descriptions of specific interventions (formal CME courses) designed to improve physician performance and/or alter patient outcomes

### 3) Subjects

Functional populations or groups of health professionals in which physicians formed at least 50% of those observed

### 4) Outcomes

The objective observation of physician performance or behavior and/or health care (patient) outcomes for at least 75% of participants in the study

### 5) Data analysis

Provision of sufficient data on which to perform statistical analyses

# The Evidence to Date

## Primary Interventions

### Formal learning activities

Despite the solid historical and functional place of traditional CME in the learning patterns of physicians, and the obvious popularity and belief in its efficacy, there are important questions about the effectiveness of such events or courses and about the ways in which they operate to alter physician competence or performance. There are a wide variety of studies of a descriptive or cohort-analytic and even controlled trial nature which illuminate various components of the effective formal CME intervention. This cluster of literature sources, by no means exhaustive, is nonetheless instructive.

### Needs assessment

The first set of studies pertains to needs assessment. In randomized controlled trials, workshops or small group learning experiences that incorporated knowledge testing and needs assessment strategies succeeded in improving physician performance.[15,16] In other trials, White,[17] Inui,[18] and Hillman[19] described the use of medical audits and questionnaires used to determined educational needs: these studies improved competence and performance of physicians (and, in one instance, patient outcomes). Similarly, the Self Evaluation Program of the College of Family Physicians of Canada was used as the basis for an effective program on rubella prevention[20] in British Columbia. In contrast, lectures in lipid control were ineffective in changing physician performance despite the use of chart audits as a needs determining tool,[21] stimulating questions about the role of belief about the efficacy of physician-directed cholesterol-reducing measures.

The question of subjective needs assessment is important, given the practice of most CME providers of using the perceptions of clinicians about important subjects or topic areas to plan CME events. Such a practice is acceptable by ACCME guidelines,[2] is practical, and assumes that physicians know what they need to know. But do they? Some authors have questioned the reliability of such assessments. Weinberg,[22] for example, developed a 4-hour course in cardiopulmonary resuscitation based on pre-course assessments of competence on the part of intended participants, both nurses and physicians. The correlation between actual and perceived levels of knowledge and skill were considerably different, but similar measurements after the course displayed a closer correlation between actual and perceived levels of competence, suggesting enhanced self-assessment ability as a result of course training. Innovative programs have been designed to assist physicians in the assessment of their competency. The OSCME, described by Craig,[23] is an example of such an intervention. Here, in the context of a standard refresher course for physicians, registrants passed through a number of clinical simulation "stations," each used to prompt physician self-assessment of learning needs.

Based on real clinical performance, two authors illustrated the use of chart audit as an effective pre-course means to determine learning objectives for CME interventions. For example, in long-term care, Elzarian[24] determined the need for a change in the use of bowel preparations. Jennett et al,[15] in the ambulatory care setting, used chart audit to assess family physicians' learning needs in cardiovascular disease and cancer care. Both confirm the effectiveness of programming based on such objectively determined needs, establishing a baseline for improvement in health care delivery.

### Instructional design

The next, perhaps largest, issue in considering the effectiveness of formal CME, and perhaps the largest, is related to the instructional design of such interventions. Many authors have described innovative ways in which the traditional lecture format may be augmented and the achievement of learning objectives may be enhanced. Perhaps the earliest documented use of learning aids was by McGuire[25] in 1964: a program on auscultatory skills was augmented by a cardiology sound-simulator, an effective tool when measured by physician self-reports, audit, and examination. A more sophisticated simulation of cardiac disease processes has been described by Gordon[26] in a large group CME setting. In more standard current use, CPR, ACLS, and ATLS courses exemplify the use of mannequins and other practice-simulations in an effective demonstration of skill improvement.[27,28]

The use of mannequins and other simulations to re-create real practice situations has prompted, in the CME setting, a debate over the efficacy of other means to simulate the clinical environment: the problem-based learning (PBL) approach. A major review of problem-based learning by Schmidt et al[29] confirms its theoretical advantages: activation of prior knowledge by PBL techniques facilitates the subsequent processing of new information; PBL enhances subsequent retrieval of knowledge; and matching the context of the PBL experience to that of practice enhances recall. Discussion of the effectiveness of this method, based on empiric evidence, has occurred across the continuum of medical education—in the undergraduate setting, prompted by the articulation of this concept by Barrows et al,[30] and, in CME, stimulated by his use of standardized patients in the neurology bedside clinic.[31]

Several studies of PBL in CME merit discussion. Over 20 years ago, Collett[32] found course satisfaction in a program which used lectures and case studies. Greenberg and Jewett[33] compared PBL and traditional formats, indicating an improvement in the PBL group in performance and knowledge gain over the didactic group. This study suffered from methodological problems, however, including nonrandomization to groups, and led to the development of a randomized controlled trial designed with a similar purpose. This last study[34] compared a large group didactic session; large group case discussion; and small group, PBL intervention in common family practice topics. Using practice-based, undetected standardized patients, the authors found no significant between-group differences, suggesting that the effectiveness of the small group PBL experience may be diluted by the 1-day format, inadequate potency of the intervention, unfocused discussion, or other problems related to the development of group cohesion, trust, and function.

Further teasing apart the question of the influence of small group learning versus large group activity, Rodney and Albers[35] reported greater early facility in sigmoidoscopy skills among small group participants, perhaps reflecting their increased participation. However, participants in the large group displayed greater rates of performing complex procedures, suggesting a different focus, content of discussion, or mix of patient problems encountered in the teaching sessions.

In addition to the literature relevant to PBL techniques, there exists a significant number of articles examining the use of instructional devices to augment or buttress learning in course participants. In nursing CE for example, Andrusyszyn compared short-term and long-term knowledge gain following lectures either augmented or not by audiovisuals, a common ingredient in virtually all CME programs.[36] While short-term outcomes were similar between groups, analysis revealed that the difference in scores between the post-test and longer term retention test was significantly lower for the non-augmented participants, indicating an influence of audiovisuals on post-course retention.

Other authors have employed innovative methods in the design of short courses: visits to clinical settings or practice sites such as occupational medicine facilities[37]; reading retreats[38]; computer-assisted instruction[39]; and, using family members of persons suffering from diseases which comprise the topic of CME courses in the context of a CME event.[40] Raising questions about altering physicians' motivation, Purkis[41] examined the use of the "commitment for change" instrument, an apparently effective tool in encouraging physicians to make a change in their practices relative to the content of the program attended. Finally, no studies were found comparing outcomes by varying the course duration.

While many of these maneuvers have been studied in before-after or qualitative studies, little evidence exists for the impact of these measures on either physician performance or health care outcomes in randomized controlled trials. What evidence there does exist in randomized controlled trials of workshops, or conferences, may be found in those interventions which were designed to assist physicians in patient education or health counseling, exemplifying instructional methods of apparent success in changing physician behavior. These studies[42-47] in pediatrics and smoking cessation used demonstration and role-playing, allowing the physician to "rehearse" new management strategies.

## Other primary interventions

In contrast to those activities which are considered "formal," and those elements integral to that activity, there are a host of other useful CME strategies. The following list of such interventions is not meant to be exhaustive, nor is the use of references in each subject area. Rather, the objective of the ensuing paragraphs is intended to furnish the reader with a sense of the wide variety of strategies encompassed by the phrase, "continuing medical education," and a sense, derived from the literature, of the effect of such interventions.

### Printed material, journals, reading

Perhaps second only to formal CME as an important learning method has been the use of journals and other mailed materials; these are ubiquitous, easily stored, and, with increasing ease, readily retrievable. Randomized, controlled trials have demonstrated little or no demonstrable effect on physician performance of mailed materials when used by themselves.[5] For example, the study of Evans et al[48] study of unsolicited mailed materials affected knowledge levels of physicians but did not alter the control of hypertension in their patients. However, in one randomized controlled trial, printed materials were as effective as chart review, feedback and patient information in altering prescribing practices[49]; and in a descriptive study, Harvey et al[50] showed a significant change in the appropriate prescribing of an antibiotic after the institution of a newsletter.

It is likely that print materials act as part of the educational "background noise," or among the many impactors on performance described in studies of physician performance change.[51] They do not appear to act independently. Journal reading, as a particular subset of the phenomenon of mailed materials, has been studied from the perspective of its influence on clinical decision making by Bergman and Pantell.[52] Here a before-after study revealed that, following reading a journal article relevant to a particular problem, physicians significantly increased their estimates of patients acquiring the disease entity described.

The problem of information overload, the degree to which physicians are besieged by a seemingly overwhelming volume of journals, has been pursued by Covell and colleagues[53] who discovered that only 30% of practitioner offices are set up in such a way that answers to clinical problems may be met during the patient visit. Further, Williamson et al determined that less than one in three physicians personally searched the literature, while the majority claimed that the volume of literature was unmanageable and applied no critical appraisal techniques to their reading of the literature.[54] At an even more basic level, a Scottish survey revealed that only 28% of physicians read the major family practice journal.[55]

Remedies to correct these problems have been the subject of several approaches. These include journal summaries or reviews, reported by Benseman and Barham[56] in New Zealand; strategies to screen and critically appraise articles[57-59]; organizing the literature into a readily retrievable home or office-based library; journal clubs[60]; and the burgeoning field of informatics, ie, computer-assisted searching in a problem-based format by electronic means.[61]

### Practice guidelines/clinical policies

Since the majority of practice guidelines are configured and distributed as printed materials, and since they possess few enabling or reinforcing attributes, they are considered as a primary intervention. As such, the evidence for their effectiveness in changing physician or patient outcomes by themselves is weak. For example, the dissemination of clinical policies or practice guidelines alone had no effect on repeat cesarean section rates.[62] In lipid lowering studies, guidelines needed extensive support from educational activities and quality assurance[63] to effect practice changes. Other studies have confirmed the general lack of effect of guidelines in infection control procedures[64] and mammography screening.[65]

A significant issue in the effectiveness of guidelines is the extent to which they are "owned" by the practicing physician, most often trained to be an autonomous and rational independent practitioner. Authors have indicated that physicians must set their own standards for practice in a sensible and flexible format[66,67]; and that planners must develop a specific adoption method.[68] Costanza et al[65] articulated three components of such a plan to enhance physician compliance with clinical policies: by improving physician attitudes about the benefits of the policy; by building on the medical community's consensus regarding the appropriateness and importance of the guidelines; and by targeting the poorest compliers with special messages or programs. In an example of such a strategy, the Royal College of Radiologists Working Party[69] induced changes in hospital referral practices by introducing clinical guidelines, enhanced by monitoring and peer review.

### Academic detailing persons

Soumerai and his colleagues have noted an increasing number of studies describing programs to improve physician prescribing behavior,[70] the result of the availability of powerful, new drugs and increasing interest in expanding cost-effective drug coverage in both public and private insurance programs. One example of an external influence on physicians' learning, perhaps to a greater extent than acknowledged, is the pharmaceutical representative. A study by Avorn et al[71] demonstrated that physicians' beliefs about the efficacy of drugs were derived more from advertisements and detail visits than from the scientific literature. Rovers,[72] however, indicated that many of the usual dissemination interventions are probably ineffective; a personal relationship with the physician is necessary to modify prescribing behavior consistently.

A modification of the detail visit has also been described by Avorn and Soumerai[73] as "academic detailing," the visiting of a physician by an individual, often a pharmacist, employed by a nonpharmaceutical source, such as an insurance carrier. The purpose of these visits is to decrease the prescription of dated, harmful, or inefficacious medication. Ray and colleagues[74] noted long-term improved prescribing practices in an office setting following such visits. Using a randomized controlled trial design, Avorn and Soumerai[73] have confirmed the evidence for the strength of this maneuver, although the inclusion of patient education materials, or providing feedback to physicians on prescribing behaviors, warrants consideration of this maneuver as a secondary intervention.

### Audiovisual resources

Lewis et al[75] studied the effect on competence of primary care physicians in AIDS care in a randomized controlled trial. Here, either printed, audio, or video educational materials were used by physicians. While demonstrating an increase in knowledge, the authors held that it was unrelated to the use of these educational materials. In contrast, Bowman[76] used office-based simulated patients to study the effect of printed material and audiotapes on the care of sexually transmitted disease on primary care physicians. Physicians who used the learning resources before the simulated patient visit performed better in every dimension, eliciting more information, displaying better patient interaction skills, and meeting more of the educational goals. In addition, there are many descriptive studies of audiovisual resources, including videotapes, teleconferencing (using audio or video methods), and computer-assisted AV resources, a small sample of which complement this section.

Interactive learning resources appear to improve performance. For example, Gask and colleagues,[77] in a descriptive study of a videotape intervention, demonstrated improved interviewing skills through videotaping with simulated patients. Further,

Premi[78] has described the effective use of videotape playback in the training of family medicine residents. Several systems of audio and video conferencing exist in North America and elsewhere to disseminate information and to provide systems of distance education. These have been reviewed by Davis and colleagues,[79] in their description of an Ontario system. Benschoter[80] provides another example of such a system in Nebraska. In contrast to the energy required to develop and maintain such systems, virtually no studies of the programmatic effectiveness of these systems exist relative to performance change or patient outcomes.

**Computer-aided instruction**

There have been a large number of reports of computer-assisted instruction in the teaching setting, and in such diverse fields as birth defects,[81] combat trauma life support,[82] respiratory radiology,[83] and neonatology.[84] In general, these studies are descriptive, detail features of the program, or declare satisfaction on the part of the program participants.

Godwin[85] noted that computers are increasingly common in physicians' offices. Initially based on a desire to improve the efficiency and efficacy of billing and word processing functions, physicians have later discovered that computers can perform other database and learning resource functions, including drug interaction, on-line article research, and CME programs. Chao[86] provided a comparative review of what he terms "CME software," including problem simulation, testing, and informatics programs. Advantages of computerized CME included local control over the topic, time, place, and interactivity of instruction, and moreover, match of resources with learning style. Bresnitz [87] has contributed the only randomized controlled trial in the study of this learning modality, albeit in undergraduate medical education. Here, learners taking a preventive medicine course were assigned either to computer or lecture groups. While differences were found in favor of the computer group over the lecture group in some aspects of knowledge, there was no difference on mean overall grade. Students' ratings of the computer-based learning program were generally favorable.

Curless and Coover-Stone[88] noted that interactive videodisc technology, based on computer-assisted instruction, could move classroom teaching methods beyond the didactic acquisition of information to the application of knowledge and skills. Henderson et al[89] contributed one example of this methodology in the training of military physicians in trauma management, while Hekelman and associates[90] addressed the issue of meeting the demands for staff development in technical skills training through interactive videodisc modalities. Finally, in the clinical setting, computers have been used as computer-aided teaching resources[91,92] and to assist in developing diagnostic strategies.[91,93] Their more intimate involvement with the clinical setting fit Type 2 or 3 classification criteria.

# Secondary Interventions

## Information sharing plus practice-enabling strategies

The criticism aimed at that form of CME which only provides information, the domain of most traditional CME providers, appears justified: information by itself rarely changes physician practices. In general, didactic sessions, printed materials, and other unidirectional, dissemination-only strategies appear ineffective, unless augmented by strategies which enable change in the practice setting. There are a wide variety of maneuvers fulfilling the criteria of these more complex enabling interventions: patient education strategies, elements in the patient encounter, and consultation with colleagues provide useful examples.

### Patient education materials

Patient education materials were effective in changing physician performance in most randomized controlled trials, when coupled with academic detail visits,[73] printed materials, or workshops,[44] but not when used with printed materials.[73] Among the effective studies, in smoking cessation, Kottke and associates[44] randomized participants to three groups: a workshop group which received free patient education materials and a 6-hour training workshop; a materials group which received only free patient education materials; and a control group. The training program with patient education materials marginally increased the smoking cessation activities of physicians and, 1 year later, improved the probability of a "quit" smoking attempt on the part of patients. However, the long-term cessation rates of patients were not different between groups of physicians.

More clear cut, positive outcomes were noted by Terry[94] in HIV testing in a multispecialty group practice. Here, a randomly selected group of family practitioners was provided with patient education resources, in addition to information about HIV antibody-testing guidelines and their own patient counseling practices. Chart audits showed: a doubling of the documentation of patient counseling; a minor increase in obtaining informed consent in HIV testing; and a decrease in overall test ordering.

Carey[95] described a trial comparing health professional education to patient education on the prescription and use of hypnotic and sedative drugs. In an Australian tertiary care hospital, staff education had a considerable impact on the administration or prescription of these drugs by nurses and doctors, while the education of patients resulted in an increase in drug knowledge but little impact on the immediate use of hypnosedatives in hospital. However, a mailed survey conducted 3 months after hospital discharge displayed a significant reduction in relevant drug use among patients exposed to the educational campaign. Finally, while most patient education strategies include the use of printed materials, Alberts[96] described a more comprehensive public education program, including interviews on television and radio, and newspaper articles. This campaign, coupled with physician education strategies, resulted in a significant increase in early stroke referrals to a relevant facility.

**Factors in the patient encounter**

There are several ways in which information driven by the patient encounter may be used by the physician in a manner which has the potential for altering practice performance.

*Information about specific patients*

The first of these has to do with information about specific patients, derived from health status questionnaires or interviews prior to the visit with the physician. This strategy demonstrated positive effects on physician performance in the management of depression in one randomized controlled trial,[97] but failed to change patient outcomes in another study of the functional status of patients.[98] Tierney and colleagues have studied the use of post-visit, computer-driven information about laboratory information[99,100] related to the cost or predictive value of tests ordered by the physician: both of these randomized controlled trials, displayed positive, though not universal, performance changes in the number of tests and total test costs.

*Questions in practice*

Another strategy is described by Jennett and her coworkers[101] who reported a 1-year experience with an information networking system between 47 rural practitioners and an academic center. Physicians were invited to phone in nonemergency clinical questions specific to daily practice needs to a telephone answering service located in the medical school library. Educational materials and article reprints were mailed in response to questions.

**Encounter forms/algorithms/flow charts**

Unlike clinical guidelines, policies, or protocols, encounter forms, flow charts, or algorithms attempt to digest the often cumbersome information presented in guideline format, easily employed checklists used at the time of the patient encounter. They may be in print or computerized form.

There are numerous examples of the former. Protocols or clinical algorithms, coupled with workshops, changed physician management in a randomized controlled trial of family physician education.[102] A descriptive example of management strategies using a clinical protocol is supplied by Packer,[103] who demonstrated that audit, didactic sessions, and a protocol of the treatment of emergency room patients presenting with acute knee injuries encouraged casualty officers to seek the help of more senior members of staff and reduced the time taken to definitive diagnosis and treatment. Similar findings were reported by Town et al in the treatment of acute asthmatics seeking emergency care.[104] Finally, protocols were helpful in enabling a staged reduction of diazepam prescribing among outpatients.[105] Protocols have also been used as a method of history-taking. Lilford,[106] for example, used structured questionnaires, both computerized and paper-based, in taking an antenatal history in a university hospital setting. These structured questionnaires provided more and better information and appeared to improve the physicians' perception of risk factors. A computerized system, however, offered no advantage over the simpler paper format. Similarly, Dietrich,[107] in a randomized controlled trial, used flow sheets, a 1-day conference, and the introduction of an office systems facilitator, and demonstrated improved cancer screening and preventive services.

Computerized protocols were studied by Margolis[108] in primary care pediatrics. While length of patient's visit, completeness of data collection, antibiotic use, and appropriateness of clinical plans improved, the project was discontinued after several weeks because the instrument appeared to be too cumbersome for routine use by physicians. Wexler[93] studied pediatric patients without diagnosis at admission who were randomized to either a study or control group. The study group included the use of a computer program which predicted a probable diagnosis for patients. Time to diagnosis, number of consultations, and inappropriate laboratory tests, although less in the experimental group, did not achieve statistical significance. Similarly, DeDombal and colleagues[91] compared three methods of support for inexperienced staff in their diagnosis and management of patients with acute abdominal pain: structured data collection forms; real-time computer-aided decision support; and computer-based teaching packages. Use of any one of these modalities improved the diagnostic accuracy of participating doctors and decreased admission rates of patients with nonspecific abdominal pain, perforation rates in patients with appendicitis, and negative laparotomy rates. The use of structured forms plus computer feedback resulted in better performance than the use of forms alone.

## Consultation with colleagues

Surveys confirm that consultation, either with peers or members of another discipline, form an integral part of the physician's learning strategies.[109] There have been several studies of this phenomenon. Muzzin,[110] for example, using ethnographic methods, established some of the parameters for effective consultation, including mutual respect and the potential for interaction. The role of consultation with colleagues has also been studied by comparing group and solo practices. For example Radecki and Rendenhall[111] demonstrated that primary care physicians in group practice tended to provide more patient education than solo physicians; and Lewis et al[75] showed a higher rate of competence in group practice in AIDS-related illness. The educational role of the consultant, trained as an opinion leader or educational influential, is discussed in greater detail below.

### Information-sharing plus reminders and feedback

Interventions or strategies which provide information and which reinforce the desired change appear to effectively overcome many of the logistical and sociological barriers to implementing optimum physician performance.[112] Feedback was used in 23 randomized controlled trials of CME interventions, of which most effected positive performance change when used alone or when used in conjunction with didactic presentations, workshops, academic detail visits, and/or printed materials.[5] Two randomized controlled trials[62,113] exhibited no change in patient outcomes with feedback, while one showed improvement using feedback to physicians relating to patient hospital discharges.[114] Reminders were also commonly used in randomized controlled trials, with uniformly positive results in changing physician performance and with mixed results in changing patient outcomes.[5]

An example of much of the general CME literature using feedback, Gurwitz[115] reported that the excessive use of H2 antagonists in geriatric patients may be reduced by educational measures coupled with feedback on prescribing behaviors. The latter, feedback phase appeared necessary to maintain the change. Like feedback, the use of reminders about specific performance, when coupled with other educational means, has been widely studied. McPhee et al[116] randomly assigned 40 primary care physicians in community-based practices to either a cancer prevention reminders group (which received computer-generated lists of overdue screening behaviors, supplemented by cancer education materials) or to a control group. Significant differences in performance scores were noted between intervention and control groups. Cummings, in randomized controlled trials of smoking cessation,[45,46] employed stickers on the charts of smokers as a reminder for the physician to counsel smokers. These studies demonstrated changes of some magnitude in physician performance but failed to display consistent, sustained changes in patient smoking behavior. The question of which of these two methods, reminders or feedback, is more useful, was examined by McPhee[117] who assigned 62 internal medicine residents to receive cancer screening reminders (computer-generated lists of overdue tests at patients' visits), audit with feedback (monthly seminars about screening and feedback about their performance rates), or no intervention (control). Reminders increased physician performance in six of seven tests, while audit with feedback achieved changes in four of seven tests. This illustrates the marginal superiority of reminders over feedback has been confirmed by a review of randomized controlled trials of CME interventions,[5] which noted the increased logistical effort necessary to achieve such a system and the necessary practice-based linkages required to achieve it.

### Information-sharing plus practice enabling and reinforcement

There were two types of interventions found in this category: those that used a mixture of intervention strategies, and those with single-maneuver strategies. Among the randomized controlled trials, those interventions which used a mixture of methods from all three preceding categories comprised the majority (eight of 17 interventions).[5] They produced positive results in all seven assessments of physician performance, and in three of five analyses of health care status. In addition, there were two single-intervention, relatively coherent maneuvers within this category: opinion leaders and chart review.

## Complex interventions

Elegant examples of complex, multiphasic interventions are found in the studies of smoking cessation and diabetes management.[42-47,118] Of these, Wilson and his associates[43] demonstrated a programmatic approach to the education of physicians about smoking cessation. This intervention comprised the following components: didactic sessions and printed materials; interactive, role-playing workshops which permitted rehearsal of practice behaviors; practice-enabling strategies such as patient education materials; and reminders and feedback on performance. This intervention produced impressive changes in physician performance but resulted in only small differences in patient outcome. Another example of a multifaceted strategy is provided by Vinicor and coworkers in the management of diabetes,[118] who added consultation with specialists to a menu of change strategies similar to those used in the smoking cessation trials.

## Opinion leaders

The effectiveness of opinion leaders or educational influentials in changing behavior and health care outcomes has been demonstrated in Lomas and colleagues'[62] randomized controlled trial designed to effect a reduction in cesarean section rates following vaginal births. This intervention demonstrated superiority over the simple dissemination of practice guidelines in the same topic area. Earlier, Stross[119-121] established the potential of the educational influentials to alter physician performance in the management of arthritis and respiratory disease; patient outcomes assessed in one of these studies were not altered.[121] Similarly, in the nursing education literature, Seto and her colleagues[122] demonstrated that both didactic educational methods and opinion leaders were necessary in the introduction of innovative care practices such as new catheter techniques.

## Chart review

Finally, chart review, when employed by a faculty member or supervisor, improved physician performance in three randomized controlled trials.[5] Chart review, studied by others from the perspective of competency assessment[123,124] and (under the rubric of chart-stimulated recall) from that of a CME intervention,[125] appears an effective and encyclopedic instrument, incorporating elements of information-sharing, reminders of desirable practices, feedback to the physician, and the opportunity for performance-enabling suggestions. A comprehensive description of the methodology is provided by McMillan et al[126] in an urban tertiary care setting. This study had these objectives: to determine whether physicians adhere to guidelines for the management of neonatal hyperbilirubinemia; to explore factors which influenced physicians' decisions to investigate and manage this condition; and to display the effect of either an educational intervention or clinical recall interview on compliance with the guidelines. Using a retrospective chart audit, the authors demonstrated increases in the proportion of infants receiving phototherapy in accordance with the criteria after chart-based interviews. Decisions to investigate and treat with phototherapy were also affected by clinical and parental factors.

# Implications for Practice:  The Provision of Evidence-based CME

It is clear that short courses, the traditional way in which undergraduates have been taught, and the major tool of CME planners, remains a firm pillar of CME for the majority of physicians undertaking the responsibility of ongoing professional learning. It is equally true that there are other significant, effective CME interventions and strategies which, when taken in the context of a new holistic view of CME, can effect significant change in physician performance and in health care outcomes.

It is the intent of this section to synthesize the findings presented above, with a view to improving the delivery of continuing medical education based on the best evidence available to date. This section will thus focus on the program developer's role in this exercise, and will consist of findings and implications in pre-program planning or needs assessment, and the design of short courses and other programmatic strategies categorized here as primary interventions. These are displayed in Figure 12.1. Broader, global recommendations about undergraduate training and CME organization will preface this section, and a brief discussion of evaluation will conclude it.

## Organizational Implications for the Continuum of Medical Education

It appears necessary to replace the notion that formal, planned courses are the sole vehicle for physician learning with a more global or holistic practice and practitioner-based view of "CME." To do so requires attention to two further, broad organizational principles germane to formal teaching methods: the first has to do with a dependence on formal teaching in the undergraduate setting; the second, with the accreditation of CME in North America.

### Lessons for undergraduate education

The extensive use of formal teaching methods in undergraduate curricula, while efficient and productive in the delivery of some types of information, fosters several harmful notions in the recipients of such a lecture-based, didactic approach. First, these perceptions about learning include that it is passive and is transferred from the knowledgeable "expert," usually the specialist, to the unlearned novice.  Second, that knowledge is relatively static and often based on opinion rather than data; and that, once transferred, it necessarily leads to improved competence or performance

## Figure 12.1

## Evidence-based CME interventions
A model to enhance intervention impact

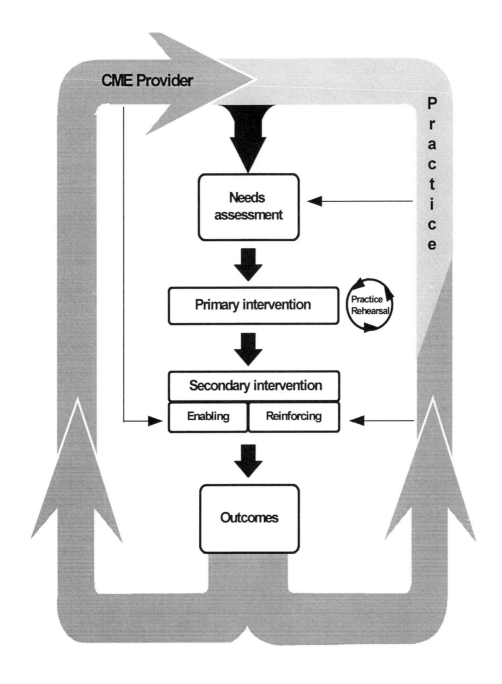

in the practice setting. Third, perhaps most dangerously, that teaching, done in lecture halls away from the practice site, is something different than learning in a patient-centered context. Finally, the sum of these experiences produces the mind-set in the traditionally taught graduate that "CME" must be an extension of this undergraduate learning experience.

This is not the first call for a strategy to correct the dependency on traditional approaches by the introduction of innovative curricula in medical schools. In fact, there exists in North America a distinct movement towards small group, problem-based teaching methods. However, those who work in the area of CME and physician learning may be the most credible witnesses to the ineffectiveness of the traditional approach to didactic learning and are thus best able to articulate the components of such an undergraduate system, based on real-life experience with practicing physicians.  Driven by the considerable evidence about CME, such a system would have as its objective the creation of the following abilities or competencies in its undergraduate learners: to perform accurate, objective self-assessments of learning needs; to establish self-directed learning projects based on these needs; to choose and utilize appropriate resources to meet these needs (from didactic sessions, where appropriate, to independent study methods); to recognize the need for, and select from, aids to facilitate the incorporation of learned strategies into the practice setting; and finally, to evaluate, in a systematic and critical manner, one's learning, practice patterns, and patient care outcomes.

## Accreditation issues

The second broad area in need of organizational reform comprises these twin elements—the system responsible for the accreditation of CME providers, and the CME credit system of physician-consumers. Both of these, heavily dependent on the provision of, and attendance at, formal CME events, need to plan extensive and coordinated restructuring of their guidelines with an emphasis on the learner and the needs of his or her patients, practice, and self. While this book cannot direct such a reform, it can point to the beginning of model programs, the evaluation of which may give direction to those responsible for accrediting CME in organizational settings. One example of such a systematic attempt to correct past identified weaknesses and to blend the accreditation of CME provider with the needs of the learner is the Maintenance of Competence Program (MOCOMP) of the College of Physicians and Surgeons of Canada.[127] Other concepts relative to accreditation are considered in Chapter 13.

The following paragraphs develop implications from this literature review for the design, execution, and evaluation of CME programs. (See Figure 12.1).

## Program Planning and Needs Assessment in the Design of CME Interventions

Mazmanian's[128] survey of providers of CME relative to their planning processes early in the last decade provides both a conceptual framework for an overview of common practices in the planning of formal programs, and a basis on which some recommendations may be made.

First, the planning activities of CME providers appear to be highly pragmatic, directed by the realities of each planned event and the perceptions of the planning committee members.[128] This traditional, subjective planning practice is thrown into some question by the findings of this chapter's literature review. Based on this review, more effective planning activities might include: assessments of practitioner beliefs about clinical areas; appraisals of knowledge as well as skills and attitudes in relevant clinical domains; exercises to improve the abilities of physicians in self-assessment; and, finally, the regular, systematic incorporation of objective data into the needs-assessment process by the use of charts, practice profiles, utilization data, and other means.

Second, a particularly troublesome question arises when attempts are made to create programs based on true need and also attract participants: namely, to what extent can the CME provider develop teaching in an area in which there is defined need, but no expressed "want" for instruction? Such needs may be determined by peer- or utilization-review organizations, by government or governing bodies, and by other professional or societal organizations. Examples are numerous, including instruction in human sexuality, assessed by the use of standardized patients in the US,[129] and malpractice risk reduction now mandated by the State of Florida.[130] Answers to this question must incorporate societal expectations, professional responsibilities, and personal goals, in addition to the development of strategic CME partnerships, tying CME providers with performance or health care monitoring activities and agencies such as hospital quality assurance programs or peer review organizations.

Third, discussions of needs assessment are incomplete without including references to the goal or mission of program planning. Among the many steps which program planners take in developing courses, Mazmanian[128] describes two basic underlying planning constructs. The first, classical model stresses the assessment of learning needs in order that clear end-point objectives are developed. The weight of evidence of this chapter supports the notion that CME outcomes are enhanced when there is clarity of expected changes.[51] Thus, it is important that both CME providers and consumers articulate clearly formed visions of end points to be achieved by CME participation. This strategy—matching desired performance outcomes with instructional techniques—may make the difference between successful and unsuccessful formal CME interventions. The other planning model, labelled "naturalistic" by Mazmanian, is more pragmatic, dependent on planning contingencies, and is process- rather than outcome-oriented. This planning process lends itself more to a discussion of learner- or practice-centered needs and characteristics, than on program planner goals.

# Dissemination, Instruction, and Considerations for the Adoption of Changes

From the evidence presented in this chapter, there appears to be a direct relationship between the intensity and complexity of the intervention and the numbers of studies with positive outcomes. In those studies which permit comparisons and judgments about efficacy, interventions using only predisposing elements to disseminate information were less apt to induce physician performance change and registered no positive health care outcomes. In contrast, those studies that used enabling and/or reinforcing elements were more effective in changing such outcomes.  Thus, re-designing CME programs, activities, or strategies incorporating this evidence, to enhance clinical performance and to adhere to the structure imposed by adult learning theory, forms a necessary part of the restructuring of CME.  Added to the widely used models of instructional plan development, based on adult education principles,[131] incorporating instructional objectives (knowledge acquisition, skill building, or attitudinal change), appropriate format,  instructor(s), learning re-sources, content, size of the "audience," and the practical considerations of a primary intervention are those follow-up, practice-linked methods considered here as secondary interventions. In short, in the case of formal CME planning, it is important to think of the learning "event" as well beyond the 1 or 2 days which are the duration of most courses or conferences.

## The primary intervention

First, to attract physicians to new formats within formal CME settings requires that physicians understand and want to participate in these opportunities. One way to accomplish this is the introduction of relevant clinical issues presented by problem-based techniques into curricular approaches. Instructional aids, such as audiovisuals, printed materials, and other devices, also appear to be useful in augmenting the physicians' learning patterns: they most likely reinforce learning, and impede decay of knowledge. Adapting these instructional devices to clinical experiences would appear to improve learning and enhance the possibility of transfer of knowledge to the practice setting. Other useful formats include those which facilitate learning and which provide the learner-participant with an opportunity to practice new skills and receive feedback on their performance.  Examples of such formats include small-group case discussion, peer review exercises in clinical settings, and particularly, role-playing or practice-rehearsal strategies. These methods invite attention to the size of audience which might best facilitate discussion and practice. While not calling solely for small-group learning experiences, the message of the literature to CME planners is this: if the goal of programming exceeds information sharing, transferable and effective learning may vary inversely with group size.

Second, there are a wide variety of other primary CME interventions or strategies which deserve attention and use by CME providers. Two broad examples are explored here—the computer and the innovative use of human resources. The computer appears as an extraordinarily effective method for the dissemination of new information, retrieval, and storage of up-to-date biomedical data, learning and testing new knowledge, providing diagnostic and management aids, and accomplishing reminder and feedback tasks. It is imperative that CME providers permit and encourage physician training in computer skills as a first step to the learning world which this method affords. Human resources, employed as the academic detail person, opinion leader, and peer mentor, also appear as effective, innovative learning facilitators. The academic detail visit, while difficult to separate from other maneuvers such as feedback and printed materials, appears to be an effective change agent, and worthy of implementation by CME providers, perhaps in consort with insurance carriers, state/provincial bodies, or the corporate sector. So, too, the selection, training, and activation of opinion leaders in selected clinical or geographic areas deserve consideration. Finally, peer mentors skilled in chart review and educational process for individualized or small group activities, appear as excellent intervention choices for the innovative, evidence-based CME provider.

## The secondary intervention

The final principle to be considered in course design is the addition of materials and methods that enable or reinforce the change in the practice-setting tools of the so-called secondary intervention. There are two major, practical aspects to this principle: materials and methods provided during the execution of a course or other formal intervention; and those which follow it. First, the incorporation of practice-useful devices during a course has been best exemplified by the smoking cessation projects. Here, participants are given chart stickers to flag appropriate charts, flow sheets or algorithms to append to charts of smoking patients, and patient education materials. Each of these practice-enablers may be easily adapted to other clinical topic areas and distributed as course materials. It is clear that these facilitators of behavior change have a strong impact on physician practices when they are used consistently.

Second, while not the usual domain of the CME provider, follow-up feedback on practice performance, reminders of desirable clinical behaviors, and ongoing patient education are all examples of CME program strategies that reach into the practice of the physician long after the "event" is over. Here, in particular, the usefulness of practice feedback is supported by both the health services research and adult education literature. These methods—audit and feedback, computer or paper-based reminders, and patient education—all require new linkages to be forged on both organizational and educational levels, between CME providers and clinical practice organizers. Such linkages, readily established in HMOs, for example, are the important work of the future-thinking CME provider.

# From Program Evaluation to CME Research: Evidence-based CME Delivery

It is important that CME providers select evaluation tools and strategies, matching the importance of their questions and the desired or appropriate level of outcome, along with the amount of error they can tolerate in the answers. While there are times when a happiness index will be sufficient to find out whether participants found a program useful, more frequently, researchers, CME providers, and others in the health care delivery system must work together to design and carry out selected, fruitful evaluation procedures. This collaboration will help to bridge the gap between practice and research, and close the loop between needs assessment, program implementation, and evaluation. It will also move CME from empirically based teacher-centered activities to those which are more learner- and even patient outcome-based, rooted in evidence of efficacy. Finally, and with equal importance, such a process empowers and enfranchises the CME planner, placing him or her firmly in the environment of health care delivery—from planning, to implementation, to evaluation of outcomes.

A movement to close this loop is shown diagrammatically in Figure 12.2, which outlines a three-phase educational model, from needs assessment, through program development, to evaluation, the standard planning and development fare of the CME provider. We call for a more thoughtful evaluation of these phases, their implementation, and outcomes in the context of improving health care. Such a focus, called "provider analysis" in this figure, leads the planner through an iterative process to a more research-oriented mode to plan and evaluate new interventions.

## Figure 12.2

## The Iterative loop applied to CME:
Moving from course evaluation to CME research

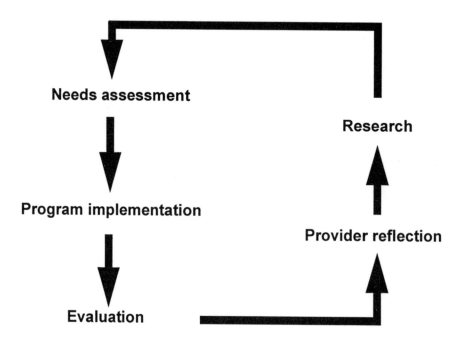

Needs assessment

Program implementation

Evaluation

Research

Provider reflection

# Implications for Research: Toward a Science of CME

There are wide-ranging recommendations for further research in CME, which arise from the current literature and their implications for practice. They are clustered in five groups, paralleling the recommendations above: program needs assessment; instructional design; learner-specific issues; program follow-up and practice-linked strategies; and finally, research methodologies, practices, and directions.

## Needs Assessment

First, it is clear at a global level that appropriate needs assessment is the sine qua non of effective CME planning. However, global certainties give way to more specific questions. We need to know much more about: practitioners' beliefs about clinical decision making; how to assess attitudes and perceptions of efficacy in relevant clinical domains; and exercises to improve the abilities of physicians in self-assessment. Similarly, while there exist a host of relevant, objective practice methods—chart review, audit, utilization review, insurance-carrier data, to name a few—there are a number of questions which these methods generate. For example: Which method is best in which clinical areas?; Which methods reflect practice performance best?; What is the sensitivity and specificity of these tests in the determination of physician competence?; and Which methods are most cost effective?

Penetrating questions arise from a consideration of subjective needs assessment and the means by which these may be made to more closely match those determined by objective means without losing inherent motivation. Efforts in the area of improved self assessment ability are of merit and deserve further testing in the setting of the practicing clinician. In addition, the question of the role of undergraduate training in the realm of self assessment speaks to the need for continued examination of problem-based and other pre-graduate learning/curricular techniques, particularly long-term studies of physician outcomes one to several decades after graduation.

## The Design of Courses

Second, there are a host of questions which arise from the design of formal CME courses and programs which call for a thorough examination of the educational literature for guidance.

- Does the use of audiovisual materials enhance learning "uptake"? Does their use decrease decay of knowledge?

- To what extent does linking practice-based learning approaches or case material to audiovisual or printed materials facilitate immediate learning and, later, practice-based recall?

- What are the specific effects of pacing and sequencing of instructional units relative to learning and recall?

- To what extent do effective learning formats and resources depend on the clinical area being discussed?

- What is the educational role of the "commitment for change" activity? Does it reinforce the transfer of knowledge disseminated to practice? Does it improve motivation to make the change? What is the boundary between the CME intervention and responses induced by the learner? What is the effect of group size? Does effectiveness in programming depend on group interaction and case discussion in order to focus the learner's attention on transfer knowledge to practice?

- What role does practice rehearsal play in transferring knowledge to practice?

- What about the place of learning? Does learning in a location at or near the practice site (eg, a hospital ward or clinic setting) facilitate transfer of knowledge to practice at a greater rate than learning at a distant site such as a university?

## Testing Other CME Interventions

Many research questions are prompted by the wide variety of other learning and practice change strategies discussed above. A partial list follows:

- Is the use of academic detailing a viable mechanism for future CME delivery? Are academic detail visits equally effective in changing drug prescribing habits between classes of physicians or in different classes of pharmaceutical preparations?

- How do opinion leaders effect change in the practice environment? What are the particular skills of the effective peer mentor?

- What are the effective training methods for opinion leaders or peer mentors involved in chart review? What academic "credentials" do they require to impact on physician behavior?

- What is the role and feasibility of "in-office" technology for CME purposes? What are the elements of printed materials or other dissemination strategies that are effective? Can these incorporate components of flow charts or other patient education materials which have been shown to be effective change agents?

- How can patient education be incorporated into CME exercises and programs? To what extent does the effectiveness of such materials depend on their dissemination in concert with physician learning?

- Is small group learning applicable to the 1-day, traditional learning format? How long, and in what circumstances, does optimal group functioning occur? What are the elements of such functioning?

- How can practice guidelines be best adapted for practice use? Are the elements of effective guidelines the same across all clinical areas? To what extent does a sense of ownership over guideline development affect their use by clinicians?

- What are the elements of computer training necessary to incorporate computers skills in the practice life of physicians?

There are also a series of questions which arise from a consideration of the interface between primary and secondary interventions, and between that of the learning resource and the learner.

The structure of both primary and secondary interventions is essentially communicative, formed of the successful transmission of a message by the sender and a predictable response from the receiver.[132,133] This understanding of program planning and CME opens questions regarding expectations of CME, physicians, and planners. What may be expected from short courses? What may be expected from carefully coordinated and sustained communications between learning resources such as opinion leaders, or peer mentors and physicians, engaged in solving practice problems? Can larger, more complex changes be achieved through an extended course of interventions promoting smaller, simpler changes?

Finally, there is need for research on convergence of media and learning.[133-135] Research and development on audit and feedback, computer and paper-based reminders, and patient education are likely to lead to higher quality communicative technology for the more effective design of interventions promoting change.[133-137] The use of such communicative or teaching aids in both primary and secondary interventions is deserving of further careful application and evaluation.

## Issues Relevant to the Learner and Learning Environment

Much of the literature devoted to CME, though rich in details of the intervention or the demographics of the physician population studied, is sparse in describing the qualitative details of the learning process. More information can be gathered through structured interviews of physicians attending formal courses, to determine which aspects of course format, learning site, or learning resources affect learning and change. Such an approach further tests the hypotheses generated by adult and continuing professional educators and reinforces the work of health service researchers. Two particular issues require attention.

First, what is the role of formal CME in creating a climate for physician change? It is clear that most if not all of the physicians in CME studies have volunteered their participation, have accepted the relevance of the subject area of the CME intervention, and are therefore at a stage of readiness to change or learn. Studies of non-volunteer physicians may be necessary to indicate whether formal CME is effective in creating a climate in which preparedness for change, or perception of the change's importance, may be altered.

Second, does participation in setting clinical criteria in a formal CME process effect change in practice? How does belief in self-efficacy or efficacy of treatment affect clinical practice following CME interventions? This is particularly relevant in the area of practice guidelines or computer strategies. Work in this area deserves closer scrutiny, compelling us to examine questions about how physicians' beliefs effect performance and forcing closer examination of the interaction between the practice context, the physician learner, and the patient.

## Post-program Follow-up

Developing mechanisms to help physicians transfer their learning into practice is a new frontier for CME providers. Reminders, feedback, and practice aids have proven to be effective enablers of change in physician performance and health care outcomes. Research questions regarding integration of these techniques into CME programs and then into practice deserve exploration. Of practical and researchable proportions is this core question: What particular practice aids are useful in which types of clinical problems or settings? Other subsets of this question include: Could practice aids function as objective, practice-audit, needs-assessment tools? Are practice aids more useful and utilized when the physician has a role in designing them? To what extent do practice auxiliary staff members play a role in the use of practice aids? Are reminders more effective than feedback in only preventive practices? Are there ways in which performance feedback may be made to have longer lasting effects?

## Research Methods, Practices, and Directions

This review reveals the need to address several broad, important issues in the research of CME interventions.

The first has to do with the questions of research methodology. In the final analysis, there is much to be learned from a review of the literature currently available to the student of CME about the nature and effectiveness of this traditional and important pillar of physician learning. While the nature of the literature sources are numerous and varied, so also are the limitations to its interpretation. On the one hand, the biomedical, quantitative study of interventions provides a comparative environment in which to study outcomes relevant to specific formal courses in an environment relatively free of contamination and cointervention. There are, however, several difficulties with the execution of such studies, including: lack of detail of physician populations; non-blinding of assessors; a dependence on volunteer physicians, limiting the generalizability of findings to physicians likely to be at or above their peers in performance; and a dearth of qualitative details of potential help in the delineation of physician management patterns, learning processes, or forces for and impediments to change. In addition, there may be publication bias in which negative or inconclusive studies may not be submitted for publication.

On the other hand, while the qualitative literature provides us with a wealth of learner-centered data, it offers an almost exclusively subjective perspective, with potential for bias and often generated by clinicians unskilled in educational research. To compensate for deficiencies in both methods, and to build on their strengths, a merger of research designs and etiologies is called for to answer the basic questions of CME and physician learning in the context of the formal CME phenomenon. Such a fusion of research methodologies, coupled with the energy of the practice-motivated CME provider, will do much to improve the research in CME and enhance its outcomes.

Second, both providers and consumers of CME need to be aware of the clear lesson derived from this review: that CME is more effective when it incorporates practice-based enabling and reinforcing strategies, and that adequate needs assessment leads to increased potential for change. Further, there are several specific interventions which appear to be highly promising and which deserve further testing and use, particularly chart review, opinion leaders, academic detail visits, computer-based strategies, and multiphasic activities. Older methods which remain in use despite evidence concerning their relative impotence also deserve study. Journal reading, for example, is clearly an important mode of learning for most physicians, but not studied to any extent, and certainly not by quantitative performance or patient-outcome methods. Third, the clinical domain of most CME studies appears to be determined more often by its simplicity of measurement (blood pressure, for example), by its cost (eg, investigations) or by its relevance to a new pharmaceutical product (eg, nicotine compounds) than by its clinical imperative. While not discounting the importance of these domains or topic areas, the weight of evidence of this chapter calls for the development of a research agenda which would include, as a first priority, studies which assess the effects of CME interventions on major causes of morbidity and mortality.

Finally, the belief that "there is a serious weak link in the chain of research that is required to create new knowledge and bring it into effective use in medical care"[10] is reiterated here. This belief compels researchers and providers of CME alike to embark on a concerted and coordinated program of further examination of those modalities which effect physician learning and change; and to develop an improved, evidence-based delivery system of continuing medical education. Such a movement would take the medical profession and its growing discipline of CME beyond the teacher-dominated scenario, reflected in the quote which begins this chapter, into an era of patient- and learner-linked CME.

## References

1.  Nowlen PA. *A New Approach to Continuing Eduction for Business and the Professions.* New York, NY:  Collier MacMillan Pub; 1988:23.

2.  Accreditation Council for CME. *Guidelines for the Accreditation of Continuing Medical Education Providers.* Lake Bluff, Ill: 1990.

3.  Richards RK. *Continuing Medical Education Perspectives, Problems and Prognosis.* New Haven, Conn:  Yale University Press; 1978.

4.  Davis DA, Delmore T, Bryans AM, Williams JI, Dunn E, Krauser J, Scott DJ, Heron A. Continuing medical education in Ontario. *Ann of the Royal College of Physicians and Surgeons of Canada.* 1983;16:136-141.

5.  Davis DA, Thomson MA, Oxman AD, Haynes RB.  Evidence for the effectiveness of CME: a review of 50 randomized controlled trials. *JAMA.*  1992;268:1111-1117.

6.  Green L, Kreuter M, Deeds S, Partridge K. *Health Education Planning: A Diagnostic Approach.*  Palo Alto, Calif: Mayfield Press; 1980.

7.  Bertram DA, Brooks-Bertram PA.  The evaluation of continuing medical education: a literature review. *Health Educ Monogr.* 1977;5:330-362.

8.  Lloyd JS, Abrahamson S.  Effectiveness of continuing medical education: a review of the evidence. *Eval Health Professions.* 1979;2:251-280.

9.  Stein LS.  The effectiveness of continuing medical education: eight research reports. *J Med Educ.* 1990;56:103-110.

10. Haynes RB, Davis DA, McKibbon A, Tugwell P.  A critical appraisal of the efficacy of continuing medical education. *JAMA.* 1984;251:61-64.

11. Beaudry JS.  The effectiveness of continuing medical education: a qualitative syntheses. *J Continuing Educ Health Professions.* 1989;9:285-307.

12. McLaughlin PJ, Donaldson JF.  Education of continuing medical education programs: selected literature, 1984-1988. *J Continuing Educ Health Professions.* 1991;11:65-84.

13. Dixon J.  Evaluation criteria in studies of continuing education in the health professions: a critical review and a suggested strategy. *Eval Health Professions.* 1978;1:47-65.

14. The McMaster Group on CME Research. *The Research and Development Resource Base in CME.* Hamilton, Ontario: McMaster University.

15. Jennett PA, Laxdal OE, Hayton RC, et al.  The effects of continuing medical education on family doctor performance in office practice: a randomized control study. *Med Educ.* 1988;22:139-145.

16. White CW, Albanese MA, Brown DD, Caplan RM.  The effectiveness of continuing medical education in changing the behavior of physicians caring for patients with acute myocardial infarction. *Ann of Intern Med.* 1985;102:686-692.

17. White CW.  An evaluation of the composition of the audience on the effectiveness of continuing education in changing physician knowledge and behavior. *Conf on Research in Med Educ.*  Assoc Am Med Coll. 1982;21:216-221.

18. Inui TS.  Improved outcomes in hypertension after physician tutorials: a controlled trial. *Ann Intern Med.* 1976;84:646-651.

19. Hillman RS.  The effect of an educational program on transfusion practices in a regional blood program. *Transfusion.* 1979;19:153-157.

20. Page GG. The effect of continuing medical education programs on clinical practice: fact or fantasy. *Med Educ.* 1979;13:292-297.

21. D'Ilvernois JF. Computer-assisted instruction for retraining family doctors in hypertension and hyperlipoproteinemia. *Med Educ.* 1979;13:356-358.

22. Weinberg AD. Perceived ability vs actual ability: a problem for continuing medical education. *Conf on Research in Med Educ.* 1977;16:79-84.

23. Craig J. The OSCME (opportunity for self-assessment CME). *J Cont Educ Health Prof.* 1991;11:87-94.

24. Elzarian EJ. Educational approaches promoting optimal laxative use in long-term-care patients. *J Chronic Dis.* 1980;33:613-626.

25. McGuire C. Auscultatory skill: gain and retention after intensive instruction. *J Med Educ.* 1984;39:120-131.

26. Gordon MS. A cardiology patient simulator for continuing education of family physicians. *J Fam Pract.* 1981;13:353-356.

27. Gass D, Curry L. Investigations in CPR Training. *Conf on Research in Med Educ.* Washington, DC: Assoc Am Med Coll. 1980;189-193.

28. Bennett JR. Advanced trauma life support: a time for reappraisal. *Anaesthesia.* 1992;47:798-800.

29. Schmidt HG, Norman GR, Boshuizen HPA. A cognitive perspective on medical expertise: theory and implications. *Academic Medicine.* 1990;65:611-621.

30. Barrows HS, Williams RG, Moy RH. A comprehensive performance-based assessment of fourth-year students' clinical skills. *J Med Educ.* 1987;243:1148-1150.

31. Tamblyn RM. Bedside clinics in neurology: an alternate format for the one-day course in continuing medical education. *JAMA.* 1980;243:1148-50.

32. Collett LS. Change in attitude as an index of effectiveness for short courses in continuing medical education. *J Med Educ.* 1970;45:237-242.

33. Greenberg LW, Jewett LS. The impact of two teaching techniques on physicians' knowledge and performance. *J Med Educ.* 1985;60:390-396.

34. Heale J, Davis D, Norman G, Woodward C, Neufeld V, Dodd P. A randomized controlled trial assessing the impact of problem-based versus didactic teaching methods in CME. *Conf on Res in Med Educ.* Washington, DC: Assoc Am Med Coll. 1988;27:72-77.

35. Rodney WM, Albers G. Flexible sigmoidoscopy: primary care outcomes after two types of continuing medical education. *Am J Gastroenter.* 1986;81:133-137.

36. Andrusyszyn M. The effect of the lecture discussion teaching method with and without audio-visual augmentation on immediate and retention learning. *Nurse Ed Today.* 1990;10:172-180.

37. Gauvain S. Continuing medical education: assessment of courses. *J Roy Coll Gen Prac.* 1970;19:223-227.

38. Pitman GI. Tennessee reading retreats: physicians find pastoral setting perfect for CME. *Am Coll Phys Obs.* 1983;4:16.

39. Cordell BJ, Greaf WD. Computer-assisted instruction: is it right for you? *J Cont Ed Health Prof.* 1988;8:97-105.

40. Appolone C. An epilepsy workshop for professionals. *Epilepsia.* 1979;29:127-132.

41. Purkis IE. Commitment for change: an instrument for evaluating CME courses. *J Med Educ.* 1982;57:61-63.

42. Maiman LA, Becker MH, Liptak GS, Nazarian LF, Rounds KA. Improving pediatricians' compliance-enhancing practices: a randomized trial. *AJDC.* 1988;142:773-779.

43. Wilson DM, Taylor DW, Gilbert JR, et al. A randomized trial of a family physician intervention for smoking cessation. *JAMA*. 1988;260:1570-1574.

44. Kottke TE, Brekke ML, Solberg LI, Hughes JR. A randomized trial to increase smoking intervention by physicians. *JAMA*. 1989;261:2101-2106.

45. Cummings SR, Richard RJ, Duncan CL, et al. Training physicians about smoking cessation: a controlled trial in private practices. *J Gen Intern Med*. 1989;4:482-489.

46. Cummings SR, Coates TJ, Richard RJ, et al. Training physicians in counseling about smoking cessation. *Ann Intern Med*. 1989;110:640-647.

47. Cohen SJ, Stookey GK, Katz BP, Drook CA, Smith DM. Encouraging primary care physicians to help smokers quit. *Ann Intern Med*. 1989;110:648-652.

48. Evans CE, Haynes RB, Birkett NJ, et al. Does a mailed continuing education program improve physician performance? results of a randomized trial in antihypertensive care. *JAMA*. 1986;255:501-504.

49. Meyer TJ, Van Kooten D, Marsh S, Prochazka AV. Reduction of polypharmacy by feedback to clinicians. *J Gen Intern Med*. 1991;6:133-136.

50. Harvey KJ, Stewart R, Hemming M, Naismith N, Moulds RFW. Educational antibiotic advertising. *Med J Aust*. 1986;145:28-32.

51. Fox RD, Mazmanian PE, Putnam RW. *Changing and Learning in the Lives of Physicians.* New York, NY: Praeger Pub; 1989.

52. Bergman DA, Pantell RH. The impact of reading a clinical study on treatment decisions of physicians and residents. *J Med Educ*. 1986;61:380-386.

53. Covell DG, Uman GC, Manning PR. Information needs in office practice: are they being met? *Ann Intern Med*. 1985;103:596-599.

54. Williamson JW, German PS, Weiss R, Skinner EA, Bowes F. Health science information management and continuing education of physicians: a survey of US primary care practitioners and their opinion leaders. *Ann Intern Med*. 1989;110:151-160.

55. Gordon MD. Helping general practitioners to keep up with the literature: evaluation of an RCRCGP initiative. *Med Educ*. 1984;18:174-177.

56. Benseman J, Barham PM. Coping with information overload: the development and evaluation of a journal review service. *Med Educ*. 1984;18:446-447.

57. Haynes RB, McKibbon KA, Fitzgerald D, Guyatt GH, Walker CJ, Sakett DL. How to keep up with the medical literature: I. why try to keep up and how to get started. *Ann Intern Med*. 1986;105:149-153.

58. Haynes RB, McKibbon KA, Fitzgerald D, Guyatt GH, Walker CJ, Sackett DL. How to keep up with the medical literature: III. expanding the number of journals you read regularly. *Ann Intern Med*. 1986;105:474-478.

59. Haynes RB, McKibbon KA, Fitzgerald D, Guyatt GH, Walker CJ, Sackett DL. How to keep up with the medical literature: III. expanding the number of journals you read regularly. *Ann Intern Med*. 1986;105:474-478.

60. Langkamp DL. The effect of a medical journal club on residents' knowledge of clinical epidemiology and biostatistics. *Fam Med*. 1992;24:528-530.

61. Haynes RB. Organizing and accessing the literature. *Acad Med*. 1989;65:673-686.

62. Lomas J, Enkin M, Anderson GM, Hannah WJ, Vayda E, Singer J. Opinion leaders vs audit and feedback to implement practice guidelines. *JAMA*. 1991;265:2202-2207.

63. Troein M, Selander S. Dissemination and implementation of guidelines for lipid lowering. *Fam Prac*. 1991;8:223-228.

64. Dajczman E. Survey of infection control precautions: a comparison to recommended guidelines. *Can J Infect Control*. 1992;7:7-12.

65. Costanza ME, Stoddard AM, Zapka JG, Gaw VP, Barth R. Physician compliance with mammography guidelines: barriers and enhancers. *J Am Board Fam Pract.* 1992;5:143-152.

66. Linton AL, Peachey DK. Guidelines for medical practice: the reasons why. *Can Med Assoc J.* 1990;143:485-490.

67. Putnam RW, Curry L. Impact of patient care appraisal on physician behaviour in the office setting. *Can Med Assoc J.* 1985;132:1025-1029.

68. Grol R. National standard setting for quality of care in general practice: attitudes of general practitioners and response to a set of standards. *Br J of Gen Prac.* 1990;40:361-364.

69. Royal college of radiologists working party. Influence of the Royal College of Radiologists' Guidelines on hospital practice: a multicentre study. *Br Med J.* 1992;304:740-743.

70. Soumerai SB, McLaughlin TJ, Avorn J. Improving drug prescribing in primary care: a critical analysis of the experimental literature. *Milbank Q.* 1989;67:268-317.

71. Avorn J, Chen M, Hartley R. Scientific vs commercial sources of influence on the prescribing behavior of physicians. *Am J of Med.* 1982;37:4-8.

72. Rovers JP. The doctor's, the druggist's, and the detail rep's dance. *Can Fam Phys.* 1991;37:100-104.

73. Avorn J, Soumerai SS. Improving drug therapy decisions through educational outreach. *N Engl J Med.* 1983;308:1457-1463.

74. Ray WA, Schaffner W, Federspiel CF. Persistence of improvement in antibiotic prescribing in office practice. *JAMA.* 1985;253:1774-1776.

75. Lewis CE, Freeman HE, Kaplan SH, Corey CR. The impact of a program to enhance the competencies of primary care physicians in caring for patients with AIDS. *J Gen Intern Med.* 1986;1:287-294.

76. Bowman MA. The effect of educational preparation on physician performance with a sexually transmitted disease-simulated patient. *Arch Intern Med.* 1992;152:1823-1828.

77. Gask L, Goldberg D, Lesser AL, Millar T. Improving the psychiatric skills of the general practice trainee: an evaluation of a group training course. *Med Educ.* 1988;22:132-138.

78. Premi J. An assessment of 15 years' experience in using videotape review in a family practice residency. *Acad Med.* 1991;66(1):56-57.

79. Davis D, Lindsay E, Fallis F, Willison D, Biggar J. Telemedicine for Ontario. *Can Med Assoc J.* 1985;137-138.

80. Benschoter RA. Satellite system addresses rural health problems. *J Biocommun.* 1992;19:26-30.

81. Buyse ML, Edwards CN. The birth defects information system: a computer-based information resource for diagnostic support, education, and research. *Am J Perinatol.* 1987;4:8-11.

82. Henderson JV, Pruett RK, Galper AR, Copes WS. Interactive videodisc to teach combat trauma life support. *J Med Sys.* 1986;1:271-276.

83. McEnery KW. Interactive instruction in the radiographic anatomy of the chest. *Comp Meth Prog Biomed.* 1986;22:81-86.

84. Tinsley L, Easa D. Pulmonary diseases in the neonate: a computer-assisted instruction. *Comp Meth Prog Biomed.* 1986;22:93-101.

85. Godwin M. Community hospital integrated computer systems. *Can Fam Phys.* 1991;37:56-60.

86. Chao J. Continuing medical education software: a comparative review. *J Fam Pract.* 1992;34:598-604.

87. Bresnitz EA. A randomized trial to evaluate a computer-based learning program in occupational lung disease. *J Occup Med.* 1992;34:422-427.

88. Curless E, Coover-Stone YJ. Simulating clinical situations: interactive videodisc. *Dimen Crit Care Nurs.* 1987;6:248-254.

89. Henderson JV, Pruett RK, Galper AR, Copes WS. Interactive videodisc to teach combat trauma life support. *J Med Sys.* 1986;10(3):271-276.

90. Hekelman FP, Phillips JA, Bierer LA. An interactive videodisk training program in basic cardiac life support: implications for staff development. *J Contin Ed in Nurs.* 1991;21:245-247.

91. De Dombal FT, Dallos V, McAdam WAF. Can computer-aided teaching packages improve clinical care in patients with acute abdominal pain? *Br Med J.* 1991;302:1495-1497.

92. Umlauf MG. How to provide around-the-clock CPR certification without losing any sleep. *J Contin Ed in Nurs.* 1991;21(6):248-251.

93. Wexler JR. Impact of a system of computer-assisted diagnosis. *AJDC.* 1991;129:203-205.

94. Terry P. The result of an educaitonal intervention for physicians providing HIV-antibody testing and counseling. *Minn Med.* 1992;75:37-39.

95. Carey DL. An attempt to influence hypnotic and sedative drug use. *Med J Aust.* 1992;156:389-396.

96. Alberts MJ. Effects of public and professional education on reducing the delay in presentation and referral of stroke patients. *Stroke.* 1992;23:352-356.

97. Magruder-Habib K, Zung WK, Feussner JR. Improving physicians' recognition and treatment of depression in general medical care. *Med Care.* 1990;28:239-250.

98. Rubenstein LV, Calkins DR, Young RT, et al. Improving patient function: a randomized trial of functional disability screening. *Ann Inter Med.* 1989;111:836-842.

99. Tierney WM, McDonald CJ, Hui SL, Martin DK. Computer predicting of abnormal test results effects on outpatient testing. *JAMA.* 1988;259:1194-1198.

100. Tierney WM, Miller ME, McDonald CJ. The effect on test ordering of informing physicians of the charges for outpatient diagnostic tests. *N Engl J Med.* 1990;322:1499-1504.

101. Jennett PA, Parboosingh IJ, Maes WR, Lockyer JM, Lawson D. A medical information networking system between practitioners and academic. *J Cont Educ Health Prof.* 1990;10:237-243.

102. Putnam RW, Curry L. Impact of patient care appraisal on physician behaviour in the office setting. *Can Med Assoc J.* 1985;132:1025-1029.

103. Packer GJ. Effect of an algorithm on the treatment of knee injuries. *Injury.* 1992;23:270-272.

104. Town I, Kwong T, Holst P, Beasley R. Use of a management plan for treating asthma in an emergency department. *Thorax.* 1990;45:702-706.

105. Ray WA, Blazer DG II, Schaffner W, Federspiel CF, Fink R. Reducing long-term diazepam prescribing in office practice. *JAMA.* 1986;256:2536-2539.

106. Lilford RJ. Effect of using protocols on medical care: randomised trial of three methods of taking an antenatal history. *Br Med J.* 1992;305:1181-1184.

107. Dietrich AJ. Cancer: improving early detection and prevention: a community practice randomised trial. *Br Med J.* 1992;304:687-691.

108. Margolis CZ. Computerized algorithms and pediatricians' management of common problems in a community clinic. *Acad Med.* 1992;67:282-284.

109. Hart G. Peer consultation and review. *Aust J Adv Nurs.* 1989;7:40-46.

110. Muzzin LJ. Understanding the process of medical referral. *Can Fam Phys.* 1992;38:301-307.

111. Radecki SE, Mendenhall RC. Patient counselling by primary care physicians: results of a nationwide study. *Patient Ed Counsel.* 1986;8:165-177.

112. Eisenberg JM. Sociologic influences on decision-making by clinicians. *Ann Intern Med.* 1979;90:957

113. Gullion DS, Tschann JM, Adamson TE, Coates TJ. Management of hypertension in private practices: a randomized controlled trial in continuing medical education. *J Contin Educ Health Prof.* 1988;8:239-255.

114. Restuccia JD. The effect of concurrent feedback in reducing inappropriate hospital utilization. *Med Care.* 1982;20:46-62.

115. Gurwitz JH. Reducing the use of $H^2$-receptor antagonists in the long-term-care setting. *J Am Geriatr Soc.* 1992;40:359-364.

116. McPhee SJ, Bird JA, Fordham D, Rodnick JE, Osborn EH. Promoting cancer prevention activities by primary care physicians. *JAMA.* 1991;266:538-544.

117. McPhee SJ, Bird JA, Jenkins CN, Fordham D. Promoting cancer screening: a randomized, controlled trial of three interventions. *Arch Intern Med.* 1989;149:1866-1872.

118. Vinicor P, Cohen SJ, Mazzuca SA, et al. DIA-BEDS: a randomized trial of the effects of physician and/or patient education on diabetes patient outcomes. *J Chronic Dis.* 1987;40:345-356.

119. Stross JK, Bole GG. Evaluation of a continuing education program in rheumatoid arthritis. *Arthritis Rheum.* 1980;23:846-849.

120. Stross JK, Bole GG. Evaluation of an educational program for primary care practitioners on the management of osteoarthritis. *Arthritis Rheum.* 1985;28:108-111.

121. Stross JK, Hiss RG, Watts CM, Davis WK, MacDonald R. Continuing education in pulmonary disease for primary care physicians. *Am Rev Respir Dis.* 1983;127:739-746.

122. Seto WH, Ching TY, Yuen KY, Chu YB, Seto WL. The enhancement of infection control inservice education by ward opinion leaders. *Am J Infect Control.* 1991;19:86-91.

123. Tugwell P, Dok C. Medical record review. In: Neufeld VR, Norman GR, eds. *Assessing Clinical Competence.* New York, NY: Norman G. Springer; 1985:142-182.

124. Davis DA, Norman GR, Premi J, et al. Attempting to ensure physician competence. *JAMA.* 1990;263:2041-2042.

125. Parbooshingh J, Avard D, Lockyer J, Watson M, Pim C, Yee J. The use of clinical recall interviews as a method of determining needs in continuing medical education. *Conf Res Med Educ.* 1987;26:103-108.

126. McMillan D, Magnan L, Lockyer J, Akierman A, Parboosingh J. Effect of educational program and interview on adoption of guidelines for the management of neonatal hyperbilirubinemia. *Can Med Assoc J.* 1991;144:707-712.

127. Parboosingh J, Maes W, Lockyer J, Bauer J. Teaching physicians to use a literature retrieval service for clinical information: a feasibility study. *Ann Roy Coll Phys Surg Can.* 1986;19:273-277.

128. Mazmanian PE. A decision-making approach to needs assessment and objective setting in continuing medical education. *Adult Educ.* 1980;31:3-17.

129. Russell NK, Boekeloo BO, Rafi IZ, Rabin DL. Using unannounced simulated patients to evaluate sexual risk assessment and risk reduction skills of practicing physicians. *Acad Med.* 1991;66:S37-S39.

130. Fore RC, Bouis PJ, Runnels JM. Mandatory risk management in CME: 2 years' experience. *J Flor Med Assoc.* 1988;75:379-381.

131. Mazmanian PE, Martin KO, Kreutzer JS. Professional development and educational program planning in cognitive rehabilitation. In: Kreutzer JS, Wehman PH, eds. *Cognitive Rehabilitation for Persons with Traumatic Brain Injury.* Baltimore, Md: Brookes Publishing; 1991:35-51.

132. Bretz R. *A Taxonomy of Communication Media.* Englewood Cliffs, NJ: Education Technology Publications; 1971:23.

133. Broadhurst AR, Darnell DK. An introduction to cybernetics and information theory. In: Sereno KK, Mortensen CD, eds. *Foundations of Communication Theory.* New York, NY: Harper and Row Publishers; 1970:59-72.

134. Peck J. The power of media and the creation of meaning: a survey of approaches to media analysis. In: Dervin B, Voight MJ, eds. *Progress in Communication Sciences.* Norwood, NJ: Ablex Publishing Corporation; 1989:145-182.

135. Krendl KA. two roads converge: the synthesis of research on media influence on learning. In: Dervin B, Voight MJ. *Progress in Communication Sciences.* Norwood, NJ: Ablex Publishing Corporation; 1989:9:105-122.

136. Simpkin JD, Brenner DJ. Mass media communication and health. In: Dervin B, Voight MJ. *Progress in Communication Sciences.* Norwood, NJ: Ablex Publishing Corporation; 1986:275-297.

137. Paisley W. New media and methods of health communication. Presented at the Conference on Effective Dissemination of Clinical and Health Information; September, 19, 1991; Tucson, AZ.

# Chapter 13

# Beyond Accreditation and the Enterprise of CME:

## An Alternative Model Linking Independent Learning Centers and Health Services Research

*Paul Mazmanian*
*Willard Duff*

# Beyond Accreditation and the Enterprise of CME:

## An Alternative Model Linking Independent Learning Centers and Health Services Research

*Distinct differences and similarities of continuing medical education (CME) providers are obscured. This is not only because the diversity of CME providers has been inadequately studied, but also because accreditation of CME providers places heavy emphasis on the administrative and logistical features of educational program planning, with less serious attention to testing theory and CME research. The product of improved collaboration among providers, and designed to facilitate the effective utilization of health services research and expanded CME efforts, independent learning centers may enable meaningful study and improvement of systems for learning, as well as monitoring of health care and education.*

## Accreditation and the Enterprise of CME

In the United States, the Accreditation Council for CME (ACCME)[1] has generated and monitors six mixed categories of sponsors: (1) medical schools, (2) specialty medical societies, (3) voluntary health organizations, (4) state medical associations or societies, (5) hospitals, and (6) others, including for-profit corporations and not-for-profit foundations. The sponsors appear to be at the same time both aggregated for practical purposes of accreditation, yet in need of separation for more intelligible analysis and quality improvement. There is no calibrated instrument to help discern the relative frequency of qualities within or among the various providers. Rather, this accreditation system has operated historically with the good intentions of participants who often volunteer to monitor and consult regarding application of the Standards for Commercial Support of Continuing Medical Education[2] and the Essentials for Accreditation.[3]

The approach in Canada is fundamentally the same. It focuses on principles for CME,[4] which form the grist of administrative and program planning. (Hereinafter, these three will be referred to as "Standards," "Essentials," and "Principles.") The Canadian accreditation process, however, is conducted under the auspices of a single political entity, the Association of Canadian Medical Colleges (ACMC), and is integrated with the overall medical school accreditation process. Each of the 16 Canadian medical schools is an accredited CME sponsor.

## Essentials, Principles, and Standards

Both the Essentials and the Principles are rooted in Ralph Tyler's[5] curriculum development model of 1949, which included four sets of activities: (1) the assessment of learning needs, (2) the determination of learning objectives, (3) the development of instructional materials, methods, resources to enable attainment, and (4) the evaluation of the learners' progress in relation to objectives. To Tyler's curriculum model, the ACCME[3] and ACMC[4] have added requirements that the accredited sponsor: (1) maintain an organizational mission statement that includes CME and (2) assure the availability of management and other sources necessary to effectively fulfill the CME mission. The sponsor is an institution or organization assuming responsibility for CME. The overall CME program of a sponsor consists of one or more educational activities consistent with the Essentials.[3]

Complementing the Essentials, the Standards are designed so that the CME activities of accredited sponsors are scientific and educational, and presented without the influence of pharmaceutical, medical, or other commercial supporters. The purpose of CME accreditation is to assure physicians and the public that CME activities meet accepted standards of education.[3] While the CME program of the sponsor often includes more than one CME activity, the accreditation process intends that all CME activities are coherent educational offerings based upon defined needs, explicit objectives, educational content, and methods.

To many who study theory and practice, Tyler's classical model, the Essentials, and the Principles, may be seen as theory needing to be tested for value. For others, they offer guideposts for good practice, marking a common-sense road to success that needs no testing. Training of practitioners and accreditation site reviewers in the tenets of program planning may be expected logically to homogenize distinctive differences between CME providers by focusing attention on compliance with predetermined standards of program planning, while at the same time minimizing attention to meaningful research.

## The Organization and Structure of CME Providers

Three original studies relate to CME providers, organizational function, and structure. Each study involves continuing professional education offered through institutions of higher education. There is a dearth of similar research for other types of CME providers.

Moutrie[6] studied the relative centralization or decentralization of program planning in six academic health centers and their continuing education units. He identified responsibilities of the individual schools, existing organizational structures, resources, and working relationships generally required to succeed in providing CME and other continuing education activities for health science professionals. Moutrie suggested that the institutional philosophy regarding independence of individual health science colleges dominated the decisions about (and the extent to which) centralization of continuing education administration occurred. As a result, for example, academic health centers with a high sense of independence within individual colleges were apt to be less centralized in their administration of continuing education than those more integrated into the larger institution.

In his national study of university-based CME programs, Moore[7] offered a combined theory of the organization of CME and outlined three levels of development: departmental domination, autonomy, and integration. At the level of departmental domination, CME programs demonstrate few external contacts, small staff with limited differentiation, and low production. At the autonomy level of development, programs show expanded contacts external to the organizational unit, minor differentiation of job responsibilities, and larger staffs, with identifiable policies, budgets, and recognition. Expanding organizational relationships and larger, more specialized staff with extensive resources mark integrated programs.

Fox[8] described relationships between formal organizational structures and the extent of participation of clients, faculty, and program administrators in planning continuing professional education programs in six southern US land-grant universities. He found that planning which occurred solely within the context of academic colleges was characterized by less participation of representatives from the targeted audiences. Conversely, planning which occurred in university-wide delivery systems was characterized by higher client participation than in college-based program planning.

## The Size and Scope of CME

The size and scope of the CME enterprise in North America are yet to be defined in reliable and concise terms, although several studies have approached the task. In 1977, Lewis Miller[9] suggested that the annual cost of CME in the United States was about $1.9 billion, including opportunity cost to physicians. Opportunity cost was defined as that portion of profit that is given up to do something else. For his analysis, Miller assumed that physicians gave up their opportunity to see additional patients in exchange for continuing their education. Of the $1.9 billion figure proffered by Miller, three quarters was in opportunity costs to physicians. The remaining $500 million included investments by government, hospitals, medical associations, medical schools, private industry, and specialty societies. It should be noted that a large portion of Miller's aggregate costs figure was extrapolated from survey results of Iowa physicians reported by Caplan[10] in 1974, at which time the average wage used to calculate opportunity costs of physicians was $49 415.

Toward the end of the 1970s and throughout the 1980s, descriptions of continuing medical education in the United States typically included the number of CME activities held during a year and CME requirements for relicensure, recertification, or membership in professional societies. Semiannual fact sheets[11,12] were published and distributed by the American Medical Association (AMA), and listings and counts of courses were published annually in the *Journal of the American Medical Association.*

Other approaches to assessing the size of the CME enterprise also have been tried. With data from the annual survey of the Liaison Committee on Medical Education (LCME), Wentz,[13] reported revenue exceeding $80 million for 121 US medical schools offering continuing medical education during 1991. This revenue included $55 million in enrollment fees, $6.5 million from medical school subsidies, $2 million from university hospitals, $2.25 million from other institutional resources including the private practices of faculty, and $14.25 million from outside sources, including pharmaceutical, and medical device companies. The CME expenses of medical schools during that same time period were reported at $76.5 million.

An unpublished ACCME report[14] of CME revenue and expense suggests the annual cost of CME for all types of providers may have run as high as $344 million for 1992 (see Table 13.1). Specialty societies accrued income over expenses at a rate of nearly $2 for every $1 spent, while expenses of not-for-profit foundations and for-profit corporations exceeded revenue by a margin of $3 to $2. Further, medical school revenue was about $9 for every $10 spent. Hospitals attracted about $9.50 for every $10 spent, and the revenue of state societies exceeded expenses by a margin of $4 to $3.

## Table 13.1

### Continuing Medical Education Revenue and Expenses for Selected Types of Sponsors:  ACCME Projections for 1992

| Type of Sponsor | Revenue | Expense | Difference |
| --- | --- | --- | --- |
| Professional/specialty societies | $161 195 042 | $ 90 347 878 | $ 70 847 164 |
| For-profit corporations & NFP foundations | 64 954 800 | 99 709 400 | -34 754 600 |
| Medical schools | 93 571 720 | 108 559 627 | -14 987 907 |
| Hospitals | 14 431 260 | 15 482 340 | -1 051 080 |
| State medical societies | 9 842 260 | 7 572 600 | 2 269 660 |
| Totals | $343 995 082 | $321 671 845 | $ 22 323 237 |

Despite the information contained in each of these reports, there continues to be much left for explanation. How much medical school support for CME is paid from state or other taxes? What activities of specialty societies are supported with apparent profits from CME activities? Does the performance of accredited for-profit corporations and the business practices of not-for-profit foundations fit with the expressed CME mission statement of these organizations? Other than confer-ences, what are the major kinds of CME activities offered by the different types of providers?

Those who study or regulate CME organizations recognize there is little consistency in the reporting of financial data. The LCME requests CME financial information on forms different from the ACCME which, in turn, differs from survey requests of the Society of Medical College Directors of CME (SMCDCME). Achieving reporting consistency is made simpler in Canada where only medical schools are accredited providers and only two organizations (the Royal College of Physicians and Surgeons of Canada and the College of Family Physicians of Canada) maintain separate approval mechanisms for CME activities or programs.

**Table 13.2**

**Distribution of SMCDCME Medical Schools:   Conferences and Symposia Held per Year for External Physicians (1984-85, 1986-87, 1988-89, 1990-91)**

| Reporting Year | Number of Courses for External Physicians | | | Total Schools |
|---|---|---|---|---|
| | 25th Percentile | 50th Percentile | 75th Percentile | |
| 1984-85 | 16 | 32 | 52 | 47 |
| 1986-87 | 22 | 34 | 56 | 56 |
| 1988-89 | 29 | 46 | 60 | 61 |
| 1990-91 | 30 | 61 | 100 | 61 |

**Table 13.3**

**Distribution of SMCDCME Medical Schools:  Number of External Attendees for Conferences and Symposia (1984-85, 1986-87, 1988-89, 1990-91)**

| Reporting Year | Number of External Attendees for Conferences | | |
|---|---|---|---|
| | 25th Percentile | 50th Percentile | 75th Percentile |
| 1984-85 | 725 | 1829 | 4104 |
| 1986-87 | 1340 | 2757 | 4962 |
| 1988-89 | 1000 | 2078 | 3300 |
| 1990-91 | 1200 | 2039 | 3957 |

# Courses, Enrollments, Tuition, and Fees

What is the size of enrollments at CME conferences, symposia, and courses? Through its biennial survey of North American medical schools, the SMCDCME has tracked CME provided by its member schools. An analysis of SMCDCME survey results for two fiscal years, (1984-85 and 1986-87),[15] reported increased numbers of CME activities and enrollments, and higher fees. Comparable data[16,17] are reported for 1988-89 and 1990-91, and displayed in Tables 13.2 and 13.3.

A review of these data reveals several trends. First, there is constant growth in the number of conferences and symposia over the years (Table 13.3). Second, CME enrollments for selected medical school activities increased as well, but with more sluggish growth and parity of enrollment (Table 13.3). Third, from 1984-85 through 1990-91, nearly all medical schools provided larger numbers of CME activities at county medical societies and community hospitals, and (consistent with data from 1984-85) fewer than a dozen medical schools conducted conferences by telephone and by television. Fourth, the per-hour fees for medical school-sponsored conferences or seminars at primary locations increased from an average of $12 per hour to over $15 per hour.[17]

In his recent Report to the ACCME Research Committee, Duff[14] includes 214 accredited sponsors reviewed during 1992, approximately 45% of the total number of national sponsors accredited in the United States. With data acquired from reverse site surveys, interim reports of accredited sponsors, site surveys, special reviews, and initial applications, Duff reports 9 962 separate activities implemented by either direct or joint sponsorship, generating a total enrollment of 442 376 physicians.

In summary, descriptions of CME available since the 1970s suggest an active physician community taking part in a large number of teaching and learning activities. These activities have been provided by a diversity of accredited sponsors whose major programmatic effort and most visible CME product is traditional conferences. CME programs accrue revenue and expenses for themselves or their parent organizations at differing rates which may be associated with the type of sponsor, as defined by ACCME. Qualitative differences among and between programs have not been studied carefully and are not immediately apparent. How, then, is the benefit of CME participation accounted?

## The Currency of CME: How Is It Acquired? How Is It Used?

Several specialty societies (including the American College of Obstetrics and Gynecology, the American Academy of Pediatrics, the American Academy of Family Physicians [AAFP], and the College of Family Physicians of Canada) have developed separate currencies of CME. For example, the AAFP approves CME activities for prescribed and elective credits in recertification of family physicians and for membership in their professional society. Similarly, the American College of Obstetrics and Gynecology issues cognates and electives. Most of these separate systems equate roughly with courses designated as Category 1 or Category 2 within the generally understood American Medical Association Physician's Recognition Award (PRA).

The PRA Information Booklet[18] defines Category 1 activities as those which satisfy the Essentials and are designated as Category 1 by an accredited sponsor, or international conferences approved by the American Medical Association for Category 1 credit. Category 2 activities include nonsupervised personal learning activities, self-instruction, consultation, patient care review, self-assessment, medical teaching, articles, publications, books, exhibits, and CME lectures and seminars designated as AMA PRA Category 2 by an accredited sponsor. Lectures and seminars not designated for CME credit, but found by the physician-learner to be effective learning experiences, also qualify as Category 2 CME activities. These various types of continuing medical education credits are often used as currency for hospital staff privileges, relicensure requirements, or membership in medical professional or specialty societies. Occasionally, they may be exchanged for discounts on medical professional liability premiums. In general, credits are awarded for participation in continuing medical education. Rarely are the awards performance based (ie, earned in terms of evaluated learning or clinical care). Rather, evaluation most often includes attendance reports, accounts of physicians' satisfaction, and analysis of fiscal status as products of CME course offerings.

## Accreditation: Participation, Costs, Benefits and Limitations

In both Canada and the United States, questions have been raised about the system of CME accreditation.[19-24] In the United States, leaders in CME question whether it is reasonable to expect that ACCME-accredited medical schools and ACCME-accredited pharmaceutical companies are actually held, or should be held, to identical standards.[21-22] So, too, questions have been raised about the adequacy of Tyler's classical curriculum planning model[25] and the Essentials[21] in their ability to support the kind of decision making that must guide Canadian and American CME providers during the decades to come.[21]

Seven organizations comprise the ACCME. They are the American Board of Medical Specialties (ABMS), the American Hospital Association (AHA), the American Medical Association (AMA), the Association for Hospital Medical Education (AHME), the Association of American Medical Colleges (AAMC), the Council of Medical Specialty Societies (CMSS), and the Federation of State Medical Boards (FSMB).[26] Each organization contributes to the annual operating budget of ACCME. The annual operating budget of the ACCME[27] for 1992 was $396 670, paid in the following increments by each member organization: ABMS, $19 500; AHA, $19 500; AMA, $19 500; AHME, $6500; AAMC, $19 500; CMSS, $19 500; and FSMB, $6500. Survey activities fees ($271 500) and other income ($14 670) accounted for the difference.[27] In January of 1993, each of the approximately 500 ACCME-accredited organizations was assessed a $500 annual fee to help support a new system put in place to monitor compliance with the Essentials and Standards. As administrative responsibility for the ACCME moves from the CMSS to the AMA (in 1994), an additional $500 000 over 2 years will be provided by the AMA to help implement the ACCME system.[28]

In 1992, support of the accreditation system in Canada approximated $60 000, exclusive of travel and other expenses associated with site visits conducted for the joint purpose of undergraduate and CME.[29] By the end of 1993, the ACMC may split the CME and undergraduate medical education accreditation processes. The underlying rationale for the possible division of responsibilities is an apparent lack of mutual interest by reviewers. Those in CME seem disinterested in undergraduate accreditation and those interested in undergraduate medical education seem disinterested in CME accreditation.[29]

To the credit of those involved in CME accreditation, assuring the success of this system has been no small accomplishment. Nevertheless, doubts about the adequacy of the Essentials have been raised. While many believe they should be addressed,[21,30] confronting possible limitations of the Essentials may not be easy. It is widely understood that the political process associated with achieving original adoption of the Essentials was so arduous and exhausting a political endeavor, that the prospect of challenging this fundamental construct of accreditation is in itself a barrier to change.

Many ACCME-accredited sponsors seem unprepared for major challenges. They are not fully subsidized, and to offset potential fiscal deficits, they become deeply involved in the provision of conferences, with the promise of spending a little money to attract a lot more. Most sponsors expect, or are expected, to break even or to turn financial profits. Trusting the logic of the Essentials for accountability and for accreditation review, CME planners carefully document educational needs assessment, objective setting, educational design, and budgetary decisions, and demonstrate the use of data from previously administered survey instruments and financial summaries. The pragmatism of program planning is codified and elevated for accreditation. Accordingly, the prospective value of diversity among the types of sponsors fades in comparison to their preoccupation with earnings and with their logistical and administrative responsibilities for compliance with the Essentials.

Some of the heavy dependence on the Essentials may be due, in part, to the limited training of those responsible for providing leadership in CME programs. It has been estimated that over 95 percent of those responsible for carrying out continuing education for professional groups in the United States have been trained as members of the professional groups with which they work, rather than in the field of adult education.[31] Many in responsible positions are likely to argue that their common sense, developed through their formal education and practical experience, is the basis for their CME successes.[32] It should not be surprising for only a few of those administrators to see the generation or testing of theories in adult development, adult learning, or evaluation as valuable contributions to CME.

The value, too, of accreditation is not well understood. Only one study of the ACCME process has been published.[33] Its purpose was "to attempt to understand the possible impact of the accreditation process on the quality of CME." Only descriptive statistics (frequency counts) were used to describe the results.[33] Sixty percent of 480 ACCME nationally accredited CME providers responded to the ACCME-sponsored questionnaire administered in 1988. Respondents indicated that the Essentials made it easier to deal with faculty, deans, and program directors, and that the needs assessment and evaluation Essentials were at the same time both the most important and difficult to accomplish. Many respondents indicated workshops were needed to teach them how to meet the Essentials and to train ACCME surveyors.

**Table 13.4**

**Accreditation Council for Continuing Medical Education Accredited Sponsors: Numbers and Types on Probation as of December 31, 1992**

| Type of Organization | Number | No. on Probation | % on Probation |
|---|---|---|---|
| Hospitals | 5 | 0 | 0 |
| Voluntary health organization | 12 | 2 | 16.7 |
| Medical schools | 122 | 5 | 4.1 |
| For-profit corporations | 74 | 3 | 4.1 |
| Not-for-profit foundations | 60 | 2 | 3.3 |
| Professional/specialty societies | 166 | 3 | 1.9 |
| **Total** | **439** | **15** | **3.4%** |

Whether it implies a lack of training by CME providers and ACCME surveyors, poor subsidies, or some other phenomenon, a recent report of the ACCME[14] indicates the highest number of providers on probation to be medical schools (see Table 13.4). This is an oddity deserving of further study, since many sponsors believe there is a measure of latitude granted to some professional associations, learned societies, and selected other providers. Despite the bona fide efforts of volunteers trained to implement the accreditation system, doubts persist about the wisdom of trying to hold hospitals, medical schools, pharmaceutical companies, and for-profit CME companies to the same standards. There are questions about the validity of mission statements, the motives of sponsors, and the interpretation of the Essentials. These apparent conflicts in accreditation deserve resolution, because the socially constructed validity of the Essentials and of the entire CME accreditation process may be at stake.

# Reorganizing the Provision of CME

To be sure, increasingly effective initiatives are being taken to help describe CME and its influence in North America. As researchers gain data and academic stability in this regard, more coordinated efforts may be expected of organizations interested in accounting for the effects of CME. As it becomes better defined, what may be expected of CME should become clearer.

The AMA provides the most comprehensive and widely accepted working definition of CME. Recognized by the ACCME,[26] it is as follows:

> *"Continuing medical education consists of educational activities which serve to maintain, develop, or increase the knowledge, skills, and professional performance and relationships that a physician uses to provide services for patients, the public, or the profession. The content of CME is that body of knowledge and skills generally recognized and accepted by the profession as within the basic medical sciences, the discipline of clinical medicine, and the provision of health care to the public."[18]*

In its PRA information booklet, the AMA indicates further that all continuing educational activities which assist physicians in carrying out their professional responsibilities more effectively and efficiently are CME. In contrast, educational activities that do not qualify as CME also are specified:

> *"Not all continuing educational activities which physicians may engage in, however, are CME. Physicians may participate in worthwhile continuing educational activities which are not related directly to their professional work, and these activities are not CME. Continuing educational activities which respond to a physician's nonprofessional educational need or interest, such as personal financial planning, and appreciation of literature or music, are not CME."[18]*

There has been a growing concern that this historically recognized definition of CME is inadequate to describe its current and expanding nature.[30,34] It demonstrates decidedly utilitarian features, facilitating administrative convenience for providers and for regulators involved with CME. Defining CME solely within the context of work guides the lifelong learning of physicians toward vocational skills and competencies. Attention is denied to the physician as a developing adult learner with cultural or human aspirations and responsibilities. For example, the value of art appreciation is discounted, since its direct application to medicine, or to the services physicians provide, is not immediately apparent.

It is ironic that the healthy intellect of those who maintain such expansive responsibility for the health of others is summarily dismissed. A gentler, more comprehensive and learner-oriented definition of CME might can be derived from earlier work in adult education:

> *". . . a process whereby (physicians) who no longer attend school on a regular full-time basis ... undertake sequential and organized activities with the conscious intention of bringing about changes in information, knowledge, understanding, or skill, appreciation and attitudes; or for the purpose of identifying or solving personal, professional, or community problems."[35]*

This alternative definition of CME raises the question of what it means to be educated. Historically, and not without influence from the profession, this question has been answered in a social context, changing from one point in time to another. The currently predominant operating definition of CME seems more rooted in society's appetite for credentialing than in any rational strategy for educating that might be found in the curricula of modern medical schools.[36] Accordingly, those interested in health care and education might be better served by a redefined CME-- one that encourages physicians to grow more attentive to their learning and to be able to contribute directly to an improved quality of medicine through more evenly fulfilled personal, professional, and community involvement.

## Dissemination and Adoption:  A Likely Link Between CME and Health Services Research?

Health services research has grown from the need to account for health care expenditures and the utilization of resources to a focus on physician performance and on outcomes of care.[37-40]  Building upon methods of political consensus and theories of diffusion,[41-44] the generation and dissemination of clinical practice guidelines[45,46] have garnered millions of dollars in federal, professional association, specialty society, and other support since 1988.  In contrast, the process of adoption has been left comparatively unattended in health services research.  For example, having encountered the disseminated guidelines or medical innovations, what causes or prevents physicians from adopting them?  How do personal and social forces affect the likelihood of successful change in a physician's practice?  A goal of the CME enterprise has been to implement practice changes.  The role of research in CME has been to explore both that goal and the course of change in medicine.

Major new initiatives in health care quality improvement are designed to monitor patterns of care and outcomes and to improve the process of producing typical care rather than to correct unusual errors.[37,40]  Yet, hospitals and physicians are often left to their own devices in terms of educational strategies that may extend beyond quality management methods.[38,47-49]  Can adoption be facilitated?  If so, how?  Especially during the past decade, research and theory building in adult education and in CME have emphasized these and similar questions related to change, learning, and adoption of innovations.[44,50-58]

That CME resources are limited is certain.  Just how limited is unclear, since research on the organization and financing of CME currently lacks cohesiveness and depth.  What is sure is that the provision of CME is largely uncoordinated, without federal or other policies to aid in setting priorities for reasonable allocation of resources.[59]  CME activity occurs without the benefit of a single overarching concept for the enterprise, without a forged link to the quality of health care, and without a coordinated means to measure progress toward achievement of goals.  The absence of such a system and the need to be resourceful in providing and studying education and health care prompt a proposal for review and criticism.

# Independent Learning Centers: An Alternative Model for Providing and Studying CME

With few exceptions, the most extended period of time for education follows completion of medical or surgical residency. Yet, medical schools and other medical teaching institutions do not place a singularly high priority on the continuing education of practitioners. Not surprisingly, the highly focused attention of faculty and staff follows the preponderance of governmental funds dedicated to undergraduate medical education and the patient care revenues of graduate medical education.

CME continues to be a largely uncoordinated effort. Both teaching and non-teaching hospitals offer CME to help meet minimum Joint Commission on Accreditation of Health Care Organizations standards or other hospital accreditation requirements. They sometimes present CME to promote services that might pay for or fill empty hospital beds. Medical schools and specialty societies offer annual conferences designed to teach large numbers of physicians, often with the intention of generating surplus revenues to pay for activities that are not CME related. To date, federally funded peer review organizations (PROs) which maintain volumes of potentially valuable medical review data have been virtually uninvolved in CME, beyond the issuance of administrative advisories and educational referrals to selected physicians.[38,48]

Through careful utilization of their limited resources, medical schools, hospitals, specialty societies, and PROs may find themselves uniquely positioned to provide useful CME curricula for very specific needs of individual practitioners. To improve the quality of CME and to develop functional linkages between these structures, a set of locally situated independent learning centers is proposed for use by medical practitioners, educators, and health services researchers.

## The Area Health Education Model

Precedents exist for remote site or regional health and education centers. A recent review[60] of the national Area Health Education Center (AHEC) program identified three major indicators of successful AHECs: (1) the formation of a new and permanent organization with participating schools and target communities that serve to decentralize and regionalize health professions education; (2) strong linkage of the organization to health service delivery in the target area; and (3) the inclusion of key decision makers from educational, service, and other organizations in the community who maintain authority for hiring staff and making program and budgetary decisions.

The study[60] suggested that the most successful AHECs demonstrate an ability to respond to current and emerging needs by remaining neutral, flexible, and more quick to respond than is possible within the administrative bureaucracies and priorities of traditional, more narrowly focused institutions. Successful AHECs are in close communication with local communities and the health care infrastructure. They are, thus, aware of local problems and are well positioned to mobilize community resources in developing local, accessible networks when new needs arise. The researchers conclude that the future viability of such centers will depend on their ability to maintain a focus on health professions education, despite state and community pressure to provide direct services (both clinical services and public education).[60]

The notion of independent learning centers is generated, in part, from selected literature,[60-68] experience of the current authors, and the research on CME providers. These data display the following: (1) that the power of institutional philosophy regarding independence of the individual health science colleges may impede working relationships required for successful presentation of continuing education;[6] (2) that planning which occurs solely within the context of academic colleges includes less participation of the targeted group of learners;[8] and (3) that CME units may experience a kind of development leading to expanded organizational relationships, larger staffs, and more extensive resources.[7] There are many similarities between AHECs and the newly proposed independent learning centers, but there are differences as well, particularly regarding research and the form of teaching and learning activities.

## The Self-directed Curriculum of Learning Centers: Where Does it Come From?

Historically, physicians have shared skills and trained one another in regard to medical and surgical techniques. Much of the learning associated with current physician practice comes from peers who serve to reflect and advance new ideas.[69-73] In this context, independent learning centers are seen as homes, not only for facilitating such skill exchanges, but also for connecting practitioners to formally sanctioned learning resources, materials, and methods. Having been formally schooled, physicians seek more schooling, and the medical school continues to be recognized as the institution specializing in those opportunities.

Medical schools can ill afford to retreat from the communities they serve. They continue to be held in high regard with respect to validation of scientific and clinical information. But they are viewed, too (by some practitioners), as medical competitors.[74,75] Involving medical and other professors in solving community-based problems with participation of local practitioners provides a chance for the university to alleviate the competitive fears of practitioners and to become more closely attuned to the problems of community-based practice.[62,76-79] Independent learning centers provide the medical practice community with an opportunity to more easily access what has been seen as the traditional "ivory tower" culture of the medical school. In turn, the medical school receives an opportunity for its CME and other curricula to better reflect the learning needs of practitioners and the health care needs of the community. Teaching is imparting knowledge or skill which facilitates learning; learning is acquiring a new skill or insight.[80] The design of a teaching activity includes roles assigned by setting a curriculum of conditions which the physician-learner must meet. While formal schooling can link teaching to such roles, not all learning is a result of formal teaching. Practicing physicians are adults, typically problem-centered, present-oriented, and self-directed in their approach to learning.[81-85] While the proposed learning centers must provide linkage to formal teaching, they must also grant access of self-directed physician-learners to the learning resources currently falling to the domain of the medical school and university.[62-64,76-79]

From the current literature,[86-90] finding complete agreement on a concise definition of self-directed learning proves very difficult, but descriptors can be discovered to guide curriculum planning in the learning centers:

> (1) *Self-directed learners are individuals who are able to plan, initiate, and evaluate their own learning experiences with or without the assistance of others.*

> (2) *Self-direction in learning can occur in a wide variety of situations, ranging from a teacher-directed classroom to self-planned and self-conducted learning projects.*

> (3) *Although certain learning situations are more conducive to self-direction in learning than are others, it is the personal characteristics of the learner--including his or her attitudes, values, and abilities - which ultimately determine whether self-directed learning will take place in a given learning situation.*

> (4) *The self-directed learner more often chooses or influences the learning objectives, activities, resources, priorities, and levels of energy expenditure than does the other-directed learner.*[88]

Physicians are often motivated to engage in formalized learning experiences (such as conferences or seminars) to the extent that those experiences are considered relevant to the goals, problems, and issues present in their personal, professional, or social lives.[58] In contrast, the traditional medical school is organized along specialty lines, not always focused in a practical, problem-based, or interdisciplinary manner. Faculty typically design undergraduate courses to enable mastery of discrete bodies of knowledge, to be applied at some time in the future. Conversely, the strategy of locally placed learning centers provides for solution of the immediate problems of practitioners, using information not only common to their specialty, but also information from other specialists, other health care providers, and persons not directly involved in the delivery of care.

# Who Implements the Curriculum?: Shared Responsibilities

The undergraduate and graduate curricula of medical schools present basic as well as applied information for training physicians. In addition, an advisor or mentor is assigned to guide the development of the student, since the CME curriculum of a practitioner studying through an independent learning center requires such guidance. The advisor is an informed resource who helps to facilitate the learning and achievement of physicians as they master the curriculum. The advisor may be a faculty member of the medical school and a recognized agent of the learning center, assigned by mutual agreement of the learning center, the physician-learner, and the advisor. Qualified peer mentors may choose to remain outside the formal career tracks of tenure and promotion of the university, but they must meet agreed university and center criteria for continued service.

Physicians and advisors need at least the following competencies: (1) conceptual competence for understanding the theoretical foundations of the profession; (2) technical competence to perform skills required of the profession; and (3) integrative competence to mold theory and skills in the practice setting. An understanding of the importance of critical thinking, communication skills, leadership, motivation for further education, and ethical conduct are among the shared expectations of the advisor, the medical practitioner, project faculty, and others interested in the provision of high-quality education and health care.[91] All those involved in the design and implementation of learning projects must recognize that the foundation for professional competence resides on a firm understanding that all learning is ultimately linked to practice.

Advisors and learners might meet two to four times per year, reviewing performance data to help determine educational needs. In addition, essential topic areas may be selected for a 3-year cycle or course of study. A 3-year cycle is based on limited research and is suggested, as it allows generous time for completion of learning projects.[58,85] The essential areas are determined to facilitate the successful achievement of primary knowledge, skills, or attitudinal goals of the physician. They are determined directly from health services research and other patient care data. Topic areas also are selected for the sake of curiosity, personal, or social improvement, and may be completed during the same 3-year cycle. To help assure the extension of high-quality university resources, faculty who participate as advisors, researchers, or teachers through the learning centers must be considered equal partners with the medical practitioners as well as the faculty of the university.

The knowledge base of the university provides an important piece, but not all of the knowledge base, of the learning centers. Data developed for evaluating access to care and quality of service can be used to help physicians assess needs in comparison with other physicians, on a local, regional, or a more widely circumscribed basis.

Accordingly, the individualized CME curriculum depicts the physician's performance in relation to predetermined standards of care, either achieved or professed locally or regionally, or on a more national scale. The introduction of such information in assessing the physician's learning needs enables a more universal perspective in terms of educational interventions that might involve interdisciplinary health care teams. Teams of practitioners may be matched with other teams for sharing tips on office efficiency, clinical advances, or team building. Such interventions may or may not require direct teaching, service, or research involvement of academic faculty; when they do, equal value must be granted to the learning center-based activities of faculty, as tenure and promotion decisions are made within the traditional medical school.

The determination of learning needs within centers is, in summary, derived from several sources. Educational needs assessment of the practitioner involves reviewing predetermined sets of performance objectives derived from or designed by the specialty society which represents the clinical specialty of the physician. In this instance, needs are determined in relation to specified objectives, standards of care, or clinical guidelines offered to inform the practice of medicine. Epidemiological reviews of health care problems of the community in the physician's service area, in addition to the individual needs and expressed desires of the physician regarding personal or social improvement, drive the curriculum. In essence, the independent learning center defines adequate health care performance, and permits self-assessment, self-monitoring, and self-directed planning of CME activities designed to achieve specified objectives integral to the overall educative and health care performance of the individual practitioner.

## Who Controls the Curriculum?

Hegemony is leadership or predominant influence exercised by one over others.[80] This concept, when considered in relation to the spirit of self-directed learning, fosters concern, particularly in regard to the role of learning center advisors. At its most fundamental level, self-directed learning presupposes control over definitions, processes, and evaluations by those who are endeavoring to learn, and not by external authorities.[92] Advisors must recognize that self-directed learning dignifies and respects the physician-learner, and challenges the conceptual and practical connections with authoritarian forms of education. This is not to say that the advisor is without influence over learning projects. It is to stress, however, that self-conscious criticism, coupled with an understanding of health care and political issues by the learner, is essential to successful self-directed learning completed through the centers.

The planned and purposeful nature of the independent learning centers requires cautious examination.[92-95] How can learner-centered control be exercised authentically in an institution that is both socially constructed and validated? Less authentic control can easily be imagined. Such control would occur without the knowledge of physicians, and would limit them in framing or making decisions about their learning by providing a predetermined conceptual framework that excludes selected ideas of activities, defining them as self-serving, subversive, unpatriotic, or even immoral. If the range of acceptable content has been preordained so that physicians deliberately or unwittingly steer clear of things they sense are deviant or controversial, then physician learning is controlled rather than self-directed. Physician-driven learning, from this perspective, must include: (1) coming to understand the origins, functioning, and contradictions of the system, and (2) working to change or replace it with one that honors the daily activities of the physician and the advisor.[92] All those involved in the design of learning projects must recognize that a fully developed project includes a reflective awareness of how one's desires and needs have been culturally formed, and how these factors can convince one to pursue learning projects in conflict with the best interests of the physician or his or her patient.

## Currency and Credit in the Learning Center

If one accepts that documented, carefully planned CME participation is likely to be more valuable than less carefully planned and more informal CME activities, then the value of participation in learning centers-developed CME may be recorded for individuals who comply with some reasonable model of CME planning. The currency of accreditation may be acquired through careful planning with the advisor and by demonstrated progress toward achievement of mutually predetermined performance indicators. Use of performance indicators allows awards of currency based upon mutually agreed measures of outcomes or change. Such indicators might include scores on selected tests of knowledge, laboratory records to show change in test ordering for selected diagnoses, or inpatient charts that indicate physician behaviors leading to improved health outcomes such as reduced incidence of pressure ulcers in adults.[96]

Although there are other terms that can be used to designate successful completion of an academic unit or change, the term "credit" seems to be the most universally accepted. The proposed concept of curriculum is not dependent upon the use of this term (or any other) so long as what is decided upon is common to all learning experiences. If it continues to be required, the currency of credit could be used in historically accepted ways such as relicensure, hospital staff privileges, membership, or certification in professional or specialty societies.

Service must be the driving principle that guides the basis of work in continuing medical education whether the work is manifest as instruction or research. As envisaged here, the independent learning centers must maintain and enhance service to the medical community and the public. Instruction may be seen in terms of direct teaching of medical doctors or in terms of modeling and assisting the values of lifelong learning. Research in these centers may not only generate new knowledge, it may also empower teachers, advisors, physicians, and the community to develop systems that enable them to solve their own problems and to generate their own innovations. While developing, funding, and even finding CME activities to promote such progress may be difficult, they may prove to be less problematic than learning the value of the activities themselves.

# Research in the Delivery of CME

What is the research agenda in the enterprise of CME?  What are the priorities for research?

Research is diligent and systematic inquiry or investigation into a subject in order to discover or revise facts, theories, or applications.[80] Research in CME may be defined by its evolving content and by its transactions with other fields of study. Like other educational research, the methods and designs of CME research are borrowed from the social and behavioral sciences, particularly anthropology, sociology, and psychology.  Until recently, much of the CME research effort was spent proving the effectiveness of CME to justify its role in the health care and educational systems.  As might be expected, its contributions may be explained in terms of social and psychological influences on the practice of medicine, as those influences help to explain physician behavior and patient outcomes.

## A General Framework for CME Research

As research on the effectiveness of CME has become more prominent and issues more apparent, questions about how to guide the development of CME research have become more frequent.  Efforts have been made to respond with sets of major research issues, but each set must be considered for its temporary nature.  As the factors influencing health care, education, and physicians in North America shift and change in intensity,[65,97-101] the CME research agenda must respond.

There are many ways that a response may be formulated.  One conceptual framework was derived in 1989 by an interdisciplinary group of persons interested in CME research.[102] This framework offered four overlapping categories of theory and information for developing specific projects.  The categories include: (1) environmental or cultural influences, (2) the physician/patient encounter, (3) measurement issues, and (4) learning issues.  A project that fits within the first category might consider the relative importance of structural impediments to making change in a hospital-based practice.  A study of communication patterns to help determine how physicians recognize knowledge and skill deficits in their performance is an example of the second.  Testing to increase the reliability of quality-of-care indicators illustrates the third category, and predicting the best instructional methods to effect certain learning objectives falls within the fourth. This conceptual framework from 1989 acknowledges the overlapping nature of many CME research ideas.

## A More Detailed Direction for Research in CME

Another strategy for those interested in studying physicians, learning, CME, and health care is to adapt seven foci for research from the literature of general adult and continuing education,[103] adding to their number and making them specific to physicians and health care.  These foci include:  (1) historical research; (2) research on adult development and learning; (3) research on gender, ethnic and other issues; (4)

research on education related to economic and social development; (5) research on education for public policy; (6) research on learning in the clinical workplace; and (7) research on knowledge systems.

Contemporary research in CME has identifiable roots in scholarship of the 1930s.[104] Recent studies[51-52] suggest sporadic activity for several decades but a steady and rapidly increasing rate of productivity, especially during the most recent decade. Earlier descriptive studies[104-105] now share the attention of those with interest in research methods as well as generating and testing of theory.[58,106-107] As patterns of research and research questions become more readily identifiable, an updated historical perspective on research in CME may help to guide the subsequent investment of resources into CME research.

Research on adult learning and on the unique developmental perspectives of selected groups such as minorities, women, and older or younger physicians deserves further inquiry,[108-111] since it is generally understood that specific social and cultural contexts affect situational teaching and learning. Not to be overlooked, however, is the knowledge that can be gleaned from studies that involve newer imaging techniques,[112-113] cognition,[114-116] and neuropsychological dynamics of cognition and memory.[117-118] In a pragmatic sense, when analyzing the health care behavior of physicians, the biomedical foundations of such knowledge may enable more concise determinations of educational and other needs. For example, the performance of a young male physician with a previously undiagnosed mild brain injury may be expected to show signs of disrupted concentration and poor judgment[118] compared with his healthier colleagues. Yet, a carefully developed rehabilitation plan with medical intervention[119] may help considerably in restoring the physician's behavior as a competent health care provider. In terms of scholarly activity, this intrapersonal research direction seems worthy of attention in explaining behaviors left unresolved by the predominating social and psychological frameworks more globally applied to CME research and adult learning.

Research on the role of CME in assuring access to health services, careful utilization of those services, and increased quality of health care will enable administrators and policy makers to enact better-informed decisions regarding both education and health policy.[45,46,48,120] Investigation into learning that occurs in the office, hospital, or other workplace must focus on the dissemination, utilization, and quality of innovations. The medical workplace has become more highly technological and frequently is equipped with sophisticated systems of communication. The role of communications systems and communications planning in this regard must be explored. Pressure for greater responsiveness to stakeholder needs and expectations has produced radical change in traditional health care as well as communications. Planning for health care and communications systems has become more complex, driven by the necessity for more farsighted management, which is required, because changing socioeconomic, demographic, and political conditions impose unacceptable penalties on those who cling to traditional mechanisms.[120,121]

Strategic planning must be oriented toward building relationships: (1) within the health care provider system as seen in the philosophy of continuous quality improvement; (2) with those who are interested in the technology of communicating images, sound, and other data; and (3) with patients and others who pay for health care services. Developing and maintaining mutual commitment to health professional education goals may be expected to produce mutual benefits in terms of systems costs and patient care outcomes. Although disseminating, adjusting, adopting, and implementing innovations must be studied in relation to CME, such research must account for the culture which emerges with changing communications on work teams[122-126] or in the workplace itself.[127-129] The physician's response to the innovation and the technology itself must be reviewed for the social meaning that it helps simultaneously to construct and interpret.[130,131]

In the context of these issues, fundamental questions must be asked of the CME accreditation process. How reliable is the process? Does it improve the quality of CME? Can accreditation recognize the individualized learning activities of physicians? Can accreditation promote diversity among accredited sponsors? How can the accreditation process be improved? What may be expected of CME accreditation, in terms of measurable outcomes for physicians and patients? How will the CME accreditation process be evaluated?

Finally, the utilization of knowledge systems and the interaction of the individual physician with: (1) other health care professionals; (2) local, regional, and national data bases; and (3) the knowledge systems themselves must be explored. It is from the study of the natural interactions with knowledge and its application to the resolution of everyday health care problems that further research and practice in CME can become better informed. It is from this interaction that theories may be developed, pertaining to change and explaining behavior, and testing hypotheses that can be added to increase the common knowledge pool in CME and health services research.

## Paradigms of CME Research

Although other paradigms have begun to gain favor among CME and health services researchers, the most widely valued approach has come from the positivist school of thought. In this view, scientific knowledge consists of facts that could be subsumed under general laws. Scientific knowledge is gained through sensory or observational experience combined with logic.[132] The basic assumption underlying positivist research is the notion of a single, objective reality that can be observed, known, and measured. Within the positivist paradigm, researchers amass facts to describe the world, the aim being to uncover laws that will explain aspects of the objective reality. Examples of positivist research in CME[133,134] typically include determining the effects of CME as an independent variable set to influence the knowledge or behavior of physicians who participate in a CME program.

Interpretive research challenges the basic assumption of the positivist paradigm. From this school of thought, reality is not seen as an object that can be discovered and measured but rather as a construction of the human mind.  Research out of this paradigm has been called qualitative, naturalistic, subjective, and grounded theory.[132] Interpretive research focuses on process rather than outcomes.  A strength of this type of research is its methods for generating hypotheses and substantive theory.  Rather than testing hypotheses, interpretive research in CME[58,110] inductively builds abstractions, concepts, hypotheses, or theories to explain how certain phenomena occur.

The aims of critical research are enlightenment and empowerment brought about through an educational process that leads to transformative action.[132]  From this school of thought, researchers assume that society and human nature are human constructions that can be altered through progressive understanding of historically specific processes and structures.  In this form of research, the task becomes developing methodological approaches involving the subject of research in the negotiation of meaning and power, as well as the discovery and validation of knowledge. In this model, the role of the scientist is not to separate himself or herself from the current phenomenon of study, but rather to engage those on whom research is being done in self-conscious action.  Knowledge is viewed as subjective, emancipatory, and productive of fundamental social change.[132] Examples of critical research[126,135,136] may be found in literature not ordinarily associated with CME, but sometimes with other areas of study such as health services, public health, or preventive medicine.

Provision of the highest quality health care by the best trained professionals is an expectation strongly held by most North Americans,[97-101] and from examples of high-quality research in these three paradigms, studies may continue to be developed to foster change in CME, adoption of innovation, and health care.  By involving practitioners in the design and implementation of CME and health care studies that generate or test their own theories, the adoption of innovation by practitioners may be expected to occur rationally.  This expectation arises in part because of practitioners' progressive knowledge of the benefits of changing and, in part, because of their expressed influence on the political and economic processes reflecting the social attitudes and values of North Americans.  Ultimately, the success of the independent learning centers must be judged in this context, and in an empirical manner, by the medical communities and the public they serve.

## Independent Learning Centers:  A Focus for Research and Practice

Rather than commercial and governmental support scattered across disparate providers of uneven quality, focusing resources on the development and testing of independent learning centers could maximize the benefits of commercial and governmental dollars spent to support CME and health services research. With improvements on the AHEC model, a more centralized and accountable financial and performance-based system could be derived for evaluating both CME and health care. Selected hospitals might provide currently unused wards or other space to house administrative or learning resources of the independent learning centers, from which such research could be developed.

Developing the learning centers enables all those interested in CME and associated research to focus attention on perennial issues in health care and education to achieve these five objectives: (1) determine the effects of interventions; (2) extend the capabilities of health services research through the physician to the community; (3) enable research on the adult development and learning of physicians in change; (4) evaluate the effects of accreditation; and (5) study the access and quality of health care. By directing energy toward research and evaluation in cooperative independent centers of physician learning, state, provincial, or federal governments show the potential of providing appropriate channels for contributing to, and accounting for, the effects of their policies and actions. In addition, specialty and professional societies may assure themselves and the consumer public that the education required for membership and certification is designed to help maintain and enhance the quality of health care. Assurances may be delivered not only in terms of physician participation in CME, but also in the form of reportable research and health care outcomes for individuals and targeted communities. Consumers, through their governments and licensing boards, may make better-informed decisions to support activities that assure access and quality of health care. Finally, those physicians comprising the constituency of organized medicine itself may be assured that the education provided for them is prepared to help meet their needs as individuals, as members of the medical community, and as providers of health care to their patient population.

## References

1. *Accreditation: Procedural and Administrative Information.* Lake Bluff, Ill: Accreditation Council for Continuing Medical Education; 1993.

2. *Standards for Commercial Support of Continuing Medical Education.* Lake Bluff, Ill: Accreditation Council for Continuing Medical Education; 1992.

3. *Essentials and Guidelines for Accreditation of Sponsors of Continuing Medical Education.* Lake Bluff, Ill: Accreditation Council for Continuing Medical Education; 1984.

4. *Accreditation of University-based Programs of CME: Manual of Procedure.* Ottawa, Ontario: Association of Canadian Medical Colleges; 1990.

5. Tyler RW. *Basic Principles of Curriculum and Instruction.* Chicago, Ill: University of Chicago Press; 1949.

6. Moutrie RR. *The Goals, Organizational Structure, and Financing of Continuing Education Administrative Units at Selected Academic Health Centers.* (unpublished doctoral dissertation). Lincoln, Neb: University of Nebraska; 1978.

7. Moore DE, Jr. *The Organization and Administration of Continuing Medical Education in Academic Medical Centers.* (unpublished doctoral dissertation). Urbana-Champaign, Ill: University of Illinois; 1982.

8. Fox RD. Formal organizational structure and participation in planning continuing professional education. *Adult Education Quarterly.* 1981,209-226.

9.  Miller LA. The current investment in continuing medical education. In: Egdahl RH, Gertman PM, eds. *Quality Health Care: The Role of Continuing Medical Education.* Germantown, Md: Aspen Systems Corporation; 1977:143-160.

10. Caplan RM. Survey of continuing medical education in Iowa. *Journal of the Iowa Medical Society.* 1974;64:159-166.

11. American Medical Association. *Continuing Medical Education Fact Sheet.* Chicago, Ill: American Medical Association; 1987.

12. American Medical Association. *Continuing Medical Education Fact Sheet.* Chicago, Ill: American Medical Association; 1988.

13. Wentz DK. Introductory comments. Presented at the Third National Conference on CME Provider-Industry Collaboration in CME; October 8, 1992; Chicago, Illinois.

14. Duff WM. *Accreditation Council for Continuing Medical Education: Annual Report to the Research Committee, January 1, 1992-December 31, 1992.* Lake Bluff, Ill: October 29, 1992. (unpublished)

15. Mazmanian PE, Harrison RV, Osborne CE. Diversity across medical schools: programs, enrollments and fees for continuing medical education. *J Cont Educ Health Prof.* 1990;10:23-33.

16. Society of Medical College Directors of Continuing Medical Education. Survey for 1988-89: *Descriptive results. (Unpublished) Report of the Survey Subcommittee of the Research Committee.* R.V. Harrison (Chairman) Washington, D.C.: April, 1990.

17. Society of Medical College Directors of Continuing Medical Education Survey for 1990-91: *Descriptive results. (Unpublished) Report of the Survey Subcommittee of the Research Committee.* R.V. Harrison (Chairman). Washington, DC: April, 1992.

18. American Medical Association. *The Physician's Recognition Award: 1993 Information Booklet.* Chicago, Ill: American Medical Association; 1993.

19. Stearns NS, Bashook PG. Continuing medical education accreditation, evaluation and credits. *Mobius.* 1985;5:51-53.

20. Escovitz GH. It's too soon to change the system. *Mobius.* 1985;5:53-54.

21. Richards RK. CME accreditation: an overview, with two challenges. *J Cont Educ Health Prof.* 1992;12:77-81.

22. Escovitz GH, Davis DA. A bi-national perspective on continuing medical education. *Acad Med.* 1990;65:545-549.

23. Parboosingh JT, Gondocz ST. The maintenance of competence (MOCOMP) program: motivating specialists to critically appraise the quality of their continuing medical education activities. *Can J Surg.* 1993;36:29-32.

24. Educating Future Physicians for Ontario. *Executive Summary of the Component 1 Interim Report.* Hamilton, Ontario: E.F.P.O. Co-ordinating Centre at McMaster University; 1992.

25. Sork TJ. Theoretical foundations of educational program planning. *J Cont Educ Health Prof.* 1990;10:73-83.

26. Maitland FM. Accreditation of sponsors and certification of credit. In: Rosof AB, Felch WC, eds. *Continuing Medical Education: A Primer.* 2nd ed. New York, NY: Praeger; 1992:15-27.

27. Budget as reported by the Secretary (Mitchell L. Rhodes, M.D.) to the Accreditation Council for Continuing Medical Education. Lake Bluff, Illinois. December 31, 1992.

28. Page L. AMA gets accreditation contract. In: American Medical News. Chicago, Illinois: *American Medical Association.* June 14, 1993;pgs 3 and 28.

29. Personal Communication with Harvey Barkin, M.D., Secretary, Council for Accreditation of Canadian Medical Colleges. April 23, 1993.

30. Davis D, Parboosingh JT. 'Academic' CME and the social contract. *Acad Med.* 1993;68:329-332.

31. Griffith WS. Persistent problems and promising prospects in continuing professional education. In: Cervero RM, Scanlan CL, eds. *Problems and Prospects in Continuing Professional Education: New Directions for Continuing Education, no. 27.* San Francisco, Calif: Jossey-Bass; 1985: 101-108.

32. Cervero RM. Changing relationships between theory and practice. In: Peters JM, Jarvis P, et al. *Adult Education: Evaluation and Achievements in a Developing Field of Study.* San Francisco, Calif: Jossey-Bass Publishers; 1991:19-41.

33. Green JS, Cohen S, Rosner F, et al. The hidden value of accreditation of continuing medical education. *J Cont Educ Health Prof.* 1991;11:53-63.

34. Davis DA. Meta-analyses and metaphors in CME literature. *J Cont Educ Health Prof.* 1991;11: 85-86.

35. Liveright AA, Haygood N, eds. *The Exeter Papers: Report of the First International Conference on The Comparative Study of Adult Education.* Boston, Mass: Center for the Study of Liberal Education for Adults of Boston University; 1968:8.

36. Swanson AG, Anderson MB, eds. *Educating Medical Students: Assessing Change in Medical Education (ACME-TRI Report).* Washington, DC: Assoc American Med Colleges. 1992:52-60.

37. Pierson RN Jr. Peer review and CME. In: Rosof AB, Felch WC, eds. *Continuing Medical Education: A Primer.* New York, NY: Praeger; 1986:134-145.

38. Jencks SF, Wilensky GR. The health care quality improvement initiative. *JAMA.* 1992; 268:900-903.

39. Anderson GM, Grunbach K, Luft HS, Roos LL, Mustard C, Brook R. Use of coronary artery bypass surgery in the United States and Canada: influence of age and income. *JAMA.* 1993;269:1661-1666.

40. Ramsey PG, Wenrich MD, Carline JD, Inui TS, Larson EB, LoGerfo JP. Use of peer ratings to evaluate physician performance. *JAMA.* 1993;269:1655-1660.

41. Casebeer L. Updating the theoretical constructs of change. *J Cont Educ Health Prof.* 1992;12:105-110.

42. Rogers EM. *Diffusion of Innovations.* 3rd edition. New York, NY: The Free Press; 1983: 1-37.

43. *Information Dissemination to Health Care Practitioners and Policymakers: Annotated Bibliography.* Washington, DC; Agency for Health Care Policy and Research (AHCPR); 1992. U.S. Dept. of Health and Human Services Publication No. 92-0030.

44. Lockyer J. What do we know about adoption of innovation? *J Cont Educ Health Prof.* 1992;12:33-38.

45. Eddy DM. Should we change the rules for evaluating medical technologies? In: Gelijns AC, ed. *Modern Methods of Clinical Investigation.* Washington, DC: National Academy Press. 1990:117-134.

46. Field MJ, Lohr KN, eds. *Guidelines for Clinical Practice: From Development to Use.* Washington, D.C.: National Academy Press, 1992.

47. Berwick DM. Continuous improvement as an ideal in health care. *N Eng J Med.* 1989;320:53-56.

48. Institute of Medicine. *Medicare: A Strategy for Quality Assurance.* Volume I. Washington, DC: National Academy Press; 1990.

49. Yessian MR. State medical boards and quality assurance. *J Med Licensure and Discipline.* 1992;79:126-135.

50. McLaughlin PJ, Donaldson JF. Evaluation of continuing medical education programs: selected literature, 1984-1988. *J Cont Educ Health Prof.* 1991;11:65-88.

51. Haynes RB, Davis DA, McKibbon A, Tugwell PA. Critical appraisal of the efficacy of continuing medical education. *JAMA.* 1984;251:61-64.

52. Davis DA, Thomson MA, Oxman AD, Haynes RB. Evidence for the effectiveness of CME. *JAMA.* 1992;268:1111-1117.

53. Beaudry JS. The effectiveness of continuing medical education: a qualitative synthesis. *J Cont Educ Health Prof.* 1989;9:285-307.

54. Mann KV. Enhancing learning: how can learning theory help? *J Cont Educ Health Prof.* 1990;10:177-186.

55. Marsick VJ, Smedley RR. Health education. In: Merriam SB, Cunningham PM, eds. *Handbook of Adult and Continuing Education.* San Francisco, Calif: Jossey-Bass Publishers; 1989:384-396.

56. Smutz WD, Queeney DS. Professionals as learners: a strategy for maximizing professional growth. In: Cervero RM, Azzaretto JF, et al, eds. *Visions for the Future of Continuing Professional Education.* Athens, Ga: The University of Georgia; 1990:183-208.

57. Bennett NL, LeGrand BF. *Developing Continuing Professional Education Programs.* Urbana-Champaign, Ill: University of Illinois; 1990.

58. Fox RD, Mazmanian PE, Putnam RW. A theory of learning and change. In: Fox RD, Mazmanian PE, Putnam RW, eds. *Changing and Learning in the Lives of Physicians.* New York, NY: Praeger Publishers; 1989:161-175.

59. Grotelueschen AD. Investing in professional development: a need for national policy. In: Cervero RM, Azzaretto JF, et al, eds. *Visions for the Future of Continuing Professional Education.* Athens, Ga: The University of Georgia; 1990:63-78.

60. Fowkes VK, Campeau P, Wilson S. The evolution and impact of the national AHEC program over two decades. *Acad Med.* 1991;66:211-220.

61. The Learning Society: *Report of the Commission on Post-Secondary Education in Ontario.* D.O. Davis (Chairman) Toronto, Ontario; 1972.

62. Illich ID. *Deschooling Society.* New York, NY: Harper and Row Publishers; 1970.

63. Illich ID. *Medical Nemesis.* New York, NY: Random House Inc; 1976.

64. Freire P. *Pedagogy of the Oppressed.* New York, NY: Seabury Press; 1970.

65. Curry L, Mann KV. Priority issues in continuing medical education show sensitivity to change in Canadian health care. *Can Med Assoc J.* 1990;142:299-301.

66. Knox AB. Evaluating continuing professional education. In: Cervero RM, Scanlan CL, eds. *Problems and Prospects in Continuing Professional Education.* San Francisco, Calif: Jossey-Bass Publishers; 1985:61-73.

67. Wilson MP, McLaughlin CP. Leadership and management. In: *Academic Medicine.* San Francisco, Calif: Jossey-Bass Publishers; 1984.

68. Houle CO. Possible futures. In: Stern MR, ed. *Power and Conflict in Continuing Professional Education.* Belmont, CA: Wadsworth Publishing; 1983:254-263.

69. Lomas J, Enkin M, Anderson GM, Hannah WJ, Vayda E, Singer J. Opinion leaders vs audit and feedback to implement practice guidelines. *JAMA.* 1991;265:2202-2207.

70. Lomas J, Haynes RB. A taxonomy and critical review of tested strategies for the application of clinical practice recommendations: from "official" to "individual" clinical policy. In: Battista RN, Lawrence RS, eds. *Implementing Preventive Services.* New York, NY: Oxford Press; 1988:77-94.

71. Stross JK, Bole GG. Evaluation of a continuing education program in rheumatoid arthritis. *Arthritis Rheum.* 1980;23:846-849.

72. Stross JK, Hiss RG, Watts CM, Davis WK, MacDonald R. Continuing education in pulmonary disease for primary care physicians. *Am Rev Resp Dis.* 1983;127:739-746.

73. Manning PR, DeBakey L. *Medicine: Preserving the Passion.* New York, NY: Springer-Verlag; 1987.

74. Caplan R, Gallis H. Financial well-being. In: Fox RD, Mazmanian PE, Putnam RW, eds. *Changing and Learning in the Lives of Physicians.* New York, NY: Praeger Publishers; 1989:55-64.

75. Paul HA, Osborne CE. Relating to others in the profession. In: Fox RD, Mazmanian PE, Putnam RW, eds. *Changing and Learning in the Lives of Physicians.* New York, NY: Praeger Publishers; 1989:123-133.

76. Illich ID. *Toward A History of Needs.* New York, NY: Random House Inc; 1978.

77. Illich I. *Tools for Conviviality.* New York, NY: Harper and Row Publishers; 1973.

78. Hentschel D. The hybrid model for implementing the continuing education mission statement. *Continuing Higher Education Review.* 1991;55:155-167.

79. Caffarella RS, Duning B, Patrick S. Delivering off-campus instruction: changing roles and responsibilities of professors in higher education. *Continuing Higher Education Review.* 1992;56:155-167.

80. *Webster's Encyclopedic Unabridged Dictionary of the English Language.* New York, NY: Gramercy Books; 1989.

81. Kantrowitz MP. Problem-based learning in continuing medical education: some critical issues. *J Cont Educ Health Prof.* 1991;11:11-18.

82. Barrows H, Tamblyn R. *Problem-based Learning: An Approach to Medical Education.* New York, NY: Springer Publishing; 1980.

83. Verby PE. Physicians learning continuing medical education from third-year medical students. *J Cont Educ Health Prof.* 1991;11:277-282.

84. Adelson R. Adult learning. In: Adelson R, Watkins FS, Caplan RM. *Cont Educ Health Prof.* Rockville, Md: Aspen Systems Corporation; 1985:3-19.

85. Tough A. *The Adult's Learning Projects.* Toronto, Ontario: Ontario Institute for Studies in Education; 1971.

86. Caffarella RS, Caffarella EP. Self-directedness and learning contracts in adult education. *Adult Education Quarterly.* 1986;36:226-234.

87. Field L. An investigation into the structure, validity, and reliability of Guglielmino's self-directed learning readiness scale. *Adult Education Quaterly.* 1989;39:125-139.

88. Guglielmino LM. Guglielmino responds to Field's investigation. *Adult Education Quarterly.* 1989;39:235-240.

89. Candy PC. *Self-direction for Lifelong Learning: A Comprehensive Guide to Theory and Practice.* San Francisco, Calif: Jossey-Bass Publishers; 1991.

90. Fox RD. New research agendas for CME: organizing principles for the study of self-directed curricula for change. *J Cont Educ Health Prof.* 1991;11:155-167.

91. Berlin LS. Balancing liberal arts with professional education. *Innovator.* 1993;24:27-31.

92. Brookfield S. Self-directed learning, political clarity, and the critical practice of adult education. *Adult Education Quarterly.* 1993;43:227-242.

93. Habermas J. *The Theory of Communicative Action.* Boston, Mass: Beacon Press; 1987.

94. Habermas J. *On the Logic of the Social Sciences.* Cambridge, Mass: The MIT Press; 1988:43-74.

95. Bonham LA. Guglielmino's self-directed learning readiness scale: what does it measure? *Adult Education Quaterly.* 1991;41:92-99.

96. US Department of Health and Human Services, Public Health Service, Agency for Health Care Policy and Research (AHCPR). Pressure Ulcers in Adults: Prediction and Prevention (AHCPR Publication No. 92-0047). Rockville, Maryland: AHCPR; 1992.

97. Osborn JE. The nature of public health after reform. *Acad Med.* 1993;68:237-243. 98. Blendon RJ, Donelan K, Leitman R, et al. Physicians' perspectives on caring for patients in the United States, Canada, and West Germany. *N Eng J Med.* 1993;328:1011-1016.

99. Heyssel RM. Beyond 'health care reform.' *Acad Med.* 1993;68:178-182.

100. Schroeder SA. Training an appropriate mix of physicians to meet the nation's needs. *Acad Med.* 1993;68:118-122.

101. Woolhandler S, Himmelstein DU, Lewontin JP. Administrative costs in US hospitals. *N Eng J of Med.* 1993;329:400-403.

102. Davis D. *Exploring New Frontiers in CME: Notes from the Banff Conference.* Unpublished working paper. Hamilton, Ontario: Continuing Health Sciences Division, McMaster University; 1989.

103. Deschler D, Hagan N. Adult education research: issues and directions. In: Merriam SB, Cunningham PM, eds. *Handbook of Adult and Continuing Education.* San Francisco, Calif: Jossey-Bass Publishers; 1989:147-167.

104. Shepherd GR. History of continuing medical education in the United States since 1930. *J Med Educ.* 1960;35:740-758.

105. Nakamoto J, Verner C. *Continuing Education in Medicine: A Review of North American Literature, 1960-1970.* Vancouver, Canada: University of British Columbia; 1972.

106. Richards RK. *Continuing Medical Education.* New Haven, Conn: Yale University Press; 1978.

107. Crandall SJS. The role of continuing medical education in changing and learning. *J Cont Educ Health Prof.* 1990;10:339-348.

108. Crandall SJS, Volk RJ, Loemker V. Medical students' attitudes toward providing care for the underserved. *JAMA.* 1993;269:2519-2523.

109. Lurie N, Slater J, McGovern P, Ekstrum J, Quam L, Margolis K. Preventive care for women: does the sex of the physician matter? *N Eng J Med.* 1993;329:478-482.

110. Mizrahi T. *Getting Rid of Patients.* New Brunswick, NJ: Rutgers University Press; 1986.

111. Franks P, Clancy CM. Physician gender bias in clinical decisionmaking: screening for cancer in primary care. *Med Care.* 1993;31:213-218.

112. Singer HS, Wong DF, Brown JE, et al. Positron emission tomography evaluation of dopamine D-2 receptors in adults with Tourette's syndrome. *Advances in Neurology.* 1992;58:233-239.

113. Wilson JTL, Hadley DM, Wiedmann KD, Teasdale GM. Intercorrelation of lesions detected by magnetic imaging after closed head injury. *Brain Injury.* 1992;6:391-399.

114. Osherson DN, Smith EE. *Thinking.* Cambridge, Mass: The MIT Press; 1990.

115. Luria AR. *The Making of Mind.* Cambridge, Mass: Harvard University Press, 1979.

116. Luria AR. *Cognitive Development: Its Cultural and Social Foundations.* Cambridge, Mass: Harvard University Press; 1976:161-165.

117. Harrell M, Parente F, Bellingrath EG, Lisicia KA. *Cognitive Rehabilitation of Memory.* Gaithersburg, Md: Aspen Publishers Inc; 1992.

118. Parente R, Anderson-Parente JK. Retraining memory: theory and application. *J Head Trauma Rehab.* 1989;4:55-65.

119. Zasler ND. Pharmacological aspects of cognitive function following traumatic brain injury. In: Kreutzer JS, Wehman PH, eds. *Cognitive Rehabilitation for Persons with Traumatic Brain Injury.* Baltimore, Md: Paul H. Brookes Publishing Company 1991:87-93.

120. Brody EW. *Managing Communication Processes.* New York, NY: Praeger Publishers 1991:48.

121. Paisley W. New media and methods of health communication (Revised Draft, November, 1991) *Presentation prepared for the Conference on Effective Dissemination of Clinical and Health Information.* Tucson, Arizona: University of Arizona, September, 1991. Sponsored by the Agency for Health Care Policy and Research; 1991.

122. Berger CR, Gudykunst WB. Uncertainty and communication. In: Dervin B, ed. *Progress in Communication Sciences,* Volume X. Norwood, NJ: ABLEX Publishing Corporation; 1991:21-66.

123. Paisley W. Information and work. In: Dervin B, Voigt MJ, eds. *Progress in Communication Sciences,* Volume II. Norwood, NJ: ABLEX Publishing Corporation; 1980:113-165.

124. Perry S, Wilkinson SL. The technology assessment and practice guidelines forum: a modified group judgment method. *Intl J Tech Assess Health Care.* 1992;8:289-300.

125. Maynard DW. Bearing bad news in clinical settings. In: Dervin B, ed. *Progress in Communication Sciences,* Volume X. Norwood, NJ: ABLEX Publishing Corporation; 1991:143-172.

126. Guidotti TL, Peabody HDD, Scrutchfield FD. Interaction between a medical group and a school of public health: a case study of a productive affiliation. *Am J Prev Med.* 1985;1:30-35.

127. Lindberg DAB, Siegel ER, Rabb BA, Wallingford KT, Wilson SR. Use of MEDLINE by physicians for clinical problem solving. *JAMA.* 1993;269:3124-3129.

128. Bautz JB, Schectman JM, Elinsky EG, Pawlson LG. Magnetic resonance imaging: diffusion of technology in an ambulatory setting. *Intl J Tech Assess Health Care.* 1992;8:301-308.

129. Levinson W, Stiles WB, Inui TS, Engle R. Physician frustration in communicating with patients. *Med Care.* 1993;31:285-295.

130. Liebes T. On the convergence of theories of mass communication and literature regarding the role of the 'reader.' In: Dervin B, ed. *Progress in Communication Sciences,* Volume IX. Norwood, NJ: ABLEX Publishing Corporation; 1989:123-143.

131. Moyer VA. Learning critical appraisal skills at the faculty level: methods and benefits. *Teach Learn Med.* 1992;4:115-117.

132. Merriam SB. How research produces knowledge. In: Peters JM, Jarvis P, et al, eds. *Adult Education: Evaluation and Achievement in a Developing Field of Study.* San Francisco, Calif: Jossey-Bass Publishers; 1991:42-65.

133. Jennett PA, Laxdal OE, Hayton RC, et al. The effects of CME upon family physician performance in office practice: a randomized controlled study. *Med Educ.* 1988;22:139-145.

134. Cohen SJ, Stookey GK, Katz BP, Drook CA, Smith DM. Encouraging primary care physicians to help smokers quit. *Ann Intern Med.* 1989;110:648-652.

135. Budrys G. 'Keeping the faith' and market realities: physicians in an HMO. *Qualitative Health Research.* 1991;1:469-496.

136. Hopkins DR. Public health measures for prevention and control of AIDS. *Public Health Reports.* 1987;102:463-467.

# Section III

# Annotated Bibliography

**Avorn J.** Improving drug therapy decisions through educational outreach. A randomized controlled trial of academically based 'detailing.' *N Engl J Med.* 1983;308:1457-1463.

This randomized trial used Medicaid data to identify high prescribers of certain drugs. One group received printed material only and another received a visit from a pharmacist—the so-called academic detail visit. The group visited by a pharmacist was the only group with significant decreases in the three drug groups studied.

**Beaudry JS.** The effectiveness of continuing medical education: a quantitative synthesis. *J Cont Educ Health Prof.* 1989;9:285-307.

This meta-analysis of studies of CME displays positive results in physician knowledge, physician performance, and patient health status (the last effect the weakest of the three). Despite cautions in interpretation, the author notes the "returns" in these three areas given the significant investment in CME on the part of providers and participants.

**Bertram DA, Brooks-Bertram PA.** The evaluation of continuing medical education: a literature review. *Health Educ Monogr.* 1977;249:330-362.

By reviewing 65 articles about CME, the authors suggest new directions for successful implementation and evaluation of CME. The authors find that generalizations about CME are difficult to make because of inadequate methods of evaluation, insufficient program descriptions, lack of defining terms, and noncomparability among CME programs.

**Berwick DM, Coltin KL.** Feedback reduces test use in a health maintenance organization. *JAMA.* 1986;225:1450-1454.

In a crossover design, the authors describe three interventions designed to influence the rate of use of commonly ordered blood tests and X-rays among internists in a health maintenance organization. Overall use fell in a 16-week period, during which physicians received confidential feedback on their individual rates of use compared with peers (cost feedback).

**Bretz R.** *A Taxonomy of Communication Media.* Englewood Cliffs, NJ: Technology Publications; 1971.

For communication in the face-to-face situation, simple transmission by sound or light (or other direct perceptual means) is all that is required.

When distance or time is to be covered, the message must be carried by a communication medium. Instructional aids are contrasted with communication media.

**Broadhurst AR, Darnell DK.** An introduction to cybernetics and information theory. In: Sereno KK, Morensen CD. *Foundations of Communication Theory.* New York, NY: Harper and Row Publishers; 1970.

Cybernetics is a term used to describe the field of communication and control. It is a conceptual model which insists that, from the point of view of communication, the human organism is not essentially different from a machine. It emphasizes the resemblances between living organisms and man-constructed machinery and points out that, even though the components differ, in theory their operation is essentially the same.

**Chao J.** Continuing medical education software: a comparative review. *J Fam Prac.* 1992;34:598-604.

Three examples of computer software for CME are compared—Cyberlog, Patient Simulator II, and Discotest.

**Cureless E, Coover-Stone YJ.** Simulating clinical situations: interactive video-disc. *Dimen Crit Care Nursing.* 1987;6:248-254.

The authors claim that interactive videodisc technology takes classroom teaching methods beyond the didactic acquisition of information to the application of knowledge and skills. Interactive videodisc programs display additional visual and auditory responses similar to those in the clinical setting. This new technology appears to have a great impact on critical care education.

**Davis DA, Parboosingh J.** 'Academic' CME and the social contract. *Acad Med.* 1993;68:329-332.

The authors question the commitment of medical schools to their CME programs and call for academic medical centers to critically appraise their educational activities, create new knowledge about physicians' learning and change, and study the dissemination of information.

**Davis DA, Thomas MA, Oxman AD, Haynes RB.** Evidence for the effectiveness of CME: a review of 50 randomized controlled trials. *JAMA.* 1992;268:1111-1117

The authors review the impact of diverse CME interventions on physician performance and health care outcomes. The majority of the 43 studies of physician performance show positive results in some important measure of resource utilization, counseling strategies, preventive medicine, and general management. In contrast, less than half of health care outcomes studies show such change.

**Dickinson JC, Warshaw GA, Gehlbach SH, Bobula JA, Muhlbaier LH, Parkerson GR Jr.** Improving hypertension control: impact of computer feedback and physician education. *Med Care.* 1981;19:843-854.

Two interventions (designed to help physicians treat hypertensive patients) are described and evaluated in a controlled trial: (1) computer-generated feedback to facilitate identification of patients whose symptoms were poorly controlled, and (2) a physician education program on clinical management strategies, emphasizing patient compliance. All "feedback" physicians displayed changes in performance and patient outcomes.

**Dixon AS.** The evolution of clinical policies. *Med Care.* 1990;28:201-220.

The author outlines the forces which play a role in the adoption of guidelines, identifying social rather than scientific factors. Four stages in the evolution of clinical policies are identified: development, diffusion, domination, and disillusionment.

**Duff WM.** *Annual Report to the Research Committee for January 1, 1992-December 31, 1992.* Presented before the Accreditation Council for Continuing Medical Education; October 29, 1992; Lake Bluff, Ill.

Data from annual and other reports to the Accreditation Council for Continuing Medical Education, including expenses and revenue for accredited providers, are presented. The data are limited by the varying formats used by accredited organizations. This is a first and valuable attempt by the ACCME to standardize such information.

**Eddy DM.** Should we change the rules for evaluating medical technologies? In: Celigns AC, ed. *Modern Methods of Clinical Investigation.* Washington, DC: National Academy Press; 1990:117-134.

A desirable technology possesses the following features: (1) it improves the health outcomes patients care about; (2) its benefits outweigh its disadvantages; (3) its effects are worth its cost; and (4) if resources are limited, it deserves priority over other technologies. Judging the value of a newly developed medical technology is important to its ultimate success in terms of dissemination, adoption, and usefulness in the health care system.

**Escovitz GH, Davis D.** A binational perspective on continuing medical education. *Acad Med.* 1990;65:545-549.

This paper presents a review and comparison of qualitative improvements in the organization, needs assessment, educational methodology, evaluation, and research in CME in the United States and Canada.

**Evans CE, Haynes RB, Birkett NJ, et al.**  Does a mailed continuing education program improve physician performance? results of a randomized trial in antihypertensive care.  *JAMA.*  1986;255:501-504.

> A CME program mailed to physicians who treat hypertensive patients reveals no influence by the program on physician practices or on the control of their patients' blood pressure.

**Field MJ, Lohr KN, eds.**  *Guidelines for clinical practice: from development to use.*  Washington, DC: National Academy Press; 1992.

> The authors advance the following argument: scientific evidence and clinical judgement can be systematically combined to produce clinically valid, operational recommendations for appropriate care. Methods and procedures are presented for developing clinical guidelines and for determining quality, cost, and risk.  A framework for the future is offered.

**Fowkes VK, Campeau P, Wilson S.**  The evolution and impact of the national AHEC program over two decandes.  *Acad Med.*  1991;66:211-220.

> Results of this qualitative review indicate that: (1) successful area health education centers (AHECs) are well integrated into the communities they serve, and (2) the viability of such centers in the future will depend on their ability to maintain a focus on health professions' education despite state and community pressure to provide direct services (both clinical services and public education).

**Fuhrer MJ, Grabois M.**  Information sources that influence physiatrists' adoption of new clinical practices.  *Arch Phys Med Rehabil.*  1988;69:167-169.

> This author reports on information sources that influenced physicians to introduce a clinical innovation into their practices.  The relative importance (in descending order) of the information sources was: (1) discovery in the individual's own practice; (2) a meeting, lecture, or continuing education course; (3) a clinical coworker; (4) a write-up in the clinical literature; (5) the individual's own research; (6) a patient; (7) a write-up in the research literature; (8) a textbook; and (9) the representative of a drug firm or equipment manufacturer.

**Green JS, Robin HS, Schibanoff J, et al.**  Continuous medical education: using clinical algorithms to improve the quality of health care in hospitals.  *J Cont Educ Health Prof.*  1992;12:143-155.

> Clinical algorithms (as a route by which quality of care may be improved) are discussed, and their implementation in a hospital system is explored.

**Grilli R, Apolone G, Marsoni S, Nicolucci A, Zola P, Liberati A.** The impact of patient management guidelines on the care of breast, colorectal, and ovarian cancer patients in Italy. *Med Care.* 1991;29:50-63.

The impact of a national education program based on the dissemination of written guidelines for the treatment of breast, colorectal, and ovarian cancer is described. Overall, the net effect of the intervention appears to be limited in terms of actual diffusion, attributable influence, and impact.

**Haynes RB, Ramsden M, McKibbon KA, Walker CJ, Ryan NC.** A review of medical education and medical informatics. *Acad Med.* 1989;64:207-212.

Advances in technology may help physicians to manage information more effectively through more accessible, validated clinical indexes, databases of diagnostic test characteristics, computerized audits of clinical activities with feedback, expert systems, on-line access to the medical literature, and other tools of medical informatics.

**Hull AL, Cullen RJ, Hekelman FP.** A retrospective analysis of grand rounds in continuing medical education. *J Cont Educ Health Prof.* 1989;9:257-266.

An analysis of data from grand rounds activities in departments of a medical school provides information about their organization, format, and attendance.

**Illich ID.** *Deschooling Society.* New York, NY: Harper and Row Publishers; 1970.

Socially defined, the institution of school may include the control of knowledge by selected individuals. Granting access to such information and facilitating its use to solve community problems enables education to serve the values of those most in need. The institution of school should focus on the needs of individuals with research on the possible use of technology to create institutions that serve personal, creative, and autonomous action.

**Jencks SE, Wilensky GR.** The health care quality improvement initiative. *JAMA.* 1992;268:900-903.

Continuous improvement is discussed as a goal of the health care system paid through the Health Care Finance Administration and Medicare program in the United States. The authors suggest the limits of administrative action in comparison with educational interventions.

**Jennett P, Lockyer JM, Maes W, Parboosingh J, Lawson D.** Providing relevant information to rural practitioners: a study of a medical information system. *Teach Learn Med.* 1990;4:200-204.

This study describes a medical information system pilot project to assist rural physicians with their CME. The service involves the cooperation of a trained librarian and of volunteer consultants who help with the identification and screening of appropriate resources to assist physicians with answering questions raised in practice.

**Kosecoff J, Kanouse DE, Rogers WH, McCloskey L, Winslow CM, Brook RH.** Effects of the National Institutes of Health Consensus Development Program on Physician Practice. *JAMA.* 1987;258:2708-2713.

The effects of the National Institutes of Health Consensus Development Program on Physician Practice are investigated by reviewing the medical records of hospital patients throughout the state of Washington. The authors demonstrate that the conferences failed to stimulate change in physician practice, despite moderate success in reaching the appropriate target audience.

**Liveright AA, Haygood N, eds.** *The Exeter Papers: Report of the First International Conference on the Comparative Study of Adult Education.* Boston, Mass: Center for the Study of Liberal Education for Adults of Boston University; 1968.

The definition of adult education enables a definition of CME that might include family living, personal development, civic education, religious or economic education, and a vast variety of other educational programs designed primarily for individual physicians.

**Lloyd JS, Abrahamson S.** Effectiveness of continuing medical education: a review of the evidence. *Eval Health Prof.* 1979;2:251-280.

A review of the literature from 1961 through 1977 describes 47 studies which employed one or more objective methods of evaluating CME. About half of the selected studies report demonstrable improvement in at least one of the three end products following CME—physician competence, physician performance, and patient health status.

**Lockyer J.** What do we know about adoption of innovation? *J Cont Educ Health Prof.* 1992;12:33-38.

This overview of research in adoption of innovation provides a helpful framework for conceptualizing change in the delivery of health care. The author suggests that progress has been made in delineating the circumstances under which change occurs among individual physicians, and that, within a medical community, local support often is necessary for successful adoption of innovations.

**Lomas J, Haynes RB.** A taxonomy and critical review of tested strategies for the application of clinical practice recommendations: from 'official' to 'individual' clinical policy. In: Battista RN, Lawrence RS, eds. *Implementing Preventive Services.* New York, NY: Oxford Press: 1988;77-94.

What might be expected in terms of resistance to clinical practice recommendations? How might those sources of resistance be overcome? The authors provide suggestions from a review of rigorous research based on physician performance and patient outcomes. Interventions include traditional and alternative approaches to CME, including hospital rounds, academic detailing, didactic courses, educational influentials, and hotlines to experts.

**Lomas J.** Words without action? the production, dissemination, and impact of consensus recommendations. *Ann Rev Public Health.* 1991;12:41-65.

The author presents some of the methods for consensus production and a set of standards by which to judge the validity of the various approaches. Evaluating the impact of dissemination on behavior reveals promise for the impact of consensus on cognitive rather than behavioral outcomes, and the potential for combining the output of consensus with more active strategies for implementing changes in practice.

**Lomas J, Enkin M, Anderson GM, Hannah WJ, Vayda E, Singer J.** Opinion leaders vs audit and feedback to implement practice guidelines: delivery after previous cesarean section. *JAMA.* 1991;265:2202-2207.

A randomized controlled trial of physicians in community hospitals evaluates audit and feedback and local opinion leader education as methods of encouraging compliance with a guideline for the care of women with previous cesarean sections. The overall cesarean section rate was reduced only in the opinion leader education group.

**Manning PR, Clintworth WA, Sinopoli LM, et al.** A method of self-directed learning in continuing medical education with implications for recertification. *Ann Intern Med.* 1987;107:909-913.

The authors describe a method of self-directed learning for physicians that can be used to satisfy a portion of specialty board recertification requirements. It integrates contract learning (self-formulated learning plans), information brokering (linking physicians with consultants and community resources), and collegial networking by discussion groups. Proof of accomplishment allows the method to be used as part of a specialty board recertification process.

**Mazmanian PE, Martin KO, Kreutzer JS.** Professional development and educational program planning in cognitive rehabilitation. In: Kreutzer JS, Wehman PH, eds. *Cognitive Rehabilitation for Persons with Traumatic Brain Injury.* Baltimore, Md: Paul H Brookes Publishing Company; 1991:35-51.

Program planning is described in terms of organizational and communicative systems. A seven-step program-planning model is presented. The rationale, decisions, and activities for each step are specified and instructional techniques appropriate to selected learning outcomes are presented.

**McPhee SJ, Bird JA.** Implementation of cancer prevention guidelines in clinical practice. *J Gen Intern Med.* 1990;5:S116-S122

Data from several sources, including consumer and physician surveys, and medical record audits, indicate that consumers do not receive cancer screening tests as recommended by the National Cancer Institute, the American Cancer Society, and the US Preventive Services Task Force. Interventions (such as computerized reminder systems, physician audits with feedback), and patient education and reminders, can be effective in promoting performance of such screening. Interventions that target both physician and patient may be particularly effective.

**Moore DE Jr.** *The Organization and Administration of Continuing Medical Education in Academic Medical Centers.* Urbana-Champaign, Ill: University of Illinois; 1982. Dissertation.

University-based CME programs face three levels of development: (1) departmental domination, (2) autonomy, and (3) integration. These levels feature small staffs with limited differentiation and low production; larger, more specialized staffs with increased resources; and marked integration into the university community.

**Nowlen PM.** *A New Approach to Continuing Education for Business and the Professions.* New York, NY: Macmillan; 1988.

The image of a double helix describes this author's construct of the integration of continuing education into the individual professional and the culture of practice. This model identifies and analyzes those variables that most Affect individual and group performance such as skills, environmental and cultural influences, and personal dimensions.

**Paisley W.** New media and methods of health communication. Presented at the Conference on Effective Dissemination of Clinical and Health Information; November 17, 1991; Tucson, Ariz.

Increasingly, medical practitioners find that information needs are efficiently met by interactive communication technologies. They access local and distant mainframe computers to communicate with colleagues and to search databases. They use other health care databases for practice management, and optical disks for information retrieval and continuing education. In a growing number of sites, expert systems help to form diagnoses and plan treatments.

**Parrino TA.** The nonvalue of retrospective peer comparison feedback in continuing hospital antibiotic costs. *Am J Med.* 1989;84:442-448.

Attending physicians in the top 50 percentile for expenditure were notified of their status in relation to their peers on a monthly basis. Automated peer comparison feedback is not an effective method for reducing antibiotic utilization; differences in prescribing patterns between services may dictate the best strategies for improving antibiotic utilization.

**Richards RK.** *Continuing Medical Education: Perspectives, Problems, Prognosis.* New Haven, Conn: Yale University Press; 1978.

Written in the late 1970s, this small text provides a history of the organizations of CME in the United States. Its references also provide a rich background for the evolving discipline of CME. Concluding sections on forces for change in the delivery of CME and recommendations about its future organization are provided.

**Richards RK.** Physician learning and individualized CME. *Mobius.* 1984;4:165-170.

This article describes early efforts in self-planned learning by physicians. Richards reviews the research on adult learning projects and discusses future efforts that will improve individualized CME.

**Richards RK.** Physicians' self-directed learning: a new perspective for continuing medical education, I: reading. *Mobius.* 1986;6:1-13.

This paper discusses how physicians use reading is a model of CME. It describes how reading is a learning method on which physicians spend considerable time.

**Richards RK.** Physicians' self-directed learning: a new perspective for continuing medical education, II: learning from colleagues. *Mobius.* 1986;6:1-7.

This paper describes how physicians' interaction with colleagues is a major method of self-directed learning, particularly in the areas of clinical problem-solving, information-seeking, and evaluating new diagnostic and therapeutic developments.

**Richards RK.** Physicians' self-directed learning: a new perspective for continuing medical education, III, the physician and self-directed learning projects. *Mobius.* 1986;6:1-14.

The author discusses self-directed learning in the health professions. In discussing motivation, the author reviews findings concerning the role of practical motivation, cognitive dissonance, curiosity, and the need to solve a particular patient problem. Resources are discussed, as is the planning of learning projects and their outcomes.

**Schaffner W, Ray WA, Federspiel CF, Mill WO.** Improving antibiotic prescribing in office practice: a controlled trial of three educational methods. *JAMA.* 1983;250:1728-1732.

The authors describe a statewide controlled trial of three methods to improve the prescribing of antibiotics in office practice: mailed brochures, drug educator visits, and physician visits. The authors report that mailed brochures had no detectable effect, and drug educator visits had only a modest effect. The physician visits produced strong attributable reductions in the prescribing of both drug classes.

**Schön DA.** *Educating the Reflective Practitioner: Toward a New Design for Teaching and Learning in the Profession.* San Francisco, Calif: Jossey-Bass; 1987.

This book describes a new epistemology of practice. As its point of departure, the competence and artistry embedded in skillful practice—especially the reflection-in-action that practitioners sometimes bring to situations of uncertainty, uniqueness, and conflict—is seen as the core question of professional knowledge. The book describes models and examples to better understand the implications that this theory holds for improving professional education.

**Sibley JC, Sackett DL, Neufeld V, Gerrard B, Rudnick KV, Fraser W.** A randomized trial of continuing medical education. *New Eng J Med.* 1982;306:511-515.

This classic and provocative article summarizes the results of a randomized controlled trial of physicians in the evaluation of a carefully constructed educational intervention which included mailed study packages. No improvement was seen in the quality of care by the physicians in the area of their preferred topics, but improvement was observed in the quality of care given by physicians relating to the nonpreferred topics.

**Soumerai SB, Avorn J.** Principles of educational outreach ('academic detailing') to improve clinical decision making. *JAMA.* 1990;263:549-556.

Some of the most important techniques of "academic detailing" include: (1) conducting interviews to investigate baseline knowledge and motivations; (2) focusing programs on specific categories of physicians as well as on their opinion leader; (3) defining clear educational and behavioral objectives; (4) establishing credibility through a respected organizational identity, referencing sources of information; (5) stimulating active physician participation in education interactions; (6) using concise graphic educational materials; (7) highlighting and repeating essential messages; and (8) providing positive reinforcement of improved practices in follow-up visits.

**Stross JK, Harlan WR.** The dissemination of new medical information. *JAMA*. 1979;241:2622-2624.

The authors survey primary care physicians to determine their knowledge of the results of the cooperative trial of photocoagulation in diabetic retinopathy. Despite the acknowledged relevance to their practice, only 28% of family physicians and 46% of internists were aware of the study results. Findings indicate that results from clinical trials may not be disseminated to practicing physicians and, therefore, not incorporated into practice.

**Stross JK, Hiss RG, Watts CM, Davis WK, MacDonald R.** Continuing education in pulmonary disease for primary care physicians. *Am Res Resp Dis*. 1983;127:739-746.

Randomly selected community hospitals nominated educational influentials (opinion leaders) in respiratory disease, subsequently trained by self-study materials and clinical preceptorship. Inpatient chart audits in these community hospitals revealed significant improvement in the management of respiratory disease over control hospitals.

**Tyler RW.** *Basic Principles of Curriculum and Instruction*. Chicago, Ill: University of Chicago Press; 1949.

Historical roots for the Essentials of the Accreditation Council for Continuing Medical Education and the principles guiding accreditation by the Association of Canadian Medical Colleges are found in this text. Tyler is largely responsible for turning the attention of educators toward the determination of learning needs and behavioral objectives as the central issue in curriculum planning.

**Williamson JW, German PS, Weiss R, Skinner EA, Bowes F.** Health sciences information management and continuing education of physicians: a survey of United States primary care practitioners and their opinion leaders. *Ann Intern Med*. 1989;110:151-160.

This study is one of the first to question the widespread stated belief that journals are a major source of information for the practicing physician. The study examines the self-perceived problems of primary care physicians and their opinion leaders in managing health science information. Primary care physicians were interviewed using a formal telephone survey. Among the findings, less than one in three practitioners personally searched the literature when information was needed; two out of three practitioners claimed literature volume was a problem, and very few practitioners actually analyzed the scientific soundness of the literature that they did review.

# Chapter 14

# Conclusion:

## The Place of
## Research
## in
## CME

*Robert Fox*
*David Davis*

# Conclusion:  The Place of Research in CME

*In a discussion between two naval officers, a navigator overheard one of the officers say, ...*"We don't know where we're going!"*  The navigator responded that you're not lost when you don't know where you're going. You're lost when you don't know where you are.*

Definitions of complex human activities may be drawn out of the minds of philosophers and writers or in applied science, or from the body of literature and practice. Often, definitions are out of date because they no longer represent the consensus of those who study and practice in a field.  We have purposely avoided a comprehensive definition of CME until very late in this text.  This has been done, not to confuse the reader, but to indicate that considerable debate is engendered by such a taxonomic discussion, only a portion of which is useful.  Instead, we have elected to focus this book, and in particular this chapter, on the research and scholarship characterizing the literature of CME.  That literature is formed in three interwoven domains--physician learning, competency assessment, and the programs designed to effect change.

On reflection, referring to ideas encompassed within the framework of this book as "continuing medical education" or "CME" seems inadequate, particularly given the diversity of topics and problems captured in the literature.  The field is, however, fluid; and we believe that it will fall to future researchers, practitioners, and theorists in this evolving discipline to develop a comprehensive and universally acceptable phrase to encompass this field of inquiry.  Certainly, whatever phrase becomes accepted, it must embrace several notions--it must reflect that education and learning are pathways to professional development, it must allow for studies that connect learning and development over the span of activities related to the practice, and it must allow for studies of other concepts and variables that contribute to the culture of medicine and the general roles of physicians in society.

Despite difficulties in definition and nominal problems, the field of CME and its scholarly base are important.  CME occupies a place, firmly embedded and with increasing importance, between the learner and medical progress in health care (See Figure 14.1).  CME serves to connect the internal processes of learning with the performance of physicians. This text was organized to reflect the bridging function of CME and the types of scholarship that characterize each of these areas.  Section I examined the diverse and complex theories and investigations that have focused on physicians as learners.  Section II surveyed the problems of investigation of competence and performance and the critical role of learning needs assessment in the facilitation of learning and changing.  Section III reviewed the literature, both theoretical and practical, supporting the practice of CME.

## Figure 14.1

## CME systems

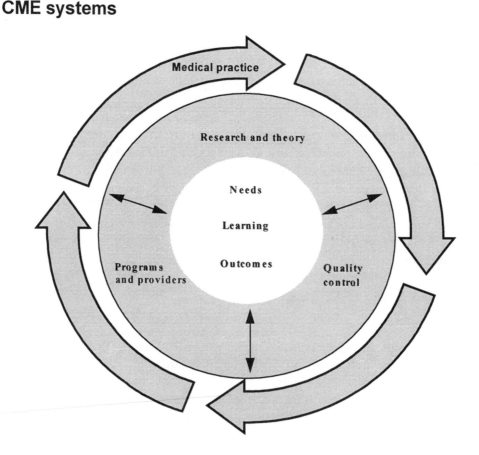

CME, however defined and described, occupies a central role in both practice and theory. Its structure possesses many of the characteristics of a semi-permeable membrane. Research into its various forms and dimensions, and its effectiveness and outcomes becomes a compelling imperative because of its role in connecting new and better CME practices with the processes of changing and learning.

# The Structure of CME

To be effective and of high quality, future CME research must be based on common understandings of the nature of CME in North America. In effect, there is a geography that can be used to describe the role of different domains of CME and their roles. These domains are: (1) the CME enterprise, including programs, activities and their providers; (2) the system of "quality control" applied to the provision of CME; and (3) the evolving research and theory related to the role of CME in physician learning. All of these domains are interconnected so that together they become the physical and ideological structure of the CME system in North America. Each domain, however, serves a unique and necessary function with the system. (See Figure 14.1) Displayed as the core of this ring is a three-phase educational model relating to the physician as learner—the determination of learning needs, the CME intervention itself, and its outcome. The "world" of medical practice surrounds the CME "ring." First, the system of CME provision, explored in Chapter 13, is composed of: industry providers (pharmaceutical houses, hospitals, and other suppliers), medical colleges and schools, professional associations (including national, international, provincial, state, and local specialty societies), regulatory agencies (including state licensing boards and government bodies), specific interest groups (such as the American Heart Association), for-profit CME providers, and others (such as the publishing industry). The purposes of CME vary within each of these organizations. In industry, for example, CME is used to promote the sales of new products or services, or reinforce the sales of older ones, by increasing the flow of product information about the problems and solutions. In some areas, the purposes of CME are more mixed; while professional associations genuinely seek to improve clinical care in their area of specialization through CME activities, profits from the associations' meetings frequently contribute to healthy annual budgets. Each of the other providers of CME also has different priorities in CME delivery, depending on organizational mission, corporate structure, and desired outcome.

The second aspect of contemporary CME is the system of "quality control." This system is marked by four features:

(1) *The Associations of CME providers.* Two key international (though primarily North American) examples are the Alliance for CME and the Society of Medical College Directors of CME. Many other groups operate at national, provincial, state, or local levels to foster CME, generally as a section of individuals within other larger, professional groups employed in medical schools, industry, professional associations, or hospitals. Such CME associations exist, at least in part, to provide professional development in CME to members. In this way, they foster understanding of the learning process, the delivery of effective programming, and the evaluation of activities.

(2) *Accreditation Systems.* Explored more fully in Chapter 13, accreditation systems in North America provide for a measure of product control and a set of principles by which to judge the quality of CME programs. Although most systems place considerable, almost exclusive, emphasis on the design of traditional courses, the existence of such a system provides a framework on which physician-learners, professional associations, licensing authorities, and CME providers may be assured of consistent, effective products. Recent innovations (eg, the accreditation system of the Royal College of Physicians and Surgeons of Canada) have been tied more closely to contemporary research and theory related to the self-directed learning of physicians as well as to their education.

(3) *Regulations.* Allied to the second set of quality-promoting activities, professional associations, states, provinces, and physician employers (such as health maintenance organizations and governments) have

enacted regulations relative to how much and what kind of participation in learning is necessary. Faced with the need for encouraging or ensuring the competence of these physicians, these bodies have developed guidelines regarding physician CME involvement, adequate support of CME programs, and the validation of specific CME interventions and activities.

(4) *Training Programs and Learning Resources.* A product of the last three decades, those involved in the discipline of continuing professional education are increasingly trained in formal, doctoral-level (PhD or EdD) programs. A relatively recent survey by the Society of Medical College directors of CME[1] indicated an approximate sixfold growth over the last 10 years in members trained in adult or continuing professional education. Other systems or strategies exist for the ongoing professional development of those involved in the production of CME, including a least one professional journal (the *Journal of Continuing Education in the Health Professions*), occasional "institutes" or brief training experiences for those interested in CME development and research, and the products of the Alliance for CME--the *primer* in CME,[2] regular workshops and meetings, and a videotape series in CME organization and delivery.

It is research in CME that makes up the third component of the CME ring. There are several major indicators of the size and nature of this research effort. First, we note significantly increased funding for research projects from government and private sources. Such projects are often the products of health services research units, government agencies, and other units, offices, or programs dedicated to research dissemination. A second indicator of increased research efforts may be found in meetings and conferences devoted in whole or in part to CME research (eg, the semiannual Research in CME Conference and Research in Medical Education Conference). A third component of CME research is found in the publication of journals in which CME research forms a focus in whole or in part. These publications, from a variety of sources, are captured in the Research and Development Resource Base in CME, funded by the professional associations, housed at University of Toronto, and described in the Preface. At the time of publication of this book the RDRB/CME contained references to over 4 500 articles, books, and monographs devoted to CME and derived from unindexed and more traditional medical literature sources. Fourth and finally, there are a small number of centers, located in medical schools and elsewhere, devoting some part of their efforts to research in CME, physician learning, and performance change. Many of these are not located in CME divisions or departments, but rather find homes in quality assurance or health service research centers.

We envisage changes over the next decade in the CME system, including a breakdown of the barriers between the three divisions—the programs and providers, quality assurance mechanisms, and the research efforts. Each division can inform and support the others, and increased collaboration will contribute to greater effectiveness.

**Figure 14.2**

**An integrated construct of physician learning**

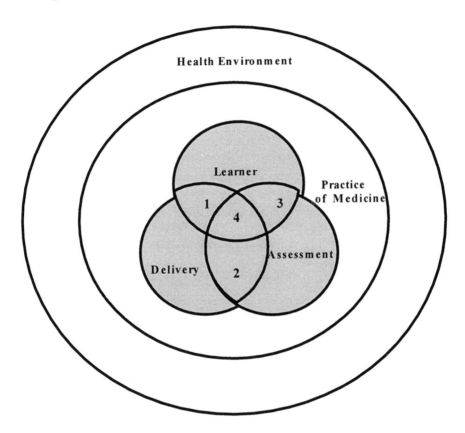

# The Function of CME:  Research and Science in Physician Learning

Experience, previous research, and logic can help researchers and scholars develop questions that link learning and education to the practices of physicians.  One starting point is to lay out a rough sketch of CME's terrain, describing defined but overlapping territories for investigation.  By displaying a reasonable topography of CME, we hope to foster projects (from the small to the comprehensive); explore each area; build better explanations, predictions, and understanding; and, thus, ease the process of investigation by suggesting the need for a more global vision, constructed from the ground up.

Three overlapping areas surrounded by a sea of professional, practice-based social, political, and economic contingencies make up this view of the content and purpose of CME.  These are displayed diagrammatically in Figure 14.2.  CME research must discover and document what, how, and why physicians learn and change; how their learning needs, competencies, and performance may be best assessed; and how better programs of education can be designed and delivered to fit into this process.

While this is research about each of the domains, it is also about the relationships and barriers. While each of these themes is presented as a section in this book, the purpose of this concluding chapter is to provide natural linkages between the sections.

# Physicians as Learners

The first area, physician learning, can be sketched with greater accuracy if we assume that, while physicians act as professionals within practice environments, they are like other adults in most ways. This assumption allows investigators to apply certain general conclusions about adults as learners. For example, both physicians and other adults process information from their environment to their short-term memory, from short-term to working memory, and from working memory to long-term memory. Physicians use cognitive "software" to process information, to reach decisions, and to guide their professional performance. They learn by association, influenced by age and experience. Some of their knowledge and skills become automatic and unconscious. Old knowledge and skills may interfere with acquiring new knowledge and skills.[3]

This process requires both facts and ideas, the content of most CME interventions. Without facts and ideas, better ways of thinking and learning lack purpose. CME evaluation research studies report that physicians foster and hold new facts and ideas, although not in a direct, linear manner. Evidence explaining how and why physicians use their knowledge, however, is more difficult to find. Other areas that need more attention include: "How are factual storehouses organized?"; "Are there hierarchies based on scenarios, critical clinical incidents, the epistemology of sciences, or medical school curricula?"; "Are there obstacles to new information?"; and "Do beliefs, attitudes, or personality attributes intervene positively or negatively in learning new information?" We need to know more about why some information lies dormant or decays while other information is quickly and frequently applied in physicians' clinical practices. Physicians are most often independent learners, but occasionally depend on others for help. The extent of dependence on others lies on a continuum. Changing physicians' clinical performances is difficult except when they are in favor of the change, have readily available means and ends, and have some control over the process.[4]

However, in meaningful ways, physicians differ from other adult learners and from each other. By the time they are admitted to medical school, physicians have shown determination, discipline, intelligence, and motivation, as noted in several chapters of this text. Through education and training, physicians have become storehouses of knowledge, and have developed relatively sophisticated skills of observing, interpreting, analyzing, and applying information. They have developed strategies for clinical interviewing, clinical reasoning, and psychomotor skills useful for such actions as performing physical examinations and surgery. Many things are learned so well they are embodied in actions: Schön[5] describes the structure of their knowledge and the ability of physicians to learn from experience as a reaction to the successes and failures of this embedded knowledge in ambiguous or unique problems.

Gagne and Glaser[3] offer another perspective on learning. They refer to learning to learn as a control process, one that shapes and determines the extent to which other thought and memory processes are developed and used appropriately. Because understanding how physicians learn is central to fostering learning in formal and informal settings, CME must develop a tradition of research related to problem solving, cognition, self-directed learning, and the adoption of innovations explored in Chapters 2 through 5. These issues and constructs, and others like them, which evaluate learning specific to the medical profession, speak eloquently to the need for further investigation and an appropriate place within a framework of the lifelong development of physicians articulated in Chapter 5. Researchers must continue to seek questions and answers on this frontier.

## Assessment Issues

A second major area of investigation explored in this book is assessment of the learner's attributes. This includes studies related to constructs such as competency (beliefs, attitudes, knowledge, skills) and performance as they relate to patient care practices or health care outcomes. Assessment is an essential element in the actions of continuing medical educators. It is the way that educational actions are connected to a reliable base of information about learners. The scope and accuracy of the assessment predicts the extent to which programs (self-directed or otherwise) are based on accurate estimates of need and outcome, the value of educational methods and techniques, and the worth of one approach over another in meeting the needs of practicing physicians. Figure 14.3 displays some of the major targets of assessment and some of the comparisons intrinsic in using measurement to inform decisions.

Chapter 7 outlines the shape and scope of competency, and lays out for the reader a map of its component parts. The chapter clarifies the terms "competence" and "performance." Competence is a construct describing the variables connected to the ability to perform; these variables are only indirectly observable. In contrast, performance is manifest and observable in transactions between physicians and patients, colleagues, and/or coworkers. Studies on assessment improve the methods and techniques of observing directly or indirectly the objects of study. Consequently, poor assessment methods and techniques project an inaccurate image of learners and their concerns, thoughts, and actions. On the other hand, excellence in assessment allows learners and educators to ground actions in valid and reliable information about health care problems, physicians' performance, competencies that contribute to performance, and factors that facilitate change and learning.

## Figure 14.3

## Assessment and program development

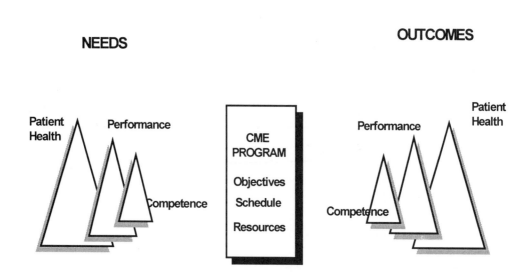

NEEDS

OUTCOMES

Patient Health

Performance

Competence

CME PROGRAM

Objectives

Schedule

Resources

Performance

Patient Health

Competence

# The Provision of CME

The third zone includes those areas of research and theory related to the design and delivery of CME. It includes program design and development, educational methods and techniques, and the organization and administration of CME units. Together, these areas of study constitute the ways and means by which CME is offered and utilized by physicians. Each of the chapters comprising the third section of this text suggests important areas of investigations that have emerged from their review of the literature related to this domain of research in CME. For example, when do lectures offer a better means for learning than simulated patients? Are real patient problems better organizing frameworks for learning to solve problems than computer or other simulations? Should CME programs be designed to become seamless components of the practice environment?

This list of questions and issues is practically endless, as planning strategies, organizational frameworks, formats, methods, and techniques are examined for their strengths and weaknesses within the realm of medicine. Investigators of the future must consider more fully the need for studies related to program design and implementation. For example, CME needs more information on the cost benefit of different methods and techniques for educating physicians. We also know too little about how to best connect instructional strategies to styles of teaching and circumstances of application. Research needs to continue to question the value and role of objectives; interactive teaching techniques; methods for teaching problem-solving and learning skills; the role of instructional media; and the compatibility of techniques to time, energy, and application.

The nature of the CME organization may itself act as a variable in the process of education. One way to begin to understand this domain is to make another assumption—all of these different CME providers are formal organizations. This allows CME scholars to apply some of the important conclusions of studies about formal organizations to those that provide CME. For example, Perrow,[6] an organizational theorist, described four concepts that also apply to the study of CME organizations—organizational goals (formal and informal intentions of the organization which predict the behavior of members of that organization), structure (the ways that units and roles within the organization are divided and organized), tasks (the actual work of the organization), and technology (the knowledge and skills that can be applied to tasks). Such elementary articulation of concepts yet to be investigated suggest that future studies should be directed towards clarifying and specifying how such variables may impact CME in all of its domains.

In addition, CME is an organization within other organizations, and the primary goals of the parent organization may differ dramatically from those of CME. For example, in medical schools, undergraduate programs, residency teaching, and biomedical research overshadow the delivery of high-quality CME, in spite of emphasis on the importance and relative equality of CME to other functions of the organization. Faculty and staff are examples of institutional resources. When they are asked to teach a group of practitioners, they are performing a formal task, one of many competing for their attention. Some tasks are relished and others are avoided, dependent in part on how faculty perceive the goals of the institution. The amount and nature of instructional methods and techniques mastered by the instructors also affect teacher performance. In this case, the performance of teachers is a function of the goals of the organization, the tasks that are assigned, and the technology available to conduct those tasks. Perrow[6] hypothesized that a decentralized organizational structure systematically affected all three of these variables. Yet this and other models of relationship affecting the CME enterprise are not evident in the literature of CME. Other valuable theories related to productivity, job satisfaction, work motivation, and leadership merit investigation in CME organizations and may be used to clarify the form and functions of the delivery of CME to physicians.

CME units and their parent organizations also operate within the context of a variety of policies, yet policy analysis plays little role in the literature of CME. Like organizational theory, policy study is an important area for exploration. Those who search here are likely to discover that, in medical schools, policies about CME compete successfully or unsuccessfully with other policies. Success may be dependent, in part, on how they are formulated and presented. They are also likely to find that policies can be either stubborn obstacles to CME or sources of power to do what needs to be done. Future research into the nature of CME policies and their relationship to both learning and program design and implementation can only clarify the factors which foster or obstruct the CME mission.

# The Interactive Effects

Just as each of these domains may be studied individually, the interactive nature of the conceptual areas should also become a focus for investigations in the future. These areas of interaction suggest major questions and issues important to the professions of medicine and education in general, and to the discipline of CME in particular. We propose general directions and several sets of questions in these areas, not to provide a comprehensive list, but rather to establish some examples of research directions.

## The Interaction of Learning and Assessment

There is a core concept in the notion of self-directed learning and in theories of motivation—that physicians, at some level of proficiency, are able to recognize their learning needs within the context of patient care and professional standards. These self-assessments are the driving force for voluntary actions that they may take to learn and change. Internal estimates of proficiency are compared to standards set by peers, regulatory bodies, patients, policies, and the literature of clinical medicine. This process establishes, in more traditional CME terminology, learner needs.

This particular aspect of competence, variably termed self-directed learning or CME skills, may be seen as a subset of skills in the assessment of competence. We see it as a necessary, but not sufficient, element in the learning physician's armamentarium, and we note that it has been explored extensively, both in this book and elsewhere. However because of its importance to the processes of learning and educating, there is a significant need to develop testable models of this process and means to enhance its development in practicing physicians.

Ideally, self-assessment should occur continuously within the context of clinical practice. Skills for self-assessment should be developed early and tested frequently throughout the medical education system. Such skills should be refined and supported by, in practice, collegial relationships with peers, consultants, and other members of the care-giver team. While owned primarily by the physician, they must be fostered by medical faculties, and altered by professional and speciality associations. While calling for the insertion of such practices into the regular practice and learning of physicians, we recognize the need to develop and test the research hypotheses inherent in such a model.

Proficiency theory, as articulated by Knox,[7] suggests a model for the process of self-assessment. The model was supported in the research of the book *Changing and Learning in the Lives of Physicians.* The model suggests that needs for learning are the result of moderate level discrepancies in competence or performance between what is and what ought to be. "What ought to be" is a function of both internal and external standards. "What is" refers to the actual level of competence and/or performance of the physician learner. We envisage increased numbers, kinds, and sophistication of standardized tools designed to assist physicians and others as they attempt more accurately to estimate level of need.

There is another focus of self-assessment broader than looking to individual competencies and proficiencies—physicians needs to develop skills in reflective practice. One potential way in which a model of self-assessment may be derived is from the model of reflective practice proposed by Schön,[5] who suggests that educational systems fail to demonstrate the basic uncertainty or unpredictability of professional practice. We would take this one step further and believe that educational systems rarely assess the abilities of trainees or graduates to manage such complex and nonroutine aspects of practice.

There are several ways in which reflection on one's clinical practices and subsequent self-directed learning might be measured. These are described in greater detail in chapter 7, and include: observation of physician learning habits, retrospective techniques used in clinical settings, structured interviews, using feedback following learning experiences, and the "triple-jump" exercise developed at McMaster University.[8]

Questions of relevance to this area of overlap include: "Can learners be taught self-assessment skills?"; "Can these be assessed at earlier stages of professional development?"; "Can they be assessed in the practicing physician in a regular, systematic, reliable, and acceptable fashion?"; and "What are the effects of specific forms of assessment on learning?"

## The Interaction Between Assessment and Programs

We can describe the area of overlap between assessment and program delivery as having two basic dimensions. The first is related to the assessment of individual and collective learner needs, and the second is related to learner or program evaluation.

The assessment of learner needs is prescribed by the principles of adult education and mandated by accreditation standards for assuring educational quality and effectiveness. It is also far more complicated in CME than in undergraduate or graduate programs. The organization of knowledge, set curricula, and the basic tasks of medicine form a somewhat inflexible foundation that determines the structure of undergraduate and graduate medical education. However, because practicing physicians are voluntary participants in CME activities, and may choose to learn in a variety of ways, accurately identifying and measuring needs allows continuing educators to take advantage of the educational and economic efficiency of formal education and group instruction. Without valid information on what is needed, opportunities to teach and to learn are missed by both physicians and CME providers. Although the literature of CME and adult education attends to the importance of this area, there are few attempts to fully develop generalizable tools for need assessment. Because of the evidence (in Chapter 12 and elsewhere) identifying strong ties between educational quality and learning needs, investigation related to better methods and techniques for accurately estimating needs should continue to be a cornerstone of CME research. First, questions in this area are in part practical or organizational: "To what extent can CME activities incorporate or be seen to include assessment principles and practices?"; "How can findings of needs assessments be consistently tied to program planning and design decisions?"; and "Can providers incorporate 'harder,' more objectively determined data into their decision making and learning activities, especially those traditionally depen- dent on the wants or perceived needs of physicians?"

Second, performance measures will be increasingly applied in the practice site as directed by the external and interrelated forces of quality assurance, concurrent quality improvement, and health economics. Though different forces exist in the US and Canadian health care systems, they are similar in their clear call for more awareness of health economic issues, and show every sign of pushing the system to monitor both process issues and outcomes. To these powerful forces are added the insurgence of the evidence-based care movement in both countries,[9] calling for strict adherence to rational management strategies based on hard evidence. The develop- ment of practice guidelines is one example of this movement. This movement can be used by CME providers and researchers to establish optimal clinical standards, allowing for more uniform template against which to assess the need for learning and change.

The second dimension of assessment and CME relates to studying the procedures for accurately evaluating programs and learner outcomes. It promises the same kinds of benefits as that of the assessment of learners' needs. Like needs assess- ment, evaluation of educational procedures inform the decisions of program design and implementation. To date, however, the majority of evaluations of CME have focused on only one set of questions—"Does CME make a difference in learning, competency, performance, or patient health?"—which only tells providers to develop or not develop CME interventions. Other program evaluation questions need more attention, such as what CME works (when, on whom, how, and why). Autopsies of failed programs will also provide useful information on why programs did not work. All of these kinds of investigations must focus on the decisions that mark the path to a CME program rather than only that the path leads to specific outcome.

## The Interaction Between CME Programs and Physicians as Learners

Much has already been written, in this book and elsewhere, about the incorporation of learner needs, practices, and styles into the delivery of CME interventions. Adult and continuing education literature from other health professional fields can guide the way of CME research. As with investigations of physician learning, an assumption is warranted—what we have learned about the efficient and effective continuing education of other adults, especially professionals, applies, in part, to the education of physicians. To some extent, all of the professions are alike and yet are all different. Evaluations of procedures for educating professionals in other fields may provide important information on ways to educate physicians. This may be especially important in such areas as ethics, patient education, medical practice management, health administration, and problem solving. For too long the literature of CME has been built on the assumption that the education of practicing physicians is unique. Investigators and scholars must work harder to see what CME has in common with continuing education for nurses, dentists, lawyers, engineers, architects, and others. A global perspective of other professions enriches CME.

Particularly valuable are investigations and literature that suggest the development of new ways to design education based on findings related to the learning process. Often referred to as "theory-to-practice," this approach is manifest in a segment of literature devoted to interpreting learning research primarily in terms of its implications for the design and development of educational programs and instructional design. One notable example of this might be the development of a text in CME that suggests ways by which newer ideas and research implies a different set of principles and practices for continuing medical educators. Other useful activities might be research-to-practice conferences, where participants suggest innovations in education based on literature. Because investigators are few and often out of direct contact with program providers, these kinds of efforts seem especially important.

## The Interactions of Learning, Assessing, and Education

It is the area of overlap of all three domains of investigation and scholarship that holds promise in developing and testing specific hypotheses based on more refined theoretical images of the relationship among learning, assessing, and education. Such studies will benefit from closer and more explicit ties to the practice environment. However, such studies must be approached cautiously and patiently to avoid certain pitfalls.

First, many questions must be answered before we understand the ultimate relationships and implications that rest in the areas of physician learning, assessment, and CME provision. We must understand each of these areas in order to predict how practice environment, educational strategy, and learning will interact. Without accounting for the likely effect of any one of the three areas, the prediction is inadequate and the results are suspect. Yet, each of the studies that may be conducted in this territory will add incrementally to the mosaic of answers that lie here undiscovered.

Secondly, it is impossible to fully understand and explain the world of CME without paying attention to the environment within which it functions. That environment includes the personal, professional, economic, political, and social forces that enable or inhibit the clinical changes CME fosters. The object of CME is most often change, whether it be changing a course of deteriorating competence, introducing an innovation, or easing the adoption of new perspectives on health care. Information and skill are usually necessary, but seldom sufficient to bring about changes in performance. Individual attributes such as differences in personalities, capabilities, satisfaction with life and career, health, and intellectual curiosity can promote or inhibit change. Desire to be more competent and the environment of clinical practice are professional forces which can drive or stall changes. Social, political, and economic forces include relationships with colleagues in the profession, pressures from medical institutions, governmental policies and regulations, and family and community roles. These forces may alter the interactions of CME organizations, programs, and physician learners. They may work singularly or in concert. They may also work against one another. They may mediate the relationship between the world of work and the world of learning. They may act to encourage participation in education while discouraging the changes that education fosters. They may act to discourage the use of education as a part of the change process. Research must recognize these contingencies to create better explanations and better predictions, especially of changes in physician performance.

Research questions arise from several sources—hypotheses and ideas which have been prompted by this book, and which deserve exploration. Having laid out the terrain of research, there are a number of ways by which questions crossing these domains may be asked. For example, how do age and stage of development, when considered as a unifying theme, affect the interplay between the learner, assessment, and CME resources? How are these factors, in light of age and experience, affected by the clinical, social, and other environments in which the physician lives and practices? Other unifying themes may be similarly derived, holding promise for the development of a comprehensive construct of physician learning and its relationship to practice.

In addition to the questions that must be asked, there are innovations that seem implicit in new directions for CME research. There is considerable potential in the idea of the learning center proposed in Chapter 13. More comprehensive than a library, more learner-centered than a traditional CME environment, and with potential for close practice linkages, such centers could become foci for CME research and the incorporation of learning into practice. Their potential prompts several practical and testable questions related to their funding, use by physicians, and ubiquity. It also prompts questions about their merit and effectiveness and the necessary conceptual shift on the part of physicians to see them (or learning itself) as much a part of their professional lives as hospital wards, outpatient clinics, and practice settings.

Finally, there are several ideas imbedded in the section on CME provision which cross boundaries and reach into the practice environment and, thus, deserve exploration. Among these are the notion of an individualized CME curriculum (chapter 10), driven by stimulation in either the practice or the learning environment, and cycling through the use of resources and ongoing assessment of learning needs. Paralleling this inclusive movement is the concept explored in Chapter 12, that CME interventions need to be considered in a light which includes traditional print and lecture media along with nontraditional, innovative, practice-linked, or practice-based interventions such as chart-stimulated review, opinion leaders or educational influentials, academic detail persons, practice reminders or feedback, and other methods. Such strategies can, in fact, bridge gaps blocking close and functional relationships between learner, assessment, and delivery systems. They deserve further testing, refining, and (passing these criteria for success) widespread use.

# Overcoming Limitations in the System

Making the changes that are necessary for informed medical practice depends on understanding the role of learning, CME programs and services, and assessment. For CME to be based on knowledge and skill, it must be built on the products of research and scholarship.  However, to build this bank of knowledge and skill, there are important barriers that must be overcome.  Some come from the perception of the profession, or from its structure, while others come from the relationship of CME to its sponsoring organization or institution (such as the academic health science centers).  Some barriers arise from debates over how to study CME.

Both research and delivery of CME suffer from the view, espoused by many (from medical school deans to physicians themselves), that anyone, regardless of training or background, can direct or provide CME activities, and further, that CME is the least important phase of the academic medical education continuum.  As a result, the role and value of CME research is misunderstood, poorly respected, or both. When CME is perceived with greater clarity, it occupies a critical role as an ethical, pleasurable, and effective mechanism for assuring appropriate changes in medical practice without waiting for new graduates.  Many of those who have responsibility for CME have no training in education, and often lack an understanding of the body of research in adult education and CME.  These problems lead to no research, or to episodic research conducted by investigators who must bootleg their projects, achieve little recognition for success, and find little or no financial support for investigations which may contribute, ultimately, to the betterment of clinical care. Systematic efforts to enhance the role of CME research should be sponsored by organized medicine.

Another factor impeding progress in understanding the CME enterprise is the relative absence of friendly funding sources for research directly related to CME. This, too, is based on a perception that CME, teaching, and dissemination all have this in common—once taught (or mailed, or lectured on), information is received; once received, understood; and once understood, directly applied to practice.  One example of difficulty in finding funding sources was the change study by Fox et al.[4] This study was sponsored by the Society of Medical College Directors of CME, depended on several funding sources, and was, essentially, research the hard way. Increasingly, however, research funds have flowed to answer, in part, the questions of CME research raised here and elsewhere.  Such funding sources derive, in part, from a changing understanding in clinical research relative to the necessity for dissemination research.  Recent examples include a multicentered trail of a CME intervention in diabetes sponsored by the Society of Medical College Directors of CME (P. E. Mazmanian, PhD, unpublished data, 1992).

A third impediment to CME research derives from the concept of CME as the product of the culture of teacher-centered undergraduate training.  In such a culture, CME is the equivalent of formal courses, and the narrow research questions which flow from such a perspective limit researchers to questions about lecture techniques. Although valuable, such questions are only a part of the whole cloth of CME and practice-based learning and change.

A fourth barrier to research in CME stems from the debate over methodology that persistently questions whether qualitative methods (case studies, ethnography, field observations, and the like) are as valuable as quantitative methods (for example, randomized trials or quasi-experimental studies). Overall, the studies upon which most of medicine is based, and the nature of biomedical research, have reached a stage of development where the experiment and accompanying statistical test is a primary avenue to truth. This is so, only because the decades of exploratory work which came first—certainly, Darwin was a scientist even if he only collected and compared specimens from a boat trip to South America. Explorations are as essential to understanding as experiments are to predictions. Both methodological approaches are helpful when used to answer the appropriate question. We would propose that CME research be more balanced between qualitative, inductive research and quantitative, deductive research. Only when sufficiently explored and described in formal investigations can the questions generated inductively be verified in deductive tests of hypotheses. Researchers must embrace both approaches to research for what they can contribute to the learning of physicians.

As there are barriers to overcome, there are also ways of pursuing the future that hold a promise of progress. First, CME research must continue to emphasize collaboration among CME organizations. The two examples of the Society of Medical College Directors of CME show that many investigators in different medical centers can work together to achieve complex projects. The concept of collaboration also applies to collaboration across disciplines. Medical performance is an interdisciplinary phenomenon involving medical science, learning, personal attributes, social relationships, economic contingencies, and organizational contexts. Although some of these aspects can be studied independently, many can only be studied from the interacting perspectives of many kinds of expertise. CME has a tradition of physicians and educators jointly investigating physician performance and change. For leaps forward in understanding, some of the research of the future must develop from the interdisciplinary perspective of teams of researchers. Some must develop from many teams at many sites collaborating in the same study.

Collaboration also applies to sharing across kinds of CME providers and others interested in the outcomes of CME. In addition to medical schools, CME is also offered by hospitals and many other types of providers represented, for example, by the Alliance for CME. Others interested in physician learning include peer review organizations, licensing bodies, and professional or specialty associations. The perspectives and the opportunities of each of these differ. Each also has common concerns. All of them need more reliable information on what, when, where, why, and especially how physicians learn.

Another way in which barriers to CME research may be overcome is to develop practical models of research strategies, such as that found in the health promotion literature.[10] Here, a framework may be identified for such research, applicable to physician learning and CME questions.

> *Phase 1: Hypothesis development addresses the question "What is the problem?" and identifies factors to be considered, such as epidemiologic*

*parameters, determinants of the clinical behavior, or dimensions of the problem.*

*Phase 2: Method development is concerned primarily with the development of potential effective intervention methods or research approaches. This may involve pilot testing, qualitative methods such as focus groups, development of measurement tools, and research protocols. Correlational techniques may be applied to study and compare factors which influence physician behavior such as educational/training differences which might affect outcomes.*

*Phase 3: Controlled intervention studies involves the evaluation of promising interventions by descriptive, before-and-after means, cohort analytic, or more controlled trial methodologies. Here the emphasis is on testing the efficacy of an intervention (ie, its ability to change physician attitudes under ideal conditions).*

*Phase 4: Defined population studies assess effectiveness, that is, the outcomes of CME and related interventions in a real-world environment, such as that of a CME provider rather than researcher. In addition, these studies test external (environmental) and internal (physician, institutional) validity.*

A further way that knowledge of physicians' learning and education can advance is by taking a longer view of the process. Much of what is known about the relationships among education, learning, and changes in performance has been learned through static or retrospective studies. The few prospective investigations have emphasized experimental or quasi-experimental methods. In the future, we would urge a longitudinal view of the role of learning and education in the practice of medicine, since we suspect that many of the changes in the practices of physicians involve long periods of time. One change may influence another. Motivation, curiosity, opportunity, and obstacles to learning may also wax and wane. Some changes in performance may be regressive and others may represent spontaneous insight possible only after reflection over many weeks or months. Things learned may be discredited over time by the culture of practice or by the practices of colleagues. These and many other ideas may grow from looking at the practices of physicians over time. Such findings could alter significantly the strategies for continuous improvement of the practices of physicians over their medical careers. Longitudinal studies of this kind require significant initial investments, but promise immediate and long-term results obtainable in no other way.

For every change that needs to be made in the work of physicians, CME can play an important part. Health care needs are changing dramatically. Relative to demographic shifts, there are needs for doctors to play a larger role in caring for a population which is shifting steadily to larger numbers of middle-aged, elderly and old-old individuals. Such population shifts translate into CME needs in chronic long-term care, geriatrics and other areas. There is a concurrent and not unrelated shift in emphasis from treatment to prevention; in such a milieu, the demand for and recognition of primary or secondary preventive care is considerable. There are several inter-digitated components to this area of research and practice—health promotion (which includes studies exploring the determinants of health and strategies to effect changes in them) illness prevention awareness, community development, and enhancing prevention practices of physicians.

Further, there are numerous shifts in the delivery of health services, requiring a focus on administration, teamwork with other professionals, cost containment, and policy making. These shifts in the political and regulatory environment in which the practice of medicine exists are delineated in the foreword of this book. Conflicts over preserving patient autonomy while acting for each patients' benefit make the ethical and legal aspects of medical practice more complicated than ever. Changes in equipment and medications, and in diagnostic and treatment technology demand change in use. Further, and more importantly, such changes require a high degree of critical appraisal and clinical vigilance—health care systems can no longer afford a plethora of tests with low specificity or treatments with low efficacy. For all of these imminent changes in the day-to-day practices of physicians, CME in some form is the most palatable change strategy. If well designed, and related to learner and practice needs, it is also the most likely to succeed.

Another shift in emphasis has occurred in the provision of care, from the strictly biomedical model, to one involving a more holistic, comprehensive management of care involving aspects of psychology, family dynamics, and cultural, ethnic and social considerations. While not accepted as its proponents originally envisaged,[11] this biopsychosocial model has nonetheless been the focus of curricular reform in undergraduate settings and texts and monographs on the subject.[12] Concurrent with this emphasis has been the generalist approach to medical education called for in the General Professional Education Program (GPEP) report,[13] stressing a decrease in the need for specialization, and the call for increased, broad-based comprehensive care provided by those trained in general medicine. Both these movements, closely related and mutually driven, call for changes in the practices and understandings of current and future physicians. As such, they speak to the imperative of new CME models, and hence, CME research in these areas.

## A New View

The history of knowledge in medicine provides an analogy that may teach us about current problems in CME. Before the Flexner report,[14] medical education was little more than a sophisticated apprenticeship system. Medical knowledge was passed to students through contact with an experienced mentor and a clinical case. What was known about medicine was accumulated from the records and impressions of practitioners and a relatively small collection of medical texts.

Yet there was a movement for change in medical education marked by the Flexner report. In addition to condemning the proprietary schools of the time, it called for medical education and medical practice based on science. By the 1930s, research was beginning to assert its value. Today, science seems to be the foundation of most decisions physicians make, although the art of dealing with ambiguity in practice has recently received renewed interest.

Until recently, the practice of CME has been based upon the accumulation of experience transmitted by word of mouth, usually about practical issues, from those with more experience to those with less. Knowing what to do in a given situation was based on what was done by experience or colleagues in a similar situation. Like early medicine, the results of practices learned in this way have been mixed, succeeding in some cases and failing in others.

In recent years, CME has begun to push for the discovery of a knowledge base to serve as bedrock for programs and practices. This book, the conference from which it arose, and the size and state of the literature in this subject area, attest to the vigor and increasing rigor of the CME research imperative. Researchers have made progress toward the time when this knowledge begins to direct practice.

It is our hope that the nature and purpose of CME will stimulate a variety of new investigations and encourage the training of new, interdisciplinary investigators. This book has attempted to describe the terrain of such investigation—the physician as learner; the assessment of competence and performance as measures of needs determination or program evaluation; and the extent, nature, and potency of CME delivery methods. Further, we have attempted to delineate questions at the interface of these areas, and to construct research agendas, models, and priorities by which they may be answered.

All of this exists in the context and crucible of two issues. First, are the purposes of CME—we see it as a change agent in the perception, competencies, and performances of individual physicians and outcomes related to their patients. From a more collective perspective, we see the objectives of CME as related to the performance of the profession in the face of societal demands.

However, as much as CME is derived from the field of adult education, so equally is it anchored to the health care system. Thus, the second construct has to do with the compelling nature of the practice environment in which we see CME as an integral part. Here, as we call for further research into the methods and means of CME, we speak equally to the need of translating what we know about physician learning from research to practice. If physicians are called on to employ the best in critical appraisal techniques, using only efficacious methods, so, too, must CME providers begin to apply such techniques to their use of physician learning strategies. Like its biomedical cousin, research in CME is useless unless applied to practice.

Although the complications of research in a field as diverse and complex as the learning and education of practicing physicians are many, the benefits are substantial. Learning and the education that contributes to learning serve as bridges for the flow of new and different information and skills. When these bridges work well, progress in medical care is made possible. When they are weakened or blocked, nothing new or better is possible, except for those changes that can be made by force or deception. Research to understand how to improve the flow of knowledge and skills from the research base to the practice of medicine is our best hope for improving the practice of medicine. However, research must also be communicated among scholars and practitioners before it can be effective. In order to be effectively communicated, it must also be organized and built on a sound foundation.

For most fields of study, research is directed by a limited number of formal explanations and predictions known as theories. The theories are, in turn, built from concepts—special words that are carefully defined based on rules of inclusion and exclusion. Once definitions are in order, variables can be identified and relationships tested. Without specificity inherent in concepts and theories, the organizing structure which connects and supports the system of research is weakened and coordination of investigations and conclusions are absent.

Research in CME has suffered from a lack of coordination, not only of the nature and direction of investigations, but also of the meaning of findings and conclusions. A major factor contributing to this has been the lack of conceptual clarity of the major ideas that organize CME as a field of investigation. The Consensus Conference at Beaver Creek was set as a means for focusing on the structure of research in an effort to more carefully and completely define the major ideas that have driven investigations in CME. It also set out an image of the future of CME research, based on shared information of its past. This chapter has sought to present this vision in global terms.

In many ways, CME is new. The perspective has changed from the study of the effects of education to the study of characteristics and conditions for learning. What is recently discovered is worth knowing, since physicians' abilities to learn new and better ways of performing their roles govern the rate of progress in medical care. We see it as the responsibility of the continuing medical educator in concert with the profession to challenge that ability, encourage learning, and facilitate progress.

### References

1. Society of Medical College Directors of Continuing Medical Education: survey for 1990-1991: descriptive results. Report of the Survey Subcommittee of the Research Committee; April 9, 1992; Birmingham, Ala.

2. Rosof AB, Felch WC. *Continuing Medical Education: A Primer.* 2nd ed. New York, NY: Praeger; 1992.

3. Gagne RM, Glaser R. Foundations in learning research. In: *Instructional Technology: Foundations.* Hillsdale, NJ: Lawrence Erlbaum and Associates; 1987:41-106.

4. Fox RD, Mazmanian PE, Putnam RW, eds. *Changing and Learning in the Lives of Physicians.* New York, NY: Praeger; 1989.

5. Schön DA. *Educating the Reflective Practitioner: Toward a New Design for Teaching and Learning in the Professions.* San Francisco, Calif: Jossey-Bass; 1987.

6. Perrow C. *Organization Analysis: A Sociological View.* Bel Mont, Calif: Cale; 1970.

7. Knox AB. Influences on participation in continuing education. *J Cont Educ Health Prof.* 1990;10:261-274.

8.  Painvin C.  The triple jump.  In: Norman G, ed.  *The Evaluation Workbook.*  Hamilton, Canada: McMaster University; 1983.

9.  Haynes RB, McKibbon A, Fitzgerald D, Guyatt GH, Walker CJ, Sackett DL.  How to keep up with the medical literature: why try to keep up and how to get started.  *Ann Intern Med.* 1986;105:149-153.

10. Green LV, Kreuter MW, Deeds SG, Partridge KB.  *Health Education Planning: A Diagnostic Approach.*  Palo Alto, Calif: Mayfield Publishers; 1980.

11. Schwartz MA, Wiggins OF.  Scientific and humanistic medicine: a theory of clinical methods.  In: *The Task of Medicine: Dialogue at Wickenburg.*  Menlo Park, Calif: HJ Kaiser Foundation Publishers; 1988:137-171.

12. McWhinney IR.  Through clinical methods to a more humanistic medicine.  In: *The Task of Medicine: Dialogue at Wickenburg.*  Menlo Park, Calif: HJ Kaiser Foundation Publishers; 1988:218-231.

13. Association of American Medical Colleges.  *Physicians for the Twenty-first Century: The GPEP Report: Report of the Panel on the General Professional Education of the Physician and College Preparation for Medicine.*  Washington, DC: Association of American Medical Colleges; 1984.

14. Flexner A.  *Medical Education in the United States and Canada: A Report to the Carnegie Foundation for the Advancement of Teaching, Bulletin No. 4.*  Boston, Mass: Updyke; 1910.

# Conclusion

## Annotated Bibliography

**Cziko GA.** Purposeful behavior as the control of perception: implications for education research. *Ed Researcher.* 1992;21:10-18.

> This article discusses the problems posed by the unpredictability and indeterminism of human behavior for educational research. A theory of purposeful behavior known as perceptual control theory is presented, providing an explicit, working model of how individuals are able to produce repeatable outcomes via variable means. It is argued that the traditional "scientific" method of educational research (which attempts to find relationships between "independent" and "dependent" variables) is, in principle, incapable of providing valid explanations of the how and why of purposeful human behavior.

**Davis D.** Meta-analysis and metaphors in CME literature. *J Cont Educ Health Prof.* 1991;11:85-86.

> This guest editorial reviews the definition and purposes of meta-analysis, discusses some of the relevant methodology, and explores the outcomes and meanings of such reviews to the field of CME research.

**Fox RD.** New horizons for research in continuing medical education. *Acad Med.* 1990;65:550-555.

> This essay describes future research and its role in investigating the three overlapping areas of CME: (1) what, how, and why physicians learn and change; (2) how better programs and education can be designed to fit into this process; and (3) in what ways the organizations that provide CME can or should differ in their policies, procedures, and resources.

**Fox RD.** New research agendas for CME: organizing principles for the study of self-directed curricula for change. *J Cont Educ Health Prof.* 1991;11:155-167.

> The paper presents a series of research questions that deal with the interrelationship of models for learning and change. Questions are addressed regarding the reasons physicians elect to change their practices, the stages experienced in self-directed curricula for change, the reasons physicians elect to engage in learning or to participate in formal education programs, and how physicians learn from experience.

**Krendl KA.**  Two roads converge: the synthesis of research on media influence on learning.  In: Dervin B,  Voigt MJ, eds.  *Progress in Communication Sciences.* Norwood, NJ: Ablex Publishing Corporation; 1989;9:105-122.

> Focusing attention on the learner's interaction with computers, the author advances the notion that people are not passively affected by technology. By their choice of task and purpose, and by their choice of what elements to attend to, they affect the way technology can affect them.  Research in this area should focus on individuals' unique approaches to the technology (independent of the specific situation and application), assuming that individuals are actively involved in media selection and use.

**Merriam SB.**  How research produces knowledge.  In: Peters JM, Jarvis P et al, eds. *Adult Education: Evaluation and Achievement in a Developing Field of Study.*  San Francisco, Calif: Jossey-Bass; 1991:42-65.

> Three paradigms are offered to interpret research in adult education: positivist, interpretive, and critical research.  Positivist research assumes a single objective reality.  Interpretive research challenges the basic assumption of the positivist paradigm.  Critical research aims to enlighten and empower those who are being studied.

**Simpkins JD, Brenner DJ.**  Mass media communication and health.  In: Dervin B, Voigt MJ, eds.  *Progress in Communication Sciences.*  Norwood, NJ: Ablex Publishing Corporation; 1984.

> The effects and outcomes of most of the mass-media communication and health research have been ultimately concerned with changing human behavior or actions in cost-effective ways.  Far less frequent are those that target behaviors that are communication variables.  The authors suggest that research should lead to an understanding of how individuals (audiences) involve mass-media communication in the health aspects of everyday living.

**Soumerai SB, McLaughlin TJ, Avorn J.**  Improving drug prescribing in primary care: a critical analysis of the experimental literature. *Milbank Q.*  1989;67:269-317.

> A thorough methodologic review of studies, targeted at the improvement of primary care prescribing practices, identified seven strategies: (1) dissemination of printed materials, (2) patient-specific medication reports, (3) group education, (4) feedback, (5) reminders, (6) one-on-one education, and (7) clinical pharmacy services.  The authors note methodologic weaknesses in many of these studies and discuss implications for further research and practice.

**Wergin JF, Mazmanian PE, Mitch WW, Papp KK, Williams WL.** *Assessing the Impact of Continuing Medical Education Through Structured Physician Dialogue.* Richmond, VA: Commonwealth University Press; 1987.

This monograph outlines an evaluation of a series of CME courses offered by the American College of Cardiology at Heart House, Bethesda, Maryland. Using practicing cardiologists as trained interviewers, the authors outline the development, validation, and implications of the structured interview technique.

# Index